Proceedings of the Symposium of the International Society for Corneal Research

Documenta Ophthalmologica
Proceedings Series volume 20

Editor H. E. Henkes

Dr. W. Junk bv Publishers The Hague-Boston-London 1979

Proceedings of the Symposium of the International Society for Corneal Research, Kyoto, May 12-13, 1978

Edited by J. François,
S. I. Brown & M. Itoi

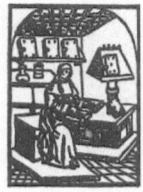

Dr. W. Junk bv Publishers The Hague-Boston-London 1979

Cover design: Max Velthuijs

© Dr W. Junk bv Publishers 1979
Softcover reprint of the hardcover 1st edition 1979

ISBN-13:978-94-009-9608-3   e-ISBN-13:978-94-009-9606-9
DOI: 10.1007/978-94-009-9606-9

CONTENTS

Jules François: Opening address.......................... VII

Jules François: Preface................................. IX

Inflammation — Immunology
Moderator: Yukihiko Mitsui

Y. Mitsui, R. Takashima, C. Kondo & K. Hirai: Stereoscopic scanning
electron microscopic observation of *Pseudomonas* keratitis...... 1

B.J. Mondino, S.I. Brown & B.S. Rabin: Corneal inflammation and
complement.. 11

N. Tanaka, T. Sasaki, I. Tanaka, N. Kinoshita & J.Y. Homma: Experimental study on the immunotherapy for the *Pseudomonas* keratitis
in rabbits... 19

M.R. Allansmith, K. Kashima & G.K. Yamamoto: Immunoglobulins in
the cornea.. 23

R.M. Hembry, J. Playfair, P.G. Watson & J.T. Dingle: Experimental
model for scleritis.................................. 29

S.P. Dhir, S. Sehgal & I.S. Jain: Cell mediated immunity in Mooren's
ulcer.. 33

T. Sasaki, E. Gotoh, K. Kamata, R. Ishikawa, R. Dokoh, M. Higuchi &
M. Inoue: Role of cell-mediated immunity in the resistance of rabbits to corneal herpes simplex virus infection 39

P. Montcourrier & Y. Pouliquen: Lymphocyte cytotoxicity against
the rabbit corneal endothelium. Morphological aspects........ 45

Endothelium
Moderator: Herbert E. Kaufman

H.E. Kaufman: The corneal endothelium.................... 51

R. Witmer, Fr. Bigar & A. Thaer: Wide-field in vivo specular microscopy.. 57

R.A. Laing, M.M. Sandstrom & H.M. Leibowitz: Clinical specular microscopy of the corneal endothelium..................... 63

T. Sato, Y. Ota, C. Kimura, T. Tanishima & S. Mishima: The endothelium of the corneal graft: Morphological and functional aspects ... 73

S. Kitano, Healing process in the alkali-burned corneal endothelium .. 83

S. Akiya, T. Oshima & M. Wada: The electron microscopic study of
Fuchs' dystrophy: the first primary case in Japan 97

Graft rejection
Moderator: Stuart I. Brown

M. Fine: Corneal transplantation and rejection 109

A.A. Khodadoust & A. Abizadeh: The fate of corneal regrafts after
previous rejection reactions........................... 115

W.J. Stark, H.R. Taylor & W.B. Bias: Keratoplasty and transplantation antigens. 123
S. Vannas, A. Tiilikainen, A. Vannas & K. Karjalainen 131
D.C. Gibbs, J.R. Batchelor, T.A. Casey, A. Werb, G. Liakos & C. Taylor: HLA matching and corneal graft rejection 139

Corneal transplantation
Moderator: Claus H. Dohlman

D.M. Maurice, J.P. McCulley & M.M. Perlman: Development in use of cultured endothelium in corneal transplantation 151
J. François, V. Victoria-Troncoso & H. Verbraeken: Post-operative control of the donor endothelium in corneal grafting by means of histochemical staining 155
W.M. Bourne: Endothelial cell loss during penetrating keratoplasty. . . 167
Y. Pouliquen, J.P. Giraud, M. Hirsch, G. Renard, M. Cordova, M. Savoldelli & O. Marquet: Chemical burn of the rabbit cornea: morphometric studies of the corneal stroma. 171
A. Kanai, M. Tanaka, T. Yamaguchi & A. Nakajima: Atypical lattice dystrophy of the cornea: a clinical and histological study 181

Epithelium
Moderator: Jules François

M. Itoi: Management of keratoconus. 193
R.A. Thoft & J. Friend: Ocular surface evaluation 201
P.C. Maudgal & L. Missotten: Histopathological study of the human herpes simplex dendritic and punctate keratitis by replica technique 211
A. Sommer, N. Emran & T. Tamba: Superficial punctate keratopathy: earliest corneal manifestation of xerophthalmia. 221
M. Reim, E. Schette, G. Scharsich, M. Seidl, H.G. Kesternich & A.W. Budi Santoso: Adenosine triphosphate, adenosine diphosphate, ascorbic acid, glutathione and lactate in experimental ultraviolet keratitis. 225
P. Vittone, R. Bertagno & M. Zingirian: The dark cells of corneal epithelium in a case of lattice-like dystrophy 233

OPENING ADDRESS

Dear Professor Itoi, Dear Doctor Brown, Ladies and Gentlemen,

It is for me a very great pleasure to welcome you very heartily on behalf the International Council of Ophthalmology. We have to congratulate and to thank very sincerely Dr. Stuart Brown for having created the International Society for Corneal Research, which becomes more and more important. It is obvious, as the cornea is the window of the eye.

It is also my pleasure to greet our honorary chairman, Professor Motokazu Itoi. I should like to thank him very warmly, as well as Professor Nakajima, Professor Mishima and their Japanese Staff for having been willing to organize this meeting and for having done it so beautifully.

The program of these two days is outstanding. The limiting membranes, the epithelium as well as the endothelium, the stroma, the corneal transplantation as well as the graft rejection will be discussed by experts in the field. Therefore, I am convinced that you will have an interesting and fruitful meeting, which will leave in your mind the best memory. I wish the greatest success to Dr. Stuart Brown and to you all.

JULES FRANCOIS

PREFACE

This book comprises the proceedings of the first meeting of the International Society for Corneal Research, held in Kyoto on May 12 and 13, 1978, on the occasion of the International Congress of Ophthalmology.

The Society was founded by Dr. Stuart I. Brown (USA), who has to be congratulated very sincerely for this idea. The cornea, window of the eye, becomes, indeed, more and more important and its diseases more and more frequent. Consequently, cornea research is of the greatest necessity not only to cure but also to prevent the various disorders of the membrane.

The scientific program of the meeting, established by Dr. Brown, was outstanding. The limiting membranes, the epithelium as well as the endothelium, the stroma, the corneal transplantation, as well as the graft rejection, the inflammations as well as the immunological aspects, were discussed by experts in the field.

The meeting, which was conducted by Professor Motokazu Itoi, honorary Chairman, and successfully organized by his Japanese colleagues, Professor Nakajima, Professor Mishima and their staff, was as interesting as fruitful and left in our mind the best memory.

I am convinced that the ophthalmologists will take a great interest in reading the various papers, which bring the latest advances in corneal pathology.

Prof. Jules François
President of the International
Council of Ophthalmology.

Docum. Ophthal. Proc. Series, Vol. 20

STEREOSCOPIC SCANNING ELECTRON MICROSCOPIC OBSERVATION OF *PSEUDOMONAS* KERATITIS

YUKIHIKO MITSUI, REIKO TAKASHIMA, CHIYO KONDO, AND KEN-ICHI HIRAI

(Tokushima, Japan)

This paper deals with stereoscopic scanning electron microscopy of *Pseudomonas* keratitis in rabbits. For this experiment we employed a technique of *Pseudomonas* inoculation which uniformly produced hypopyon keratitis in rabbits as reported elsewhere.

As you know rabbit corneas are less susceptible to *Pseudomonas*. An inoculation of this organism into the rabbit cornea by slight needle pricks rarely results in keratitis. Fig. 1-A (below) shows a rabbit cornea 48 hours after inoculation by the needle prick procedure of *Pseudomonas* suspended in saline. There is no keratitis. Fig. 1-B shows the cornea of the opposite eye of the same rabbit. For this eye, the same organism was suspended in a solution of gastric mucin and was inoculated by the needle prick procedure. Severe infiltration with ulceration is seen at the sites of the needle pricks. This experimental system seemed to be convenient in the study of *Pseudomonas* keratitis in rabbits, because the clinical findings resemble those of human cases and, in addition, the results are constant.

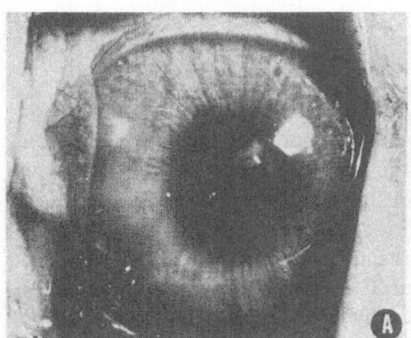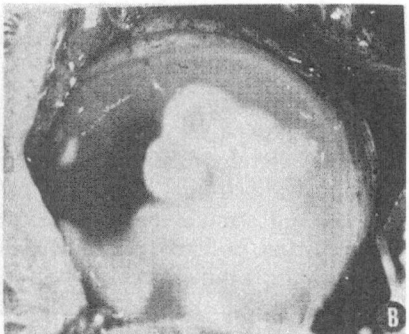

Fig. 1.

The corneas were examined chiefly by stereoscopic scanner. Light microscopy and transmission electron microscopy were used as supplementary procedures. Fig. 2 (below) shows a schematic illustration of *Pseudomonas* keratitis in rabbits at onset. At the center is an exposure of the corneal stroma by breakdown of Bowman's membrane and cell infiltrations into the stromal tissue. Surrounding this true ulceration is a wide area where what is probably Bowman's membrane is exposed by sloughing off of the epithelial layer. This area is circumscribed by the sloughing margin of the epithelial layer. This finding resembles a volcano. At the center is a crater. Surrounding the crater is a caldera with its outside somma. Around the periphery the exposed Bowman's membrane is often covered by monolayer cells. The nature of these cells will be an item of discussion. Actual pictures of these structures will be shown by slides, but stereoscopic projection is not available. Therefore, I took the liberty of circulating stereoscopic viewers.

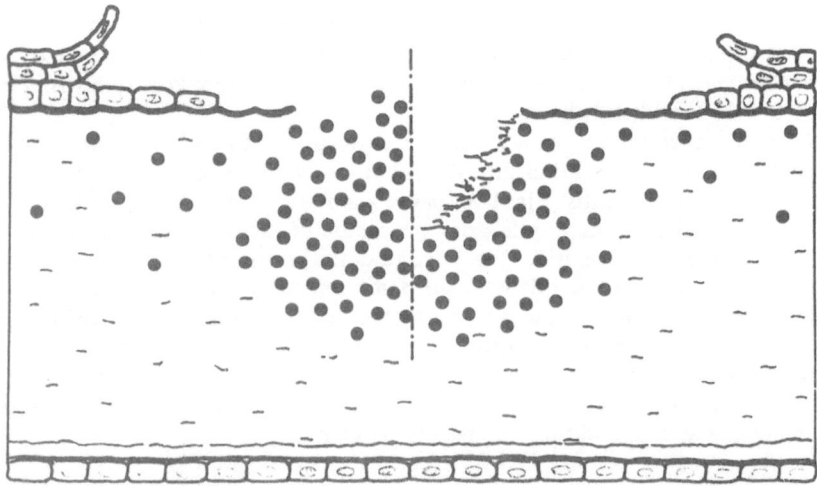

Fig. 2.

Fig. 3 (below) is a complete view of one lesion produced by one needle prick observed at a low magnification. At the center of the lesion is a true ulcer as shown by the symbol A. Here, the Bowman's membrane has broken down and the stromal tissue with cell infiltrations is exposed. In some case the exposed stromal tissue is elevated above the surface. This is due to accumulation of leucocytes in and on the necrotic stromal tissue. In other cases the ulcer shows a deep excavation. This may be due to the sloughing off of necrotic tissue. The area indicated by the symbol B is a plane where the probable Bowman's membrane is exposed. Surrounding this plane is a sloughing margin of the epithelium, as indicated by the symbol C.

Now the sloughing margin of the epithelium will be shown at a slightly higher magnification (Fig. 4) (below). You may see epithelium at the lower left part. An overhang of epithelium is seen at its sloughing margin. The upper right two thirds of the picture is a portion where the monolayer cells are arranged on Bowman's membrane.

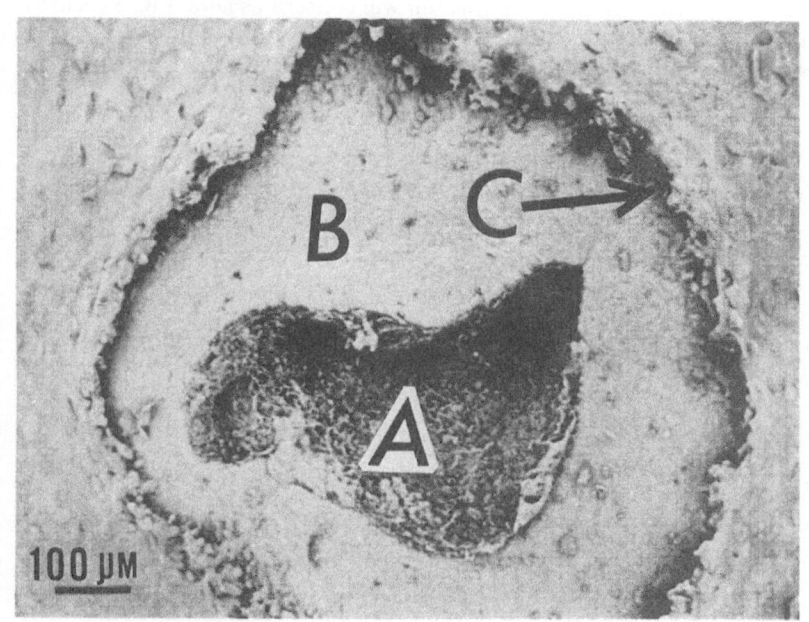

Fig. 3.

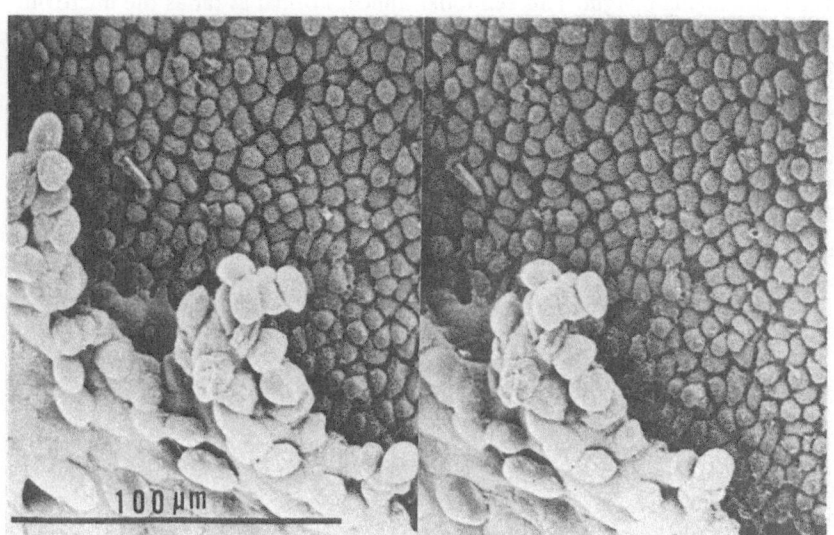

Fig. 4.

3

At first, the situation of the epithelium will concern us here. Fig. 5 (below) is a high power picture of the surface epithelial cells near the overhanging margin. The surface structure of these cells is considerably destroyed, as shown by the deformation of the microvilli.

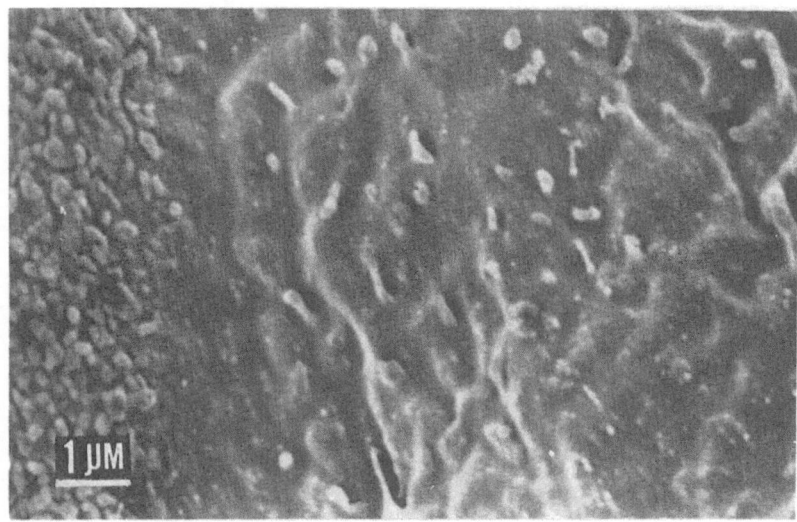

Fig. 5

Fig. 6 (below) shows a surface epithelial cell about 10 cell widths apart from the overhanging margin. This cell looks almost normal as far as the microvilli are concerned.

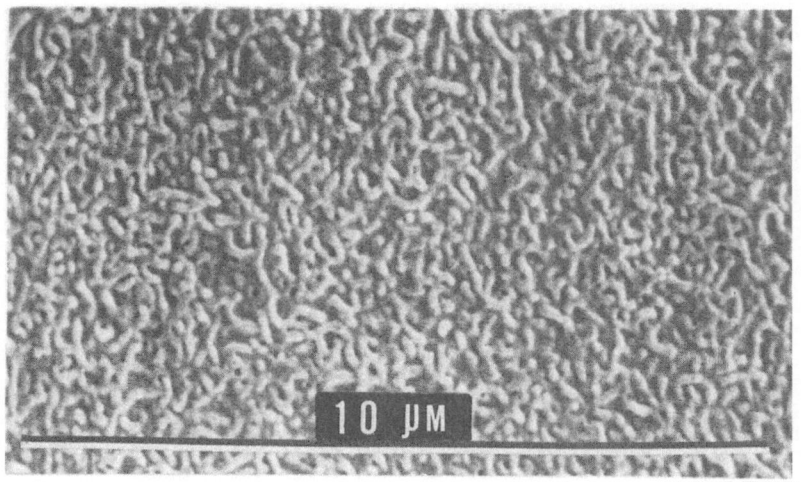

Fig. 6.

4

Now, the monolayer cells on Bowman's membrane will be shown at a higher magnification (Fig. 7) (below). These cells are mostly ellipsoidal in shape and each cell measures 5 to 8 μ in diameter. They join each other by cell processes and as will be shown later they are also anchored to the underlying tissue by cell processes. The presence of this kind of cell has been described in other kinds of corneal ulcers such as dendritic keratitis. Some investigators consider these cells to be basal cells of the epithelium and others to be leucocytes. This problem will be discussed again later.

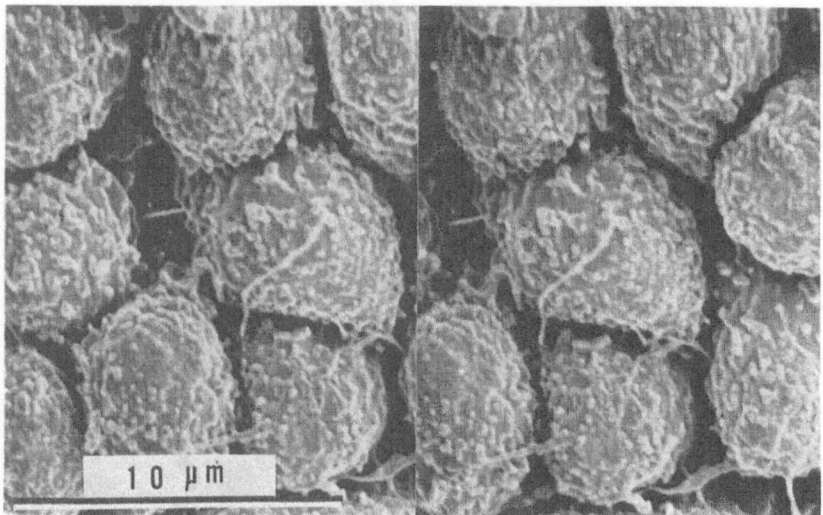

Fig. 7

Now, the finding of the exposed Bowman's membrane will concern us here. Fig. 8 (below) is a picture of the exposed membrane. According to the anotomy of rabbits, it is not certain whether the rabbit cornea has a definite Bowman's membrane or not. Therefore, it may be better to say that this is the surface of the basement membrane. However, this problem is not the present subject, so, let me call it Bowman's membrane at this moment. As shown in the picture, this membrane looks to be cribriform. By stereoscopic observations the surface of this membrane is not flat, it looks like an assembly of shallow cribriform saucers. The size of each saucer is about 5-8 μ in diameter which corresponds to the size of the monolayer cells on this membrane.

Fig. 9 (below) is a finding suggesting strongly that the saucers were underlying single monolayer cells. This is a picture of monolayer cells. At the central portion some cells are missing and cribriform saucers are seen as if one monolayer cells was anchored on each.

5

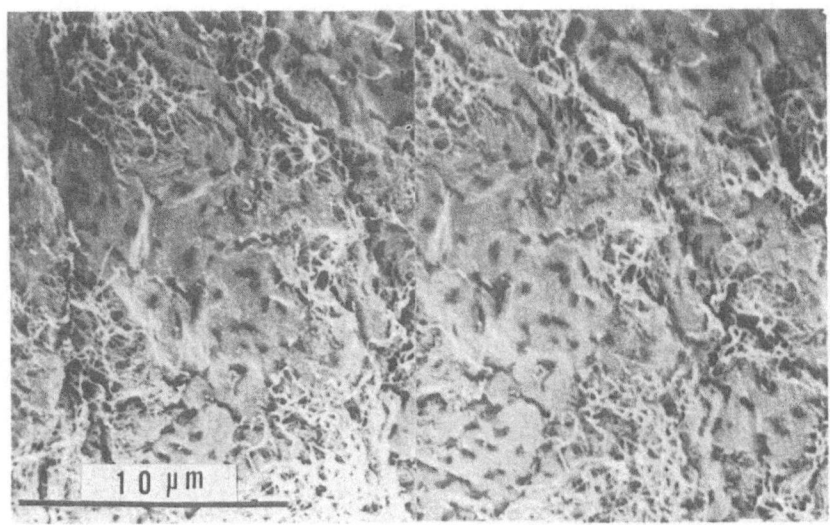

Fig. 8.

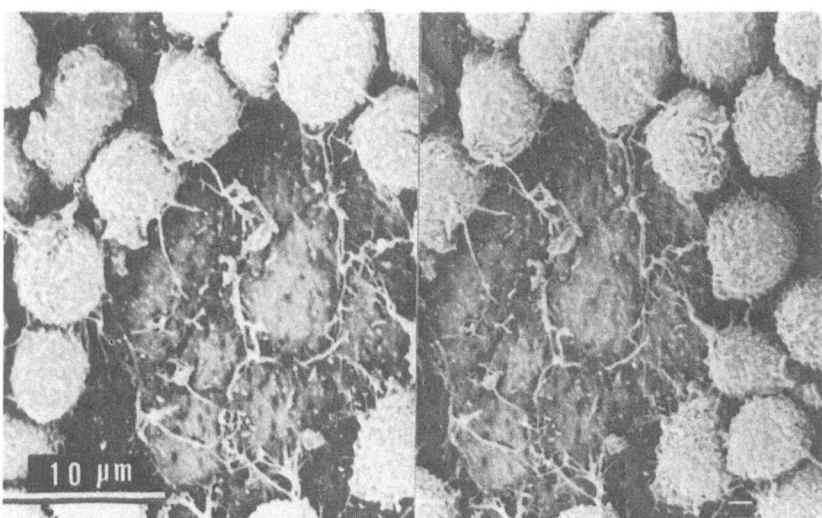

Fig. 9.

Fig. 10 (below) represents the inside of the true ulcer where the stromal tissue is exposed. The findings are complex. In the upper half, you may see many leucocytes gathered on or embedded in destroyed fibrous tissue. The lower half consists of a mass of fibrous tissue. By stereoscopic observation the lower part is deeply caved in. It is not difficult to suppose that this deep excavation and exposure of the stromal fibers are a result of throwing off of

6

the necrotic tissue as seen in the upper half of this picture. Now, the upper half and the lower half of this picture will be examined under higher magnification.

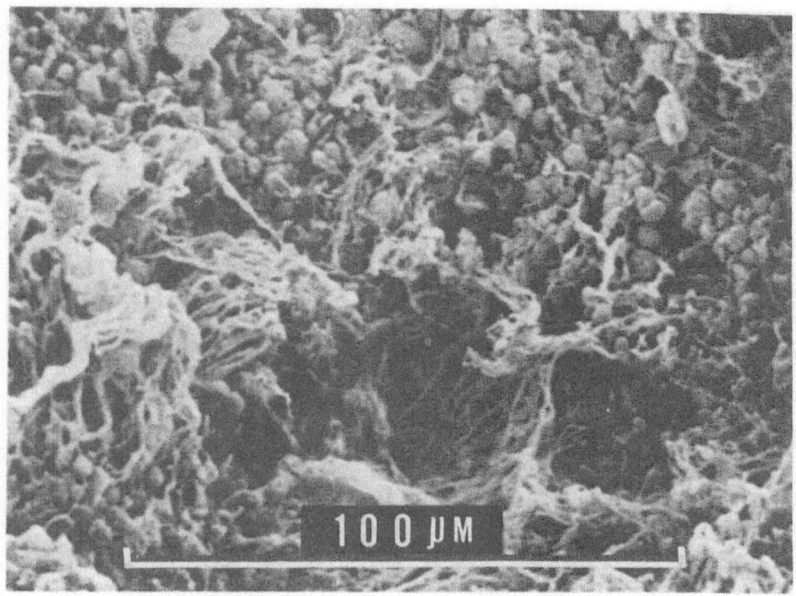

Fig. 10.

Fig. 11 (below, left) shows a high power findings of the upper half of the previous picture. Many leucocytes are seen on and in the necrotic tissue complex. The morphology of the leucocytes by scanner will be discussed again later. Fig. 12 (below, right) shows a high power findings of the lower half of the previous picture where the ulcer showed deep excavation. There is a wreck of fibrous tissues.

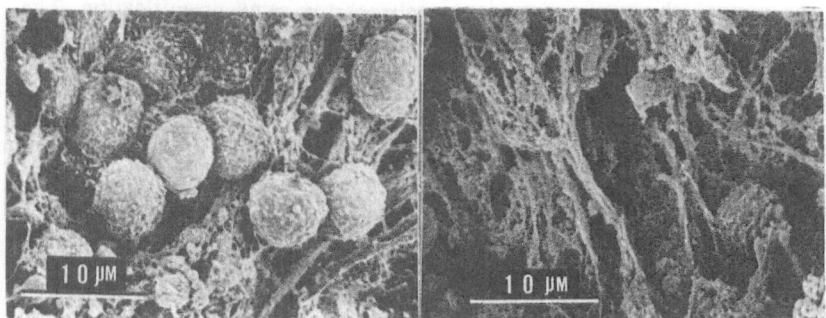

Fig. 11.   *Fig. 12.*

7

Finally we would like to discuss the nature of the monolayer cells seen on Bowman's membrane. Fig. 13 (below) shows *Pseudomonas* keratitis observed by light microscopy. Monolayer cells are constantly seen on Bowman's membrane. They are always an extension of epithelial cells as shown by this picture. Leucocytes can also be seen on this membrane but they appear individually or as a lump and never form a monolayer.

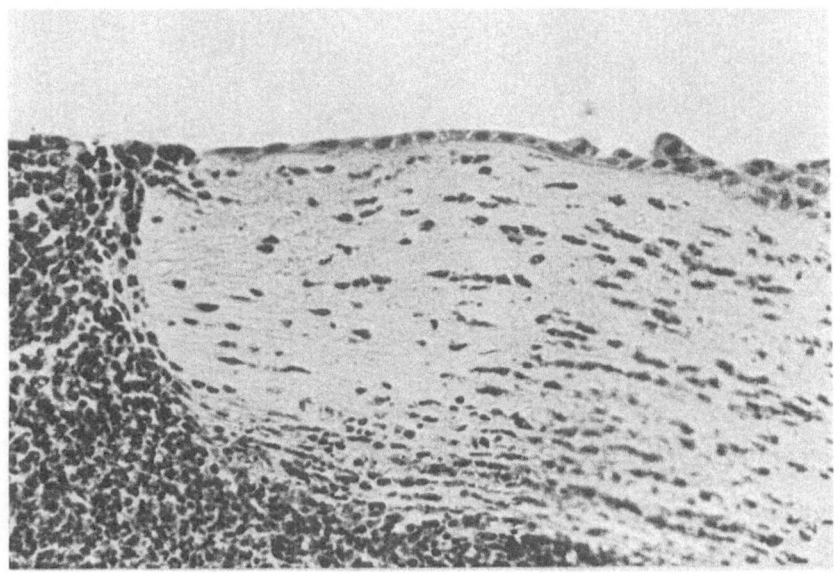

Fig. 13.

The upper left picture of Fig. 14 (below) shows a leucocyte obtained from the rabbits blood. The findings are quite the same as in the leucocytes seen in the necrotic tissue of the ulcer as shown in the lower left picture. The right picture shows the monolayer cells at the same magnification. The leucocytes bear some resemblances in appearance to the monolayer cells, but they do not join each other by cell processes even if they appear in groups, whereas the monolayer cells join with the neighboring cells and with the underlying tissue by cell processes. It is difficult to assume, therefore, that the monolayer cells are derived from the leucocytes.

Finally, artificially produced monolayer cells on Bowman's membrane will be shown. When the central cornea was frozen for half an hour *in vivo*, the epithelium sloughed off to expose Bowman's membrane. Near the sloughing margin of the epithelium, monolayer cells remain on the membrane as shown in Fig. 15 (below).

Fig. 16 (below) is a high power finding of the artificially produced monolayer cells. Their appearance is equivalent to monolayer cells seen in the

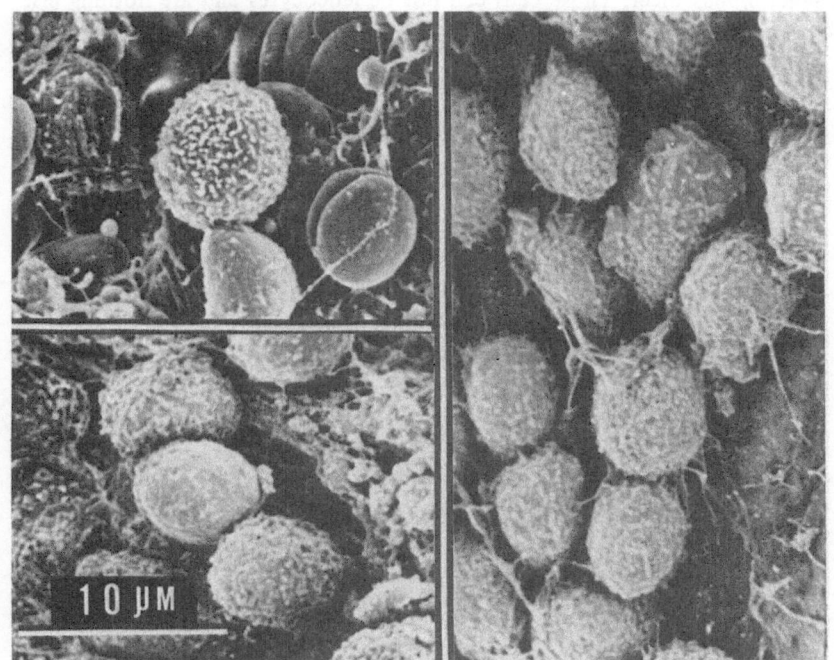

Fig. 14.

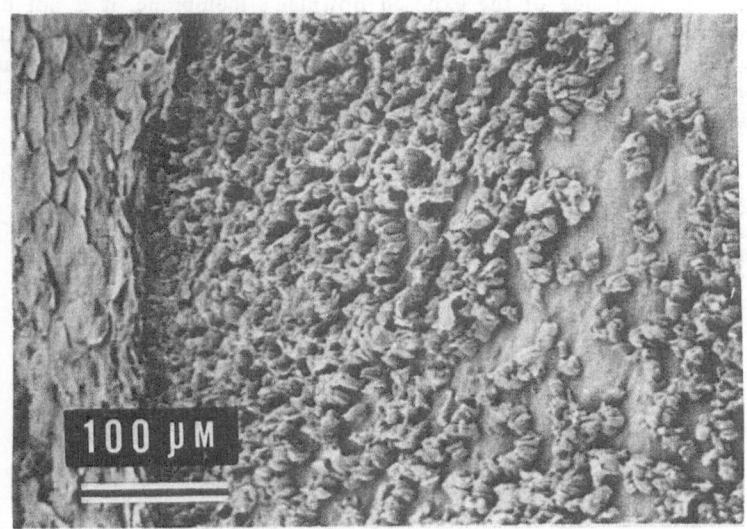

Fig. 15.

Pseudomonas ulcer. Those cells can not be leucocytes and are nothing else but the basal cells of the epithelium.

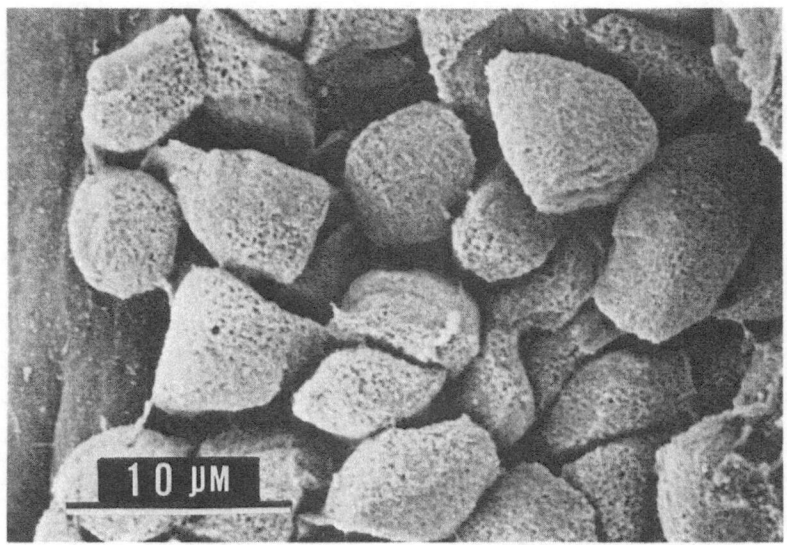

Fig. 16.

From these results, and from the fact that the monolayer cells are seen only at the epithelial side of the exposed Bowman's membrane, it is not unreasonable to conclude that the monolayer cells are in all probability the basal cells of the epithelium, and that the separation of the epithelium is apt to occur leaving basal cells on the Bowman's membrane because these cells are firmly fixed on their saucers there.

Author's address:
Department of Ophthalmology
Tokushima University School of Medicine
Tokushima
Japan

CORNEAL INFLAMMATION AND COMPLEMENT*

BARTLY J. MONDINO, STUART I. BROWN AND BRUCE S. RABIN

(Pittsburgh, Pennsylvania, U.S.A.)

INTRODUCTION

Over the past decade there have been numerous studies demonstrating the integral role of complement in the pathogenesis of various disease processes (Müller-Eberhard, 1977). Activated complement is known to mediate tissue inflammation and may also destroy cells. There are two ways in which complement is activated: the classical and the alternate pathway (Roitt, 1977). The classical complement pathway depends upon an antibody-antigen interaction which activates the first component (C1) of the classical pathway with the sequential activation of the rest of the complement components down to G9 (Fig. 1).

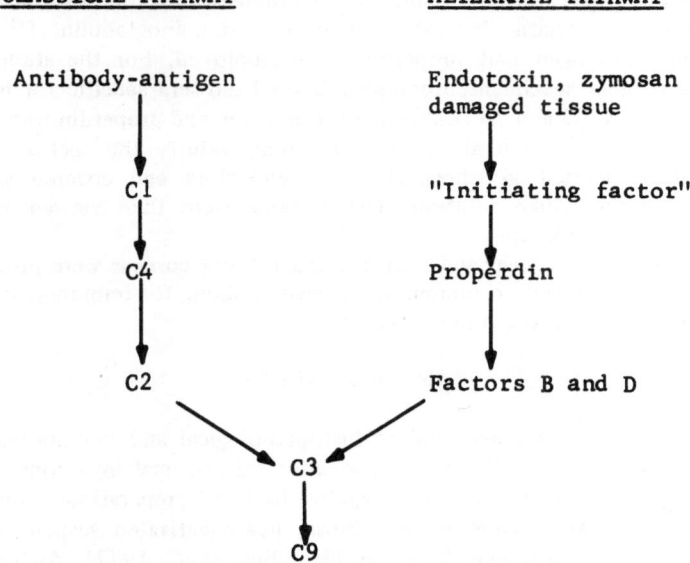

Fig. 1. Classical and alternate pathway activation of complement.

* This research was supported in part by National Eye Institute, Grant Number 1 RO1 EY02304-1.

In contrast, the alternate pathway does not depend upon an antibody-antigen interaction but is activated by microbial products such as endotoxin and zymosan and even damaged tissue. It is currently theorized that activation of the alternate pathway starts with activation of an 'initiating factor' and then leads to activation of properdin which stabilizes the enzymes of this system (Müller-Eberhard, 1977). The alternate pathway operates without activation of the first three complement components, that is, C1, C4 and C2, begins directly at the C3 component and continues thereafter as in the classical pathway. Pillemer, who originally postulated the existence of this system, suggested that the alternate pathway was involved in the very earliest host response to bacterial or viral infections before an antibody response has been mounted (Müller-Eberhard, 1977).

Today we will present evidence suggesting that both alternate and classical pathway activation of complement are operative in corneal inflammation.

MATERIALS AND METHODS

Corneal specimens from rabbits and humans were bisected for histopathological and immunopathological examination. One-half was fixed in 37% formaldehyde, stained with hematoxylin-eosin and PAS and processed for paraffin sectioning in the usual fashion. The other one-half was immediately frozen and sectioned at 4 μ on a cryostat. After air drying, the corneal tissues were overlayed with fluorescein-labeled antisera diluted 1:20 in pH 7.2 phosphate buffered saline. In the rabbit studies, fluorescein-labeled goat antisera specific for rabbit polyvalent immunoglobulin, C3 complement, fibrinogen and properdin were employed. For the studies on human corneal specimens, fluorescein-labeled antisera specific for human IgG, IgA, IgM, C3 and C4 complement, fibrinogen and properdin were used. After 30 minutes incubation at room temperature, the sections were thoroughly washed in phosphate buffered saline and covered with a 90:10 glycerin: saline solution. The sections were then viewed with a fluorescence microscope.

Normal rabbit corneas and normal human donor corneas were processed as above and showed no immunofluorescent staining for immunoglobulins, complement, fibrinogen and properdin.

ANIMAL STUDIES

Our animal investigations involved histopathological and immunopathological studies of rabbit corneas made after intrastromal injections of the following gram-positive and gram-negative bacterial preparations: complete Freund's adjuvant, viable P. aeruginosa, heat-inactivated suspensions of P. aeruginosa, E. coli and S. aureus (Mondino et al., 1977). All corneas developed dense infiltration at the sites of these centrally injected bacterial preparations. Only the corneas injected with viable P. aeruginosa and heat-inactivated E. coli and P. aeruginosa, that is, the gram-negative bacterial preparations, developed prominent ring infiltrates surrounding the centrally injected materials within 24 to 48 hours. Histopathological examination of the corneal rings revealed accumulations of polymorphonuclear leucocytes. A heavy infiltration of polymorphonuclear leucocytes was also found surrounding all the centrally injected bacterial products. We suggested that endotoxin was the factor responsible for the production of these corneal rings since purified endotoxin from either P. aeruginosa or E. coli also produced corneal rings after intracorneal injection.

We then attempted to determine if the corneal rings found in association with gram-negative bacteria were similar to the immune rings found in association with the Wesseley phenomenon. Wesseley rings develop two weeks after a single intracorneal injection of horse serum and are thought to result from antibody-antigen precipitates with the production of chemotatic factors that attract inflammatory cells to the sites of the corneal rings (Sery et al., 1962). Although corneal rings found in association with gram-negative bacteria have been labeled immune rings and even Wesseley rings in the past (Ellison and Poirier, 1976; Aronson et al., 1970), we found that they differ from Wesseley rings in several important respects. First of all, corneal rings found after intrastromal injections of gram-negative bacteria or their endotoxins developed within 24 to 48 hours. The rapidity with which the rings developed precluded the participation of antibody which requires at least one week for its formation. Although it was theoretically possible that high titers of precipitating antibodies to endotoxin were present in the rabbits we used from previous exposure to endotoxin in the gastrointestinal tract, precipitating antibody in rabbit sera was not detected before or two weeks after intracorneal injections of endotoxin using immunodiffusion techniques in which wells containing rabbit sera were exposed to wells containing endotoxin. Finally, immunofluorescent studies of the corneal rings utilizing fluoresceinlabeled goat antisera specific for rabbit polyvalent immunoglobulin failed to demonstrate immunoglobulins in them. Instead, staining for properdin and C3 complement was found. It was concluded that the corneal rings found in association with endotoxin were independent of antibody and dependent upon activation of the alternate pathway because of the presence of properdin and C3 complement. Consequently, chemotactic complement factors for polymorphonuclear leucocytes were generated without the necessity for antibody-antigen reaction.

Properdin was found not only in the peripheral corneal rings, but also in association with the heavy polymorphonuclear infiltration surrounding all the centrally injected bacterial preparations in the study, that is, S. aureus, Freund's adjuvant, P. aeruginosa and E. coli. It has been recently reported that S. aureus (Stalenheim et al., 1973) and Mycobacterium tuberculosis (Allison et al., 1976) have the ability to activate the alternate pathway. This was supported in our study by the finding of properdin in association with injections of Freund's adjuvant and heat-inactivated suspensions of S. aureus.

We concluded that bacteria in the cornea stimulate the alternate pathway of complement which results in the production of chemotactic fragments for polymorphonuclear leucocytes. This response is particularly useful to a tissue infected with destructive organisms since it provides a rapid polymorphonuclear response that does not depend upon the formation of antibody.

In another series of experiments we sensitized rabbits to heat-inactivated S. aureus by repeated subcutaneous injections of this preparation. After four months, immunodiffusion studies showed immune precipitin lines when sera taken from sensitized rabbits were reacted against wells containing heat-inactivated S. aureus. Thus, precipitating antibodies to S. aureus were raised in these rabbits. Afterward, intrastromal injections of heat-inactivated S. aureus were made in both the sensitized and control rabbit corneas. The control and sensitized rabbits developed infiltrations and ulcerations at the sites of the centrally injected material. The sensitized rabbits, however, had more conjunctival hyperemia and chemosis and more corneal infiltrate at 24 to 48 hours than their control counterparts. More importantly, corneal ring infiltrates developed within 24 to 48 hours only in the sensitized rabbits. These rings were composed of polymorphonuclear leucocytes. In the unsensitized rabbits, intracorneal injections of heat-inactivated S. aureus were associated with properdin deposition. However, the corneas of sensitized rabbits also disclosed staining for immunoglobulins and complement. In this way, an Arthus-like reaction with antibody-antigen precipitates and activation of the classical pathway of complement was produced in the sensitized rabbits.

We concluded that it was possible to demonstrate alternate pathway activation of complement in the rabbit cornea by showing properdin and C3 complement deposition in the absence of immunoglobulins in the corneal rings caused by endotoxin. We also concluded that it was possible to demonstrate classical pathway activation of complement by creating titers of precipitating antibodies to S. aureus by sensitizing rabbits to S. aureus and then demonstrating immunoglobulins and C3 complement in the cornea in association with corneal rings found after intracorneal injections of heat-inactivated S. aureus. This suggests that complement activation by either or both pathways contributes to the polymorphonuclear infiltration of corneas with bacterial infections.

HUMAN STUDIES

We then attempted to assess the clinical significance of what we found in animal studies by direct immunofluorescent studies of human corneas (Mondino et al., 1978). Four corneal specimens were obtained following perforation from bacterial or fungal ulcerations, and one corneal specimen was obtained from a donor eye with a peripheral ulcer (Table 1).

One of the corneas had a Proteus mirabilis ulceration that perforated after eight days. The cornea obtained at keratoplasty was found to contain prominent staining for properdin and C3 complement. There was no staining for C4, immunoglobulins or fibrinogen. The presence of staining for properdin and C3 complement in the absence of staining for C4, IgG or IgM suggested that alternate rather than classical pathway activation of complement was present in this ulcerated cornea. The absence of staining for

	Properdin	C3	C4	IgG	IgA	IgM
Proteus mirabilis	+	+	–	–	–	–
Aspergillus flavus	+	+	+	+	–	+
S. aureus in chronic herpetic keratitis	+	+	–	+	–	+
S. aureus in ocular pemphigoid	–	+	–	+	+	+
Donor cornea with a catarrhal ulcer	–	+	–	+	+	+

Table 1. Human corneal ulcer specimens.

fibrinogen eliminated the possibility that the staining for C3 and properdin represented a non-specific accumulation of plasma proteins.

A patient with an Aspergillus flavus corneal ulceration in his blind eye eventually perforated after five weeks. The corneal specimen obtained at the time of evisceration disclosed staining for properdin, C3 and C4 complement, IgG and IgM but not fibrinogen. Finding properdin and C3 complement suggested alternate pathway activation of complement in this case, while finding C3 and C4 complement, IgG and IgM suggested classical pathway activation of complement. Alternate pathway activity in association with fungi is well documented (Sohnle *et al.*, 1976). The chronicity of this infection presumably allowed sufficient time for the formation of antibody to the invading organisms so that classical pathway activation of complement was probably superimposed on the alternate pathway activity. The presence of immunoglobulins, however, may have accounted for alternate pathway activity on the basis of feedback loop activation by the classical complement pathway (Roitt, 1977).

A patient with chronic herpetic keratitis and a patient with ocular cicatricial pemphigoid developed chronic paracentral corneal ulcerations which eventually perforated. Ocular cultures demonstrated Staphylococcus aureus. Corneal specimens were obtained from both patients at keratoplasty. One specimen revealed properdin, C3 complement, IgG and IgM but no fibrinogen, while the other revealed C3 complement, IgG, IgA and IgM but no properdin or fibrinogen. The specimen with properdin suggested that both classical and alternate pathway activation of complement were present while in the case without properdin only classical pathway activity could be implicated.

A donor cornea with e peripheral infiltrate and ulcer suggestive of a catarrhal ulcer of staphylococcus was studied by direct immunofluorescence and was found to contain C3 complement, IgG, IgA and IgM but no properdin. It has been suggested that the catarrhal infiltrates and ulcers of staphylococcus represent an antibody-antigen reaction in the sensitized host (Smolin and Okumoto, 1977), and these findings of classical pathway activation of complement are not surprising.

15

Although the number of human corneal specimens studied is small, definite patterns are emerging which are consistent with the findings in our animal studies. There are clear indications that either alternate or classical pathway activation of complement or both can be found in human corneas with microbial infections.

SUMMARY

We found that both classical and alternate pathway activation of complement were operative in rabbit and human corneas with microbial infections using direct immunofluorescent techniques. Corneal ring infiltrates found in association with intracorneal injections of gram-negative bacterial preparations in rabbits were caused by endotoxin and were associated with the deposition of properdin and C3 complement. The finding of properdin and C3 complement in the absence of immunoglobulins and fibrinogen suggested alternate pathway activation of complement. Rabbits sensitized with subcutaneous injections of heat-inactivated S. aureus also developed corneal rings infiltrates after intracorneal injections of S. aureus. These corneal rings were associated with the deposition of immunoglobulins and C3 complement and represent an Arthus-like reaction with classical pathway activation of complement.

Human corneal specimens obtained after perforation from S. aureus, P. mirabilis and A. flavus were studied as well as a peripheral ulcer in a donor eye suggestive of a catarrhal ulcer of staphylococcus. Evidence was found for the presence of either classical or alternate pathway activation of complement or both.

Activation of complement by the alternate pathway provides a very early host response to bacterial or viral infections before an antibody response has been mounted. The role of the alternate pathway in corneal inflammation has heretofore not been stressed. When sufficient time has elapsed for the formation of antibody to an invading organism, classical pathway activation of complement may be superimposed upon alternate pathway activity and further contribute to polymorphonuclear infiltration of the cornea and destruction of invading organisms.

REFERENCES

Allison, A.C., H.V. Schorlemmer & D. Bitter-Suermann. Activation of complement by the alternate pathway as a factor in the pathogenesis of periodontal disease. *Lancet.* 2: *1001–1003*, (1976).

Aronson, S.B., J.H. Elliott, T.E. More & D.M. O'Day. Pathogenetic approach to therapy of peripheral corneal inflammatory disease. *Am. J. Ophthalmol.* 70: *65–90*, (1970).

Ellison, A. & R. Poirier. Therapeutic effects of heparin on Pseudomonas-induced corneal ulcerations. *Am. J. Ophthalmol.* 82: *619–627*, (1976).

Mondino, B.J., B.S. Rabin, E. Kessler, J. Gallo & S.I. Brown. Corneal rings with gram-negative bacteria. *Arch. Ophthalmol.* 95: *2222–2225*, (1977).

Mondino B.J., S.I. Brown, B.S. Rabin & J. Bruno. Alternate pathway activation of complement in a Proteus mirabilis ulceration of the cornea. *Arch. Ophthalmol.* 96: *1659–1661*, (1978).

Müller-Eberhard, H.J. Chemistry and function of the complement system. *Hospital Practice*. August: 33–43, (1977).

Roitt, I.M. Essentials of Immunology. 3rd edition. London, Blackwell Scientific Publications, 1977, pp. 137–146.

Sery, T.W., A.H. Pinkes & R.M. Nagy. Immune corneal rings: I. Evaluation of reactions to equine albumin. *Investigative Ophthalmology*. 1: *672–685*, (1962).

Smolin, G. & M. Okumoto. Staphylococcal blepharitis. *Arch. Ophthalmol.* 95: *82–916*, (1977).

Sohnle, P.G., M.M. Frank & C.H. Kirkpatrick. Deposition of complement components in the cutaneous lesions of chronic mucocutaneous Candidiasis. *Clin. Immuno. and Immunopath.* 5: *340–350*, (1976).

Stalenheim, G., O. Götze, N.R. Cooper, J. Sjöquist & H.J. Müller-Eberhard. Consumption of human complement components by complexes of IgG with protein A of Staphylococcus aureus. *Immunochem.* 10: *501–507*, (1973).

Author's address:
Department of Ophthalmology
University of Pittsburgh
School of Medicine
Pittsburgh, Pennsylvania
U.S.A.

17

Docum. Ophthal. Proc. Series, Vol. 20

EXPERIMENTAL STUDY ON THE IMMUNOTHERAPY
FOR THE *PSEUDOMONAS* KERATITIS IN RABBITS

N. TANAKA, T. SASAKI, I. TANAKA, N. KINOSHITA
AND J.Y. HOMMA

(Yokohama and Tokyo, Japan)

Corneal ulcer caused by pseudomonas aeruginosa is one of the most serious problems of human eye infection. This organism is found to be the most frequent causative organisms of all bacterial corneal infections seen in the Hospital of Yokohama City University in Japan in recent years (Tanaka *et al.*, 1972).

Once the corneal tissue infects with the organism, ulcer spreads over it very rapidly, destroying the tissue so seriously that if it spreads to a certain extent, it eventually leaves a scar in the cornea disturbing the vision, even with antibiotics treatment.

The purpose of present study is to establish an immunotherapy for experimental pseudomonas keratitis, using albino rabbits.

Experiment 1

The first experiment was designed to investigate their protective property by active immunization against the corneal infection.

Three kinds of immunogen were given to them to form active immunization in them. 'OEP', which stands for original endotoxin protein, is a protein portion of endotoxin, which is isolated and purified by J.Y. Homma from a pseudomonal strain. This is an antigen existing serologically in common and it has been proven by the intraperitoneal challenge that the mice vaccinated with the OEP have the protection against pseudomonas infection of all serotypes of strains (Homma, 1968 & 1971).

Protease and elastase, which were isolated from certain strains of pseudomonal aeruginosa, are purified into crystalline by K. Morihara (Morihara *et al.*, 1965 & 1977). The toxoids of these enzymes and the OEP were given to the rabbits once a week for three weeks.

Antibody response against the OEP, protease and elastase was tested by passive hemagglutination titer.

Figures 1 and 2 illustrate the antibody response of OEP and protease.

In the test of elastase, however, no antibody for elastase was noted in the present test scale of examination.

One week after the third immunization, both corneas of three of the immunized rabbits were traumatized and challenged with 10^7/ml viable cell

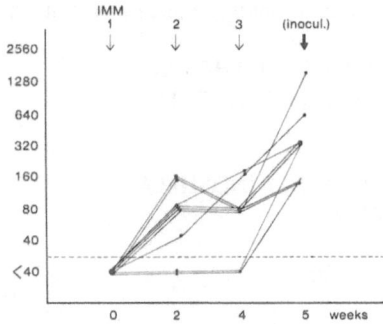

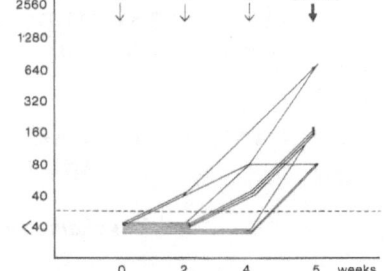

Fig. 1. Passive hemagglutination titer against OEP.

Fig. 2. Passive hemagglutination titer against protease

suspension of a strain No. 1210. This was a virulent strain which demonstrated the production of both extracellular protease and elastase in vitro study. Three rabbits without immunization were served as control. Corneal disease caused by inoculation was observed biomicroscopically for three days following inoculation and was given grade marks of 0, ±, 1 + to 4+, according to the degree of corneal opacity.

Slighter corneal disease was seen in all eyes of the immunized rabbits as shown in Table 1.

IMMUNE RABBITS Corneal Diseases						NON-IMMUNE RABBITS Corneal Diseases			
Day		1	2	3	HA titer (5th W.)	Day		1	2	3
No. 1	R	±	±	±		No. 10	R	0	1+	4+
	L	±	±	±	OEP = 160		L	0	1+	3+
					P = 160					
No. 2	R	0	1+	1+		No. 11	R	±	1+	3+
	L	0	1+	1+	OEP = 640		L	±	1+	4+
					P = 160					
No. 3	R	0	0	0		No. 12	R	1+	2+	4+
	L	0	0	0	OEP = 160		L	1+	2+	4+
					P = 160					

It has been noted that active immunization with the OEP, protease and elastase can effectively protect the cornea from pseudomonal infection.

Experiment 2

The second experiment was designed to investigate the therapeutic effect of topical use of the immune serum. The immune serum we used was obtained from the animals which we used in the experiment 1 and which had been subjected to the corneal challenge with pseudomonas aeruginosa subsequent to the immunization. Topical treatment in the form of eye drop was attempted first. The treatment started three hours after the challenge by instilling drops of the immune serum four times a day (two drops at each time) for three days. This method, however, showed no more therapeutic effect on the pseudomonal ulcer in the eyes of the experimental rabbits than on that in the eyes of the control animals receiving normal rabbit serum.

Subconjunctival application of the immune serum, twice a day for three days also showed no significant therapeutic effect either.

A further experimental attempt was made to treat them by intrastromal injection of the immune serum. Injections were given twice a day for three days, with the first one given three hours after the inoculation. All of the four corneas of the two rabbits which had received normal serum injections and which formed the control group developed severe lesions, whereas a marked suppression of the infection was noted in the eyes of the animals treated with intrastromal injection of the immune serum (Table 2).

			Day 1	2	3	7
				Treatment		
Immune Serum (OEP, P, E)	No.1	R		±	±	±
		L		1	1	±
	2	R		2	2	±
		L		±	±	±
Normal Serum	No.1	R		3	4	4
		L		±	4	4
	2	R		3	4	4
		L		3	4	4

Table 2: Treatment by intrastromal injection.

Experiment 3

The third experiment was undertaken to confirm the therapeutic effect of intrastromal injection of the immune serum.

The experiment was designed to investigate a therapeutic effect of a serum obtained from a beagle dog highly immunized with the OEP, protease and elastase. Three rabbits were used in each of the control and immune serum groups to undergo this experiment. This time the eyes of the control units were treated with phosphate buffered saline.

Both corneas were traumatized by making double crossing incisions at the central areas of their corneas for the inoculation purpose, and then two drops of viable cell suspensions containing 10 to the seventh per ml of the strain No. 1210 were applied there.

Three hours after the inoculation, the experiment animals and the control units were treated with intrastromal injections with approximately 0.03 ml of the immune serum and phosphate buffered saline respectively for two days with two injections per day. Biomicroscopic examination was conducted on their corneas for 7 days after the inoculation.

Reviewing the clinical course after the inoculation of the six eyes, severe corneal lesions were observed in the corneas treated with phosphate buffered saline, while only very slight clinical changes were noted in the corneas treated with the immune serum.

The results of the experiments show that intrastromal injection of the immune serum does have a significant therapeutic effect at least on the corneal ulcer caused experimentally by pseudomonas aeruginosa on the eyes of rabbits and that the data and information we have obtained from present experiments are very interesting and will help us a lot in explicating the pathological mechanism of the pseudomonas keratitis.

REFERENCES

Homma, J.Y. *Zeitschr. für Allg. Mikyobiol.* 8: *227* (1968).
Homma, J.Y. *Japan. J. of Exp. Med.* 41: *387* (1971).
Morihara, K. *et al. J. Biol. Chem.* 240: *3295* (1965).
Morihara, K. *et al. Infection and Immunity* 15: *675* (1977).
Tanaka, N. *et al. Ganka* 14: *269* (1972).

Authors' addresses:
Department of Ophthalmology
Yokohama City University
School of Medicine
Yokohama
Japan
and
Department of Bacteriology
Institute of Medical Science
Tokyo University
Tokyo
Japan

IMMUNOGLOBULINS IN THE CORNEA*

MATHEA R. ALLANSMITH, KAYOKO KASHIMA
AND GILBERT K. YAMAMOTO

(Boston, Mass., U.S.A./Tokyo, Japan)

INTRODUCTION

The use of immunofluorescence for detecting abnormal deposits of proteins (immunoglobulin, complement, fibrinogen) in the cornea in clinical cases is increasing. The consideration of immunologic mechanism in the cornea, especially those concerning antigen-antibody combinations, is becoming more clinically relevant. In view of these two advances in the study of immunology of the cornea, it is appropriate to review the status of immunoglobulin in the cornea prior to inflammation; that is, the normal cornea.

MATERIAL AND METHODS

Subjects

1. For immunofluorescence localization of immunoglobulins in the cornea, 15 pairs of eyes were obtained from subjects at autopsy. The patients ranged from 14 to 82 years of age and were free of eye disease as far as could be determined from their hospital records and inspection of the globes. The time between subject's death and processing of eyes ranged from 1 to 36 hours.

2. For quantitative analysis of albumin and immunoglobulin in the cornea, 10 pairs of eyes from subjects 29 to 75 years of age were studied. Eyes were removed 5 to 26 hours postmortem along with a blood sample from the heart or a great vessel.

Processing of Eyes

1. Processing of eyes for fluorescence microscopy . The globes were divided into anterior and posterior segments by a cut through the equator. The anterior segment was further divided into pie-shaped pieces by meridianal cuts. The tissues were processed by one of the three following techniques: (1) snap-frozen by dropping into isopentane cooled by liquid nitrogen, lyophilized, and then embedded in parrafin (Allansmith *et al.*,

* This work was supported by grant EY-01552 and research fellowship award EY-05213 from the National Eye Institute, National Institutes of Health.

1973), (2) snap-frozen in liquid nitrogen to prepare for cryostat sectioning, or (3) fixed in a modified St. Marie solution of 19 parts alcohol and one part glacial acetic acid for 4 hours, then embedded in paraffin. The sections, either frozen or paraffin-embedded, were cut at 4 μ, and stained with a first layer of rabbit anti-IgG, -IgA, -IgM, -IgD, or -IgE. After washing, the sections were stained with fluoresceinated goat anti-rabbit gamma globulin. The anti-albumin, anti-IgG, anti-IgA, and anti-IgM and goat anti-rabbit were commercial preparations. The stained sections were observed on a Zeiss fluorescence microscope and findings were recorded on Polaroid film for black and white, and on high-speed Ektachrome film for color.

2. Processing of eyes for quantitative determination of immunoglobulin content — Within an hour or so of enucleation, the cornea was removed from each globe by cutting at the cornea-scleral limbus, excluding all sclera. A central button of cornea was then removed with a 5-mm trephine. The remaining donut-shaped corneal ring was cut into four equal quadrants. The immunoglobulins were extracted as previously described (Allansmith and McClellan, 1975). In brief, the corneal pieces were placed in buffered saline which had been previously weighed. The saline and corneal piece were re-weighed and the difference between the first and second weights was the wet weight of the corneal tissue. The tissues were allowed to extract for 48 to 72 hours at 37°C. No preservatives were used. The eluates were trans-ferred into small, plastic, self-capping centrifuge tubes in preparation for analysis by radial diffusion. The fluids were analyzed for IgG, IgA, IgM, and albumin content by the single radial immunodiffusion technique (Mancini *et al.*, 1963). Lower limit for immunoglobulin detection was 5 mg/100 ml. The amount of immunoglobulin in each corneal piece was calculated by the following formula:

$$Ca = \frac{(W + V \cdot g) \, Cb}{W}$$

where Ca is the concentration of protein in the tissue in mg/100 ml of tissue; Cb is the concentration of protein in the eluting fluid, in mg/100 ml; W is the weight of the tissue, in grams; g is the specific gravity of the tissue, in g/ml; and V is the original volume of the eluting fluid, in ml. For pur-poses of calculation, the specific gravity of the cornea was 1 (actually it is 1.05) (Felchlin, 1926) Serum immunoglobulin albumin content was determined by radial immunodiffusion in the same way as for corneal extracts.

RESULTS

Immunofluorescence

Most of the immunoglobulins in the cornea were in the stroma (Fig. 1). IgG, IgA, IgD, and IgE were detected in all specimens and had identical patterns of distribution. Albumin was also found but seemed decreased toward the center of the cornea. The immunoglobulins were present from just beneath

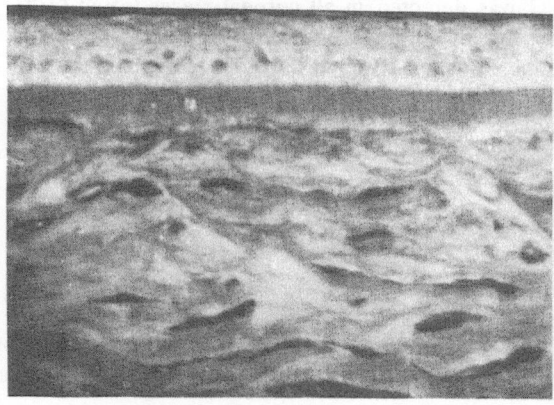

Fig. 1. Anterior cornea stained for IgG (left) and control (right). Note that stroma is brightly fluorescent on left (arrow) and non-stained on right.

Bowman's layer to Descemet's membrane (Fig. 1). The pattern in the sections was that of the collagenase lamellae: regular, linear, and parallel to the epithelium. The keratocytes were seen as autofluorescent fusiform structures devoid of immunoglobulin. Bowman's layer was consistently free of staining for all of the six proteins, as was Descemet's membrane, which was highly autofluorescent. Trace amounts of IgM were detected occasionally in the corneal stroma and seemed concentrated near the limbal edge.

The epithelium was, for the most part, free of stain. Occasionally, a cell full of immunoglobulin or albumin was seen, usually in the basal layer, but occasionally in the most superficial layers. A rough estimate indicated that 1% to 5% of cells stained for either albumin or one of the immunoglobulins.

The basement membrane of the epithelium was generally positive for all proteins except IgM. The membrane appeared as a thin line of fluorescence anterior to the dark Bowman's layer.

The endothelium was frequently lost in processing. It was our impression from several observations that the cytoplasm of the endothelial cells occasionally contained immunoglobulin.

The anterior portion of the cornea usually had a line of fluorescence at its edge, which we interpreted to possibly be tear proteins adherent to the corneal surface.

Tissues processed by the three techniques gave the same results as to demonstration of immunoglobulin and albumin.

Quantitation of Proteins

Albumin was present in all corneal pieces tested (35 of 35). The central buttons were significantly lower in albumin content than were the peripheral corneal pieces ($p < .05$). The amount of albumin in the cornea was about one-fifth that of the serum. The ratio of peripheral to central albumin in these subjects was 3:1.

25

IgG – Immunoglobulin G was detected in all corneal pieces tested (100 out of 100), ranging from a low of 107 mg/100 ml to 856 mg/100 ml, with an average of 460 mg/100 ml. Thus, on a weight basis, the cornea contained about one-half as much IgG as the serum (Fig. 2). The peripheral and central cornea contained equal amounts of IgG (p > .05).

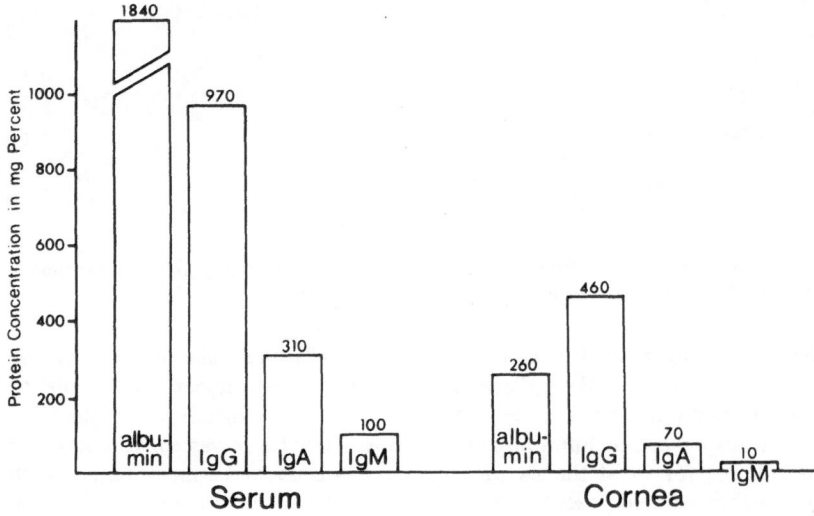

Fig. 2. Amount of albumin and immunoglobulins in serum and cornea. Numbers over bars are milligrams percent protein. Note that concentration of IgG in cornea is about one-half that of serum.

IgA – Immunoglobulin A was detected in all but two of the 100 corneal pieces. On the average, the cornea contained about one-fifth the concentration of IgA as the serum. It was evenly distributed across the cornea, as was IgG (p > .05).

IgM – We tested for the presence of IgM in most corneal pieces in seven subjects. In the remaining three, one or two corneal pieces of each subject was tested. For one subject, the concentration of IgM was higher in each of the ten corneal pieces than in that subject's serum. This did not occur in any of the nine other subjects. Also, the average IgG or IgA level was never higher in the cornea than in the serum for any subject. Because of the peculiarity of the elevated IgM in both corneas in this one subject, the data from this case were excluded from IgM comparisons of central and peripheral cornea and from calculations for average Igm content of one cornea (Fig. 2).

Of 16 of 20 central corneal pieces tested for the presence of IgM, only the subject mentioned above showed IgM. Comparison of IgM in peripheral and central cornea showed significantly less IgM in central cornea (p < .01).

DISCUSSION

The cornea has abundant immunoglobulin throughout its stroma. This agrees with an earlier conclusion that, in general, immunoglobulins are found in any ocular tissue that has enough extracellular space to accommodate them. (Allansmith *et al.*, 1973)

The distribution of the blood-derived solutes (albumin and immunoglobulins) across the cornea appears to be determined not only by the exclusion volume of the cornea, but also by the ratio of its loss across the endothelium to its rate of diffusion in the plane of the stroma (Maurice and Riley, 1970). Low molecular weight solutes pass readily across the endothelium and do not penetrate far beyond the cornea-scleral limbus. Larger molecules, such as serum albumin, are lost more slowly across the endothelium but penetrate relatively quickly in the stroma. Although they may not penetrate to the apex of the cornea, their concentration in the center is lower than at the periphery. Higher molecular weight proteins, such as IgG and IgA, will pass even more slowly across the endothelium, will spread evenly even farther into the cornea, and may approximate uniform concentration over the entire surface. Large molecules, such as IgM, will penetrate only a short distance into the stroma, if at all, and will be absent from the central cornea. A schematic representattion of our concept of the passage of albumin and IgG, IgA, and IgM into the cornea is presented in Fig. 3.

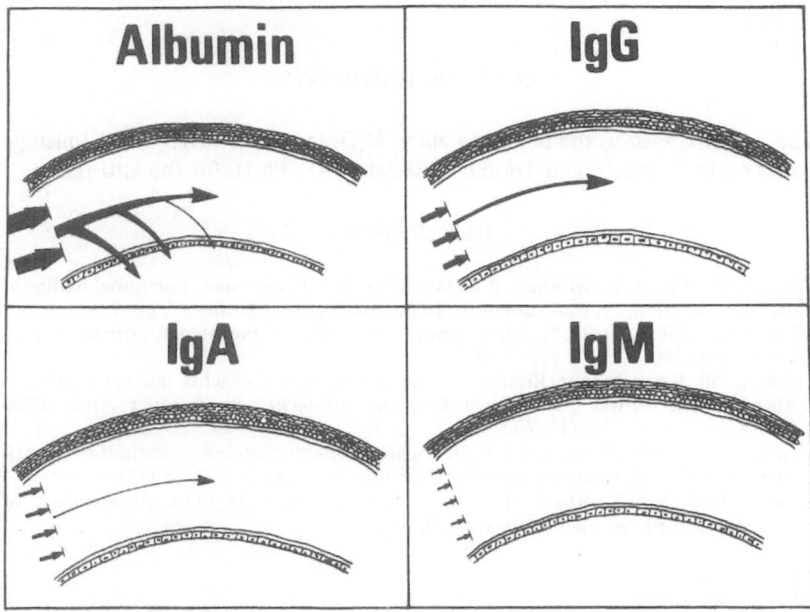

Fig. 3. Diagrammatic representation of distribution of albumin and immunoglobulins in cornea.

Quantitative relationships bear out the immunofluorescence relationships and add IgE and IgD as immunoglobulins that approximate a uniform concentration throughout the cornea.

SUMMARY

The clear cornea would seem to be poorly equipped to initiate immunologic reactions. Lymphocytes are absent from the stroma and only rarely present in the epithelium. A rare macrophage is present in the stroma. It may be that the humoral immunologic system is the main mechanism by which immunologic reactions in the cornea start. Thus, the type, amount, and distribution of antibody protein is of interest.

Fifty corneas of 25 subjects were examined to determine the amounts and location of immunoglobulins and albumin. The immunoglobulin level was determined in central and peripheral areas of 10 pairs of eyes. The other 15 pairs were used for immunofluorescent localization of the five immunoglobulin types.

IgG and IgA were present at high levels in all corneas and were distributed evenly over the central and peripheral areas. Compared to IgG, IgA was relatively impeded from entering the cornea. Immunoglobulin M was restricted to the corneal periphery. The conjunctiva at the limbus had high levels of all immunoglobulins. IgE and IgD, like the other immunoglobulins present, were distributed evenly across the entire cornea.

The humoral immune system may, be the primary line of defense for the cornea.

ACKNOWLEDGMENTS

The authors wish to thank John Fahey, M.D. for the anti-IgD and Kimishige Ishizaka, M.D., Ph.D. and Teruko Ishizaka, M.D., Ph.D. for the anti-IgE.

REFERENCES

Allansmith, M.R., C.R. Whitney, B.H. McClellan, & L.P. Newman. Immunoglobulins in the eye: Location, type and amount. *Arch. Ophthalmol.* 89: *36–45*, (1973).

Allansmith, M.R. & B.H. McClellan. Immunoglobulins in the human cornea. *Am. J. Ophthalmol.* 80: *123–132*, (1975).

Felchlin, M. Versuche zur Ermittlung des spezifischen Gewichts der verschiedenen Augenmedien mittels einer neuen Methode. *Albrecht von Graefe's Arch. Klin. Ophthalmol.* 117: *325*, (1926).

Mancini, G., A.O. Carbonara, & J.F. Heremans. Immunochemical quantitation of antigens by single radial immunodiffusion. *Immunochemistry* 2: *235*, (1963).

Maurice, D.M. & M.W. Riley. The cornea. In Graymore, C.M. (ed.): Biochemistry of the Eye. London, Academic Press, 1970, p. 56.

Author's address:
20 Staniford Street
Boston, MA 02114
U.S.A.

EXPERIMENTAL MODEL FOR SCLERITIS

R.M. HEMBRY, J. PLAYFAIR, P.G. WATSON AND J.T. DINGLE

(Cambridge, England)

INTRODUCTION

Necrotising scleral disease and the accompanying corneal complications (Watson & Hazleman 1976) is a painful destructive disease which can lead to blindness or loss of the eye. In order to investigate new methods of treatment it was necessary to produce an animal model.

Collagen damage has been shown to occur in cornea (Breebaadt & James-Witte 1959; Germuth 1962; Mohos *et al.* 1969; and others) following immune injury but in no case has progressive destruction been reported. Consden *et al.* (1971) described a method for producing a chronic progressive arthritis in rabbits and we have found that a modification of this method has enabled us to develop chronic progressive destructive corneoscleral disease in these animals.

MATERIALS AND METHODS

Mature New Zealand White rabbits were injected intra-dermally with an emulsion of 5mg ovalbumin (Sigma Grade III) in 0.25ml sterile saline and 0.25ml complete Freunds adjuvant (Difco) in 5 sites. The intra-dermal injections were repeated three times over a year to 18 months. The animals were then sedated with 1.5–2.0 ml Hypnorm (Janssen Pharmaceutrica, Beerse, Belgium) and the left eye locally anaesthetised with 0.5 ml xylocaine 2% (Astra Chemicals Ltd., Watford, U.K.).

2mg ovalbumin in 100 μl sterile saline was injected into the limbus superiorly, adjacent to the superior-rectus muscle. The injection was deemed successful if an opaque bleb was visible in both cornea and sclera. If the injection entered the aqueous humour, as judged by the relative ease of injection and the lack of bleb-formation, the animal was killed. The animals were observed and photographed regularly and killed at various time intervals after injection into the eye.

Three control groups of animals were used: (a) sensitised animals injected into the eye with 100 μl 0.9% NaCl; (b) unsensitised animals, injected into the eye with 2.0 mg ovalbumin in 100 μl 0.9% NaCl and (c) unsensitised animals injected with 100 μl 0.9% NaCl.

Serum was collected from all animals at death, and the presence of antibodies to ovalbumin was shown using Ouchterlony gel diffusion plates.

The eyes were fixed in 10% formal saline and paraffin wax-embedded sections were prepared for histological examination. Photographs were taken using Kodak Photomicrography 2483 film.

RESULTS

Table 1. Number of animals in which corneo-scleral lesion appeared.

Injection into eye	Animals sensitised to ovalbumin	Unsensitised animals
Ovalbumin 2.Omg in 100 μl 0.9% NaCl	6/8	0/4
0.9% NaCl 100 μl	0/4	0/4

OVALBUMIN SENSITISED ANIMALS, 2 MG OVALBUMIN INTO LEFT EYE ONLY

The clinical course of the ocular reaction varied in timing and severity. In general on the day after injection the corneal opacification had subsided but there was profuse mucus production, the eye congested and the lids shut. Over the next few days the congestion increased, the conjunctiva was often haemorrhagic and a dense linear white stromal corneal opacity appeared at the site of the injection. By the seventh day postinjection the generalised congestion of the conjunctiva had diminished but the cornea remained hazy and peripheral vascularisation of the cornea became evident. This was sometimes accompanied by an intense uveitis leading to a coagulum in the anterior chamber. The eyes became less congested from about two weeks and all were quiet by 2 months and remained so until the animals were killed. The corneal haze cleared by 6 weeks. In one animal in this group the eye then became quiet and clinically normal but in all the others further progressive abnormalities became obvious. In some of these animals the pupil became eccentric and the iris adherent to the peripheral cornea; this usually occurred from 3−8 weeks. Linear thinning of the limbus as judged by clinical examination and transillumination in a concentric fashion from about 2.30−3.30 was noted from as early as two weeks but only much later in others. After an interval during which the eye was entirely quiet, peripheral scleral thinning appeared $90°−180°$ from the site of the original injection. This was accompanied by minimal and sometimes no inflammatory signs. These lesions were progressive in a circumferential fashion from the original locus and did not heal. In one animal the necrotic scleral lesions did not appear until the third intralimbal injection.

SENSITISED ANIMALS, SALINE INJECTED INTO LEFT EYE

The sensitised animals were injected in the usual manner with saline at 1 o'clock. Opacification of the upper half of the cornea was produced. How-

30

ever, this had cleared within 24 hours and the eyes remained quiet up to 18 weeks.

UNSENSITISED ANIMALS, LEFT EYE INJECTED WITH 2MG OVALBUMIN

The limbus was injected in the usual manner. Opacification of the upper half of the cornea was produced. These eyes also remained quiet. However, a few localised blood vessels were noted in the cornea at the site of injection in one eye at 7 days. These regressed and all eyes were normal at the time of killing at 20 weeks.

UNSENSITISED ANIMALS, LEFT EYE INJECTED WITH SALINE

The limbus was injected as in Group I. The usual opacification of the upper cornea was produced. The cornea had cleared by 24 hours and there was no mucus discharge or congestion of the eyeball. The normal appearance of the eye persisted until the animals were killed at 20 weeks.

HISTOLOGY

In the animals with lesions the extent of the histological damage varied, but typically showed a diffuse granulomatous reaction of the sclera and adjacent cornea, containing many plasma cells and lymphocytes. The corneal stroma was thinned, the lamellar collagen fibres disrupted and oedematous with many blood vessels and lymph channels. The stromal keratocytes were abnormal throughout the cornea, being enlarged, round and vacuolated. The epithelium covering the lesion was thin, Bowman's membrane was absent and the epithelial cells were vacuolated. Descemet's membrane had been broken in several places, and repair attempted, leaving a duplicated Descemet's membrane. Adjacent to the diffuse granuloma, Descemet's membrane was also broken, the end thin and frayed and the adjacent lamellar collagen fibres very disorganised. Histological preparations of the eyes of the control animals appeared normal.

DISCUSSION

Progressive destructive scleral disease similar to that seen in man has been reproduced in rabbits by prolonged sensitisation to ovalbumin by intradermal injection. The scleral lesions appeared after an interval following intra-limbal injection of ovalbumin. The initial acute reaction occurred at the site of this injection and was accompanied by an intense corneal and sometimes uveal reaction. This settled down and between two weeks and eight months later the necrotic changes in the sclera appeared between 90° and 180° from the site of the original injection. The histological appearance of these lesions are very similar to those described by François (1970) in patients with necrotising scleritis.

31

We believe that this animal model will be useful in enabling us to study the mechanism of destruction of corneal and scleral collagen in the chronic progressive lesion and enable us to attempt new methods of treatment.

REFERENCES

Breebaardt, A.C. & J. James-Witte. Studies on experimental corneal allergy. *Amer. J. Ophthal.* 48, *37–47*, (1959).

Consden, A. Doble, L.E. Glynn & A.P. Nine. Production of a chronic arthritis with ovalbumin. Its retention in the rabbit knee joint. *Ann. Rheum. Dis.* 30, *307–315*, (1971).

François, V. Ocular manifestations in collagenoses, Vol. 23 in Advances in Ophthalmology. Karger 1970.

Germuth, F.G., A.E. Maumenee, S.B. Senterfit & A.D. Pollack. Immunohistologic studies on antigen-antibody reactions in the avascular cornea. *J. Exp. Med.* 115, *919–928*, (1962).

Mohos, S.C. & B.M. Wagner. Damage to collagen in corneal immune injury. *Arch. Path.* 88, *3–20*, (1969).

Watson, P.G. & B.L. Hazleman. The sclera and systemic disorders. Vol. 2 in Major Problems in Ophthalmology. Saunders Co. Ltd., 1976.

Author's address:
Strangeways Research Laboratory
Worts' Causeway
Cambridge CB1 4RN
England

CELL MEDIATED IMMUNITY IN MOOREN'S ULCER

S.P. DHIR, S. SEHGAL AND I.S. JAIN

(Chandigarh, India)

Mooren's ulcer is a chronic ulcer starting in the corneal periphery with a characteristically undermined edge. It progresses slowly and relentlessly until the entire cornea is involved (Duke Elder and Leigh, 1965).

The aetiology of Mooren's ulcer is obscure. Several aetiological factors have been postulated from time to time, but none of the suggestions has stood the test of time. Recently Rahi and Carner (1976) have considered Mooren's ulcer under auto-immune disorders on the basis of its pathological features.

We here present two patients of Mooren's ulcer. Cell mediated immunity (CMI) to autologous cornea was studied in one case. CMI to homologous cornea was studied in both cases, employing the Leucocyte Migration Inhibition (LMI)test.

CASE HISTORY

Case 1. KD 40 years female had been suffering from a chronic peripheral corneal ulcer for one year. She had received several lines of treatment without any benefit.

The cornea had gutter-like ulcer running all around in the mid-periphery. The cornea, peripheral to the ulcer, had superficial vascularization and was covered with epithelium. The central part of the cornea was thickened and edematous with overhanging edge on the gutter (Fig. 1). The anterior chamber was normal in depth and no evidence of iridocylitis was seen. The intraocular pressure was normal. She also had nodular goitre. Culture from the ulcer bed was sterile. Urine and stool examination did not reveal any abnormality. She was diagnosed as a case of Mooren's ulcer. The gutter in the cornea further extended towards the centre over a period of one month. A 5 mm diameter central disc of the cornea was left by the advancing edge of the ulcer. A lamellar keratectomy was performed and the central corneal disc was removed. Following keratectomy the ulcer healed rapidly. The excised corneal tissue was used as a source of autologous antigen for a LMI test. Ten ml of blood was drawn from the antecubital vein for the LMI test.

Case 2. R.K. 50 years old male was seen with the history of recurrent attacks of pain, redness and watering from the right eye from which he had

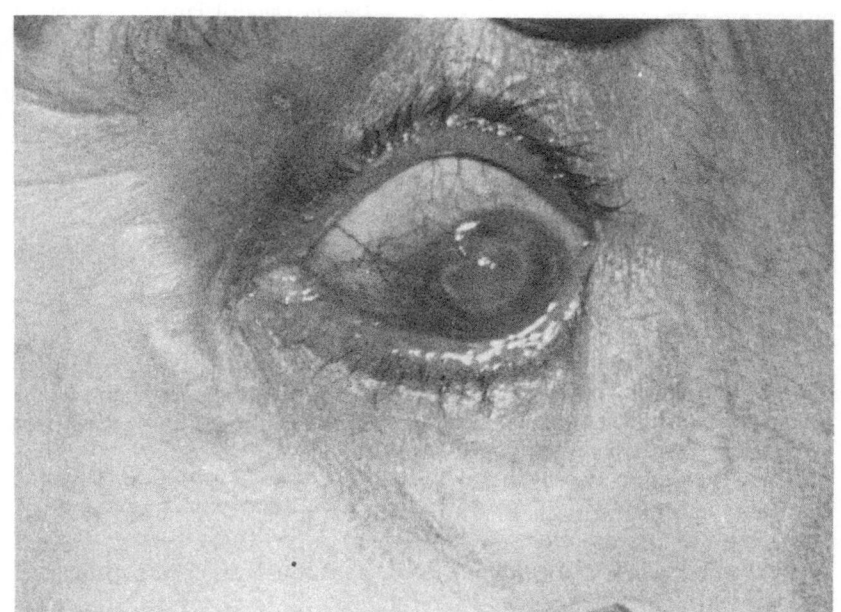

Fig. 1.

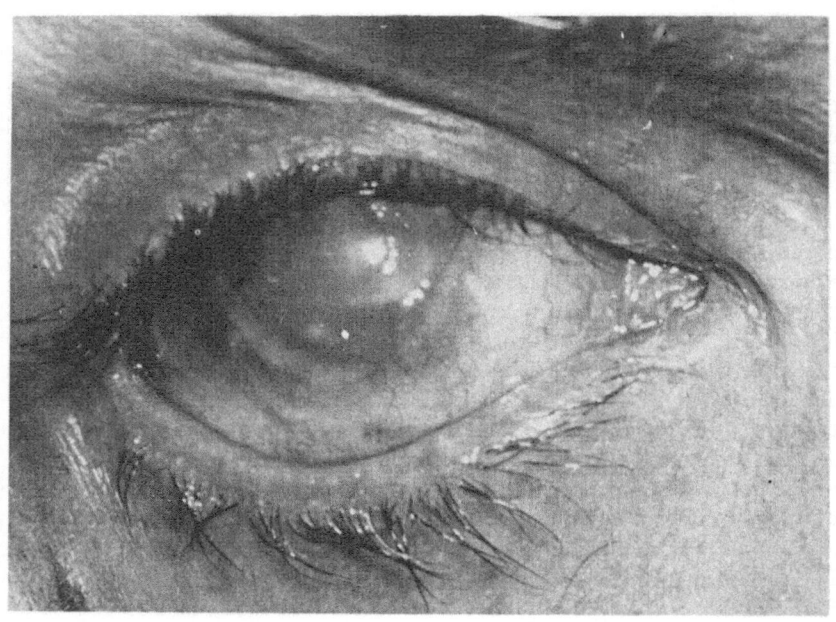

Fig. 2.

34

been suffering for ten years. He had had four such attacks, the first three subsided with treatment without much visual loss. With the onset of the present attack he had developed diminution of vision. He had received treatment in the form of drops, ointments and subconjunctival injections without any relief.

On examination, the visual acuity in the right eye was reduced to hand movements. There was moderate circum-corneal congestion. The cornea had a marginal gutter-like ulcer (Fig. 2) which stained with fluorescin only at the edges of the gutter in a few spots. The cornea peripheral to the ulcer was vascularised and covered with epithelium. The central part of the cornea was hazy and thickened with over hanging edge of the gutter. There was no hypopyon and no evidence of uveitis could be seen. He was diagnosed as a case of Mooren's ulcer. He was treated initially with atropine eye drops and framycetin eye drops without much improvement in the condition. Later he was put on betamethasone and atropine eye drops, to which he responded very favourably. The ulcer healed rapidly. Ten ml of blood was withdrawn from the anticubital vein for a LMI test. He had recurrences of attacks which were controlled with betamethasone eye drops.

LEUCOCYTE MIGRATION INHIBITION TEST

The LMI test was performed by the method of Sobang and Beudixeu (1967). Two antigens were used, autologous corneal antigen was obtained by homogenisation of corneal disc removed from patient 1. The second antigen was prepared by homogenisation of cadaver corneal disc. Leucocytes were obtained from both the Mooren's ulcer cases and from a case of chronic fungal ulcer.

The peripheral blood 't' cells were studied by a direct rosette test with sheep erythrocytes using lymphocytes purified on a fical hypaque gradient.

Table 1. Results of LMI test in corneal ulcer

Antigen	Mooren's ulcer Case 1	Mooren's ulcer Case 2	Fungal corneal ulcer
Autologous cornea	68%	N.T.	N.T.
Cadaver cornea	25%	34%	10%

* Percentage inhibition of leucocyte migration as compared to control media.

The results of the LMI test are shown in Table 1. It is seen that there was marked inhibition of leucocyte migration when autologous corneal antigen was introduced into the chamber in case 1 (Fig. 3.) Indicating that the patient's leucocytes have been sensitized to the autologous antigen, and to some extent to the homologous antigen as well. Case 2 also showed significant inhibition of leucocyte migration in the presence of homologous antigen. The patient with fungal corneal ulcer, however, did not reveal any

35

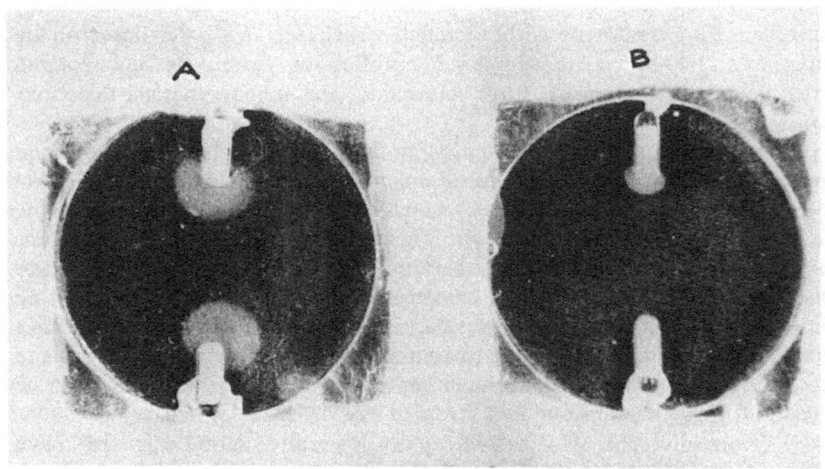

Fig. 3.

significant inhibition in the presence of homologous antigen. The 'T' cell count was normal in both cases.

COMMENTS

The demonstration of sensitization of leycocytes to autologous and homologous cornea in patients with Mooren's ulcer does support the hypothesis of breakdown of the immunological barrier between the cornea and the body due to some unknown reason. However, this barrier was found intact in the case with fungal corneal ulcer. Thus ulceration is perhaps not the explanation for this break in immunological barrier. It is possible that this break in immunological barrier has led to auto-immune reaction, setting up an inflammatory reaction at the junction of the corneal antigens and the sensitized leucocytes leading to chronic ulceration at the limbus. With ensuing vascularization this process is further carried towards the centre of the cornea until the whole of cornea was involved. It appears that this sensitization is to the superficial cellular elements of the cornea, namely epithelium. Indeed Schapp et al. (1969) have demonstrated immunoglobulin bound to the corneal epithelium as well as serum lg G auto-antibodies in a patient with Mooren's ulcer.

In experimental studies on rabbits by Khodadoust (1978) it has been shown that all three cellular elements of the cornea, i.e. epithelium, stroma and endothelium, may be involved in the corneal graft rejection process. Epithelial cell rejection begins in the vicinity of congested limbal vessels especially when there is extension of the vessels into the rim of the recipient cornea, followed by replacement with host epithelium. The intervening necrotic zone between the rejected and host epithelium is infiltrated with inflammatory cells.

36

Grunett et al. (1976) found cytotoxic lymphocytes in the peripheral blood by direct cell mediated lympholysis in corneal graft rejection cases.

There is a strong possibility that the erosion in Mooren's ulcer is initiated by auto-immune lysis of the epithelium with consequent release of collagenolytic enzymes. The histopathological findings of sub-epithelial leucocyte infiltration with ulceration of the epithelium and underlying stroma beginning at the corneal periphery also support an auto-immune theory for the occurrence of Mooren's ulcer. The clinical observation that the disease process heals, once the entire cornea is involved would be an indication of an auto-immune process to superficial corneal layers. Once the cornea is exhausted of the antigen the disease subsides. Amelioration with administration of corticosteroids (Leigh, 1962) is another pointer towards an auto-immune process.

SUMMARY

Two cases of Mooren's ulcer and one case of fungal corneal ulcer were studied for cell mediated immunity by Leucocyte Migration Inhibition test. Autologous cornea was used as challenge antigen in one case of Mooren's ulcer and homologous corneau in all three cases. Sensitization of a patient's leucocytes with Mooren's ulcer to autologous corneal antigen and to homologous corneal antigens could be demonstrated.

No such sensitization was observed in the case of fungal corneal ulcer studied. It is hypothesized that Mooren ulcer is an auto-immune disorder and due to some unknown reason the immunological barrier between the superficial corneal layers and the body breaks down.

REFERENCES

Duke Elder, S. & A.E. Leigh. in: System of Ophthalmology Vol. III, Part 2. Henery Kimpton, London, p. 915, 1965.

Grunnet, N., T. Krishtensen, F. Kissmeyer-Nielson & N. Ehlens. Occurrence of lymphocytotoxic lymphocytes and antibodies after corneal transplantation. *Acta Ophthalmologica* 54: *167–173*, (1976).

Khodadoust, A.A. The allograft rejection reaction the leading cause of late failure of clinical corneal graft failure Ciba Foundation Symposium 15 pp. 161)164, 1973.

Leigh Trans. Ophthal. Soc. U.K., 79, 439. (1959) Acta XIX Int. Cong. Ophthal. New Delhi (1962).

Rahi, A.H.S., & A. Garner. Immunopathology of the Eye. Blackwell Scientific Publications, London, p. 128, 1976.

Scaap. O.L. Feltkamp, T.E.W. & A.C. Breedbert. Circulating auntbodies to corneal tissue in a patient suffering from Mooren's ulcer (ulcer roders corneae) *Clin., Exp. Immunol.* 5: *365, 370*, (1969).

Sobang M., & G. Beudixen. Human lymphocyte migration as a parameter of hypersensitivity. *Acta Med. and Scand.* 181: *247*, (1967).

Author's address:
Department of Ophthalmology and Pathology
Postgraduate Institute of Medical Education & Research
Chandigarh
India.

ROLE OF CELL-MEDIATED IMMUNITY IN THE RESISTANCE OF RABBITS TO CORNEAL HERPES SIMPLEX VIRUS INFECTION

T. SASAKI, E. GOTOH, K. KAMATA, R. ISHIKAWA, R. DOKOH, M. HIGUCHI, AND M. INOUE

(Yokohama, Japan)

With the progress of modern immunology, much evidence (Wilton *et al.*, 1972; Rosenberg *et al.*, 1972; Lodmell *et al.*, 1973; Easty *et al.*, 1973; Lodmell & Notkins, 1974) has been produced to demonstrate the immune response of some animals and humans to the herpes simplex virus (HSV), but the host- defense mechanism and the mechanism of recurrence are as yet not clearly understood (Meyers & Chitjian, 1976).

In order to study the host-defense mechanism against HSV corneal infection, we experimented on the effect of cell-mediated immunity on host defense.

EXPERIMENT 1. THE EFFECT OF CELL-MEDIATED IMMUNITY IN THE RESISTANCE OF RABBITS TO CORNEAL HSV RE-INFECTION

Materials and methods

The experimental animals used were young, adult, female, white rabbits, weighing approximately 2.5 kg. The rabbits were divided into two groups and inoculated with HSV by different routes, by the corneal route, or by the intravenous route, in order to establish different states of immunity.

After topical anesthesia, the left corneas of ten rabbits were traumatized with a 26 gauge needle, and two drops of culture fluids of HSV infected VERO cells, were instilled.

Another five rabbits were immunized systematically with 10^8 $TCID_{50}$ of HSV by the intravenous route. Intravenous injection at the same dosage was repeated after 1 week, 2 weeks, and 6 weeks.

8 weeks after primary inoculation, the rabbits of both groups were bled from an ear artery, and the blood examined for lymphocyte transformation and neutralizing antibodies.

After bleeding, both corneas of all rabbits were re-inoculated with the same strain of HSV.

After re-inoculation, clinical manifestations were observed daily by biomicroscope until the animals had recovered.

Lymphocyte transformation tests were carried out by using cultures of washed whole blood cells according to the procedure prescribed by Scriba (1974). Heat-inactivated HSV antigen was used. Results plotted as a

39

function of stimulation index.

Measurement of neutralizing antibodies not requiring a complement was carried out by the micro method. The number of neutralizing units per sample was expressed as the reciprocal of the endpoint dilution.

Results

1. Immune responses following primary HSV inoculation.

Fig. 1 shows that the stimulation indices of rabbits inoculated by the intravenous route were lower than those of the corneal route group. It seems likely that repeated injection of the intravenous group depressed the stimulation of lymphocytes.

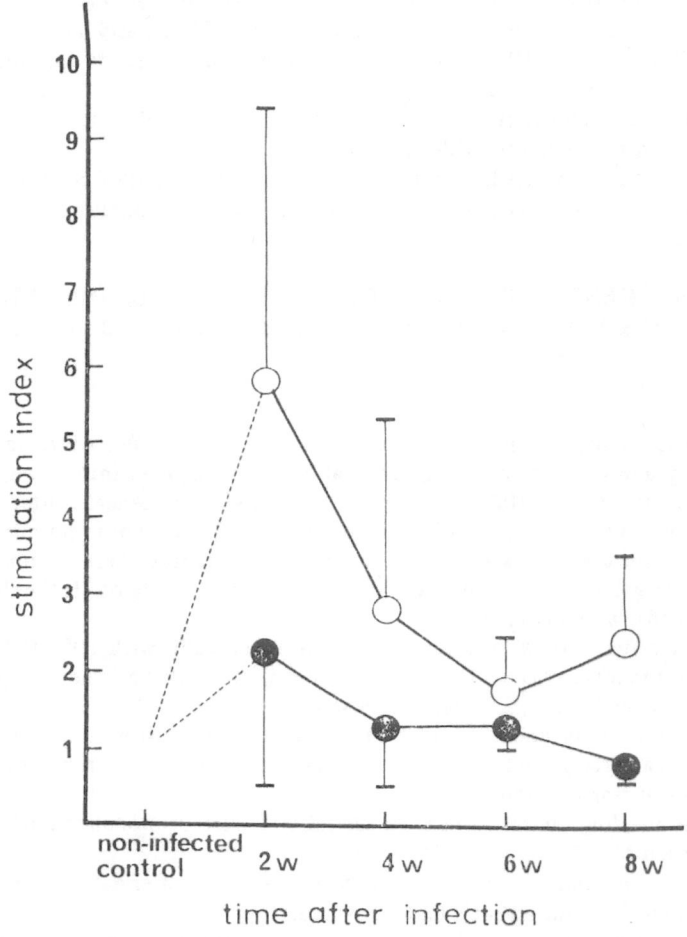

Fig. 1. Stimulation of peripheral lymphocytes after HSV inoculation. O: corneal route, ●: intravenous route.

Fig. 2. shows the stimulation index and neutralizing titer of individual rabbits at 8 weeks after primary inoculation. The intravenous group showed stimulation indices and a high number of antibodies. The corneal route group showed wider distribution.

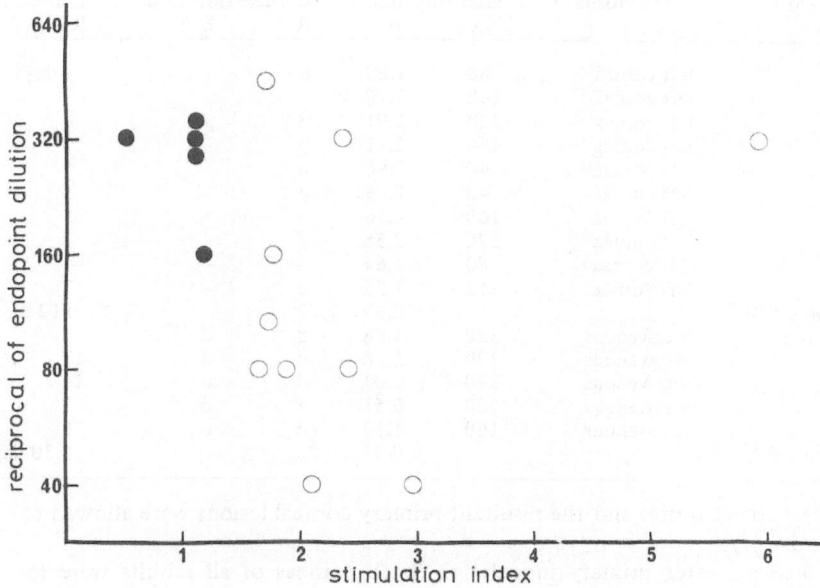

Fig. 2. Neutralizing antibody titers and stimulation of peripheral lymphocytes at 8 weeks after HSV inoculation. O: corneal route, •: intravenous route

2. Clinical picture after re-inoculation (Table 1).
Previously inoculated corneas except left cornea of rabbit No. 3 did not show evidence of re-infection.
On the other hand, the previously unaffected eyes of rabbits immunized by the corneal route manifested punctate and dendritic ulcers after re-inoculation. These ulcers were milder than the primary corneal lesions.
    Both eyes of rabbits immunized by the intravenous route developed dendritic or geographic ulcers showing stronger lesions and longer duration than those of the corneal route grous.

EXPERIMENT 2. THE EFFECT OF IMMUNOSUPRESSANTS ON CORNEAL HSV REÏFECTION

Materials and methods

The right corneas of nine rabbits were inoculated with HSV by the same procedure as was used on the original 10 rabbits which were inoculated by

Table 1. Corneal HSV re-infection and immune responses of rabbits immunized with HSV by different routes. NA: Neutralizing Antibody, SI: Stimulation Index, p' Punctate ulcer, d: dendritic ulcer, g: geographic ulcer, R: Right cornea, L: Left cornea.

Rabbit No.	Primary Virus Inocul.	at 8 Weeks after Infection		Second Corneal Infection		Duration of Corneal Ulcer	
		NA	SI	R	L	R	L
1	left cornea	80	1.89	p	–	4 days	–
2	left cornea	448	1.70	–	–	–	–
3	left cornea	320	5.91	p	p	6	4
4	left cornea	160	2.41	p	–	7	–
5	left cornea	40	2.96	p	–	5	–
6	left cornea	40	2.09	p	–	5	–
7	left cornea	160	1.76	p	–	5	–
8	left cornea	320	2.35	d	–	3	–
9	left cornea	80	1.64	–	–	–	–
10	left cornea	112	1.72	d	–	7	–
Mean ± SD			2.39 ± 1.27			512 days	
11	intravenous	320	1.08	d	d	8	8
12	intravenous	320	1.08	d	d	13	8
13	intravenous	320	1.04	d	d	14	15
14	intravenous	320	0.51	g	d	7	7
15	intravenous	160	1.17	d	d	8	5
Mean ± SD			0.97 ± 0.26			9.30 days	

the corneal route, and the resultant primary corneal lesions were allowed to heal.

4 weeks after primary inoculation, both corneas of all rabbits were re-inoculated with the same strain of HSV.

The animals were divided into three groups, one group receiving 100 mg/kg of aziathioprine per day, one group receiving 100 mg/kg of cyclophosphamide per day, and one group receiving no treatment for 4 days before re-inoculation.

Lymphocyte transformation and neutralizing antibodies were assayed both before and after the administration of immunosupressants.

Clinical manifestations were observed by biomicroscope daily until the animals recovered.

Results

1. Changes in the immune response following treatment with immuno-supressants.

The stimulation index decreased in all animals which had been treated with immunosupressants. However antibody titers did not decrease after treatment.

2. Clinical picture after re-inoculation.

The previously unaffected eyes of rabbits treated with azathioprine manifested strong geographic ulcers much like a primary infection. The eyes of most rabbits treated with cyclophosphamide manifested dendritic ulcers. These lesions were stronger than those of the control animals, and lasted longer.

42

Previously infected corneas did not show evidence of re-infection in spite of treatment with immunosupressants.

COMMENTS

The data of the first experiment indicate that in previously uninfected corneas of both groups immunized by different routes, the corneas of the corneal route group, which have higher stimulation indices, showed milder lesion than those of the intravenous route group. With the intention of confirming these facts a second experiment was carried out to examine re-infection of compromised rabbits in which cell-mediated immunity was depressed by use of immunosupressants.

The data of second experiment indicate that compromised rabbits in which cell-mediated immunity was depressed showed stronger corneal lesions than the control animals following HSV reinfection.

The experiments of R.L. Hall in 1955, M. Okumoto in 1959 and Y. Yokoyama in 1961, which showed that the corneas of animals immunized with HSV resisted re-infection, led them, at that time, to believe that intracorneal antibodies were the key factor in the defense mechanism.

As a result of our experiments, however, we believe that cell-mediated immunity is the significant factor in the resistance and recovery of rabbits immunized with HSV.

REFERENCES

Easty, D.L., et al. Tran. Ophthalmol. Soc. UK. 93: 171 (1973).
Hall, R.L., et al. Am. J. Ophthalmol. 39: 226 (1955).
Lodmell, D.L., et al. J. Exp. Med. 137: 706 (1973).
Lodmell, D.L. & Notkins, A.L. J. Exp. Med. 140: 764 (1974).
Meyers, R.L. & Chitjian, P.A. Surv. Ophthalmol. 21: 194 (1976).
Okumoto, M., et al. Am. J. Ophthalmol. 47: 61 (1959).
Rosenberg, G.L., et al. Proc. Nat. Acad. Sci. 69: 756 (1972).
Scriba, M. Infect. Immun. 10: 430 (1974).
Wilton, L.M.A., et al. Brit. Med. J. 18: 723 (1972).
Yokoyama, Y. Acta Soc. Ophthalm. Jpn. 65: 507 (1961).

Authors' address:
Department of Ophthalmology
Yokohama City University
School of Medicine
Yokohama
Japan

Docum. Ophthal. Proc. Series, Vol. 20

LYMPHOCYTE CYTOTOXICITY AGAINST THE RABBIT CORNEAL ENDOTHELIUM. MORPHOLOGICAL ASPECTS*

P. MONTCOURRIER AND Y. POULIQUEN

(Paris, France)

ABSTRACT

Inoculation into the rabbit's anterior chamber of skin-sensitized allogeneic lymphocytes (a local graft-versus-host reaction) leads to the destruction of corneal endothelium. The activated lymphocytes attach to the endothelial layer and display changes indicating motility, especially a broad cytoplasmic process (uropod). They infiltrate under the endothelial layer and work out in it their cytotoxic action. Within two or three weeks, the regenerated endothelium is quite normal. The role of thymus-dependant lymphocytes and the way the lymphocyte cytotoxicity leads to target cell death is discussed, and this *in vivo* experimental model is compared to other *in vitro* models.

INTRODUCTION

Many light and electron microscopic studies clearly showed in rejecting corneal homografts, that the immune process is mediated by lymphoid cells (Inomata *et al.*, 1970; Khodadoust and Silverstein, 1969; Polack, 1962; Porter and Knight, 1973). A reaction which can be proved to be a model for allograft rejection is the graft-versus-host reaction (Cerottini and Brunner, 1974; Grebe and Streilein, 1976) where immunologically competent lymphoid cells are grafted into a histoincompatible host unable to reject them. So it has been taken advantage of the immunological privilege of the anterior chamber of the eye (Porter and Knight, 1973) to elicit in it a graft-versus-host reaction.

Among the various different models so investigated by different authors (Kaplan *et al.*, 1975; Khodadoust and Silverstein, 1975; Prendergast and Franklin, 1971), the one of Khodadoust and Silverstein, (1975) in the rabbit, has been used to study at the ultra-structural level, the relationships between lymphocyte killer cells and corneal endothelial target cells.

MATERIALS AND METHODS

Immunologically competent lymph node cells were obtained from a pair of adult albino rabbits by an exchange of full-thickness ear skin grafts. At the time of graft rejection, a suspension of lymphoid cells were prepared from

* Supported by grants INSERM U 86, CNRS ATP 1998 and DGRST 76.7.0969.

45

the draining lymph node, and filtered by a single passage through a nylon fiber column (Julius *et al.*, 1973) in order to eliminate a maximum of adhering cells: phagocytosing cells and bursa-dependent lymphocytes. The remaining B lymphocytes (from 1,5 to 8% of filtered cells) were tested by means of direct immunofluorescence (Touraine *et al.*, 1976). Trypan blue dye exclusion test always showed a better than 97% viability. 5 x 10^6 living lymphocytes were inoculated into the anterior chamber of the skin donor rabbit eyes using a heparinized syringe.

For transmission electron microscopy, corneas were fixed in 2,5% glutaraldehyde in phosphate buffer, postfixed in 1,3% osmium tetroxide, and embedded in Epon 812. Ultrathin sections were stained with uranyle acetate and lead citrate, then observed with a Philips EM 300 electron microscope. For scanning electron microscopy, the surface of fixed and embedded specimens was washed with the Epon solvent before complete hardening, coated with gold, and observed in a Cámeca 07 scanning electron microscope.

RESULTS

An intense inflammatory reaction follows the lymphocyte inoculation into the anterior chamber, reaching its peak at days 3 to 5. Contemporaneously, a more or less severe corneal oedema develops, mainly located in the lower part of the cornea, as the cells sedimented, accompanied with a Tyndall phenomenon, and retro corneal dust-like keratic precipitates (Khodadoust and Silverstein, 1975).

An electron microscopic study first shows lymphocytes firmly adhering to the endothelial layer (fig. 1). They can be small (4 to 6 μm in diameter) and round-shaped, with fine long processes anchoring on the endothelium (figs. 2,3), or bigger (6 to 9 μm in diameter), with a more ruffled surface and large pseudopods spreading over the endothelial surface (fig. 2). A large proportion of activated motile lymphocytes develop a specialized cytoplasmic process, the caudal uropod (McFarland *et al.*, 1966) (Figs. 4, 5, 6, 7) which permits them to penetrate into the target layer (fig. 5, 6). The uropod, varying in length, contains many cytoplasmic organelles and cytofibrils, and its surface is characterized by the occurrence of endocytic vesicles and microvilli (fig. 7). The migrating lymphocytes, stopped by Descemet's membrane, detach partially the endothelial cells (fig. 6), and often establish close contact with their target. Lymphocyte surface processes sometimes appear to force progressively into the target cell. The uropod tip often develops a network of turbulent villi deep into an endothelial cell (fig. 8).

As a consequence, corneal endothelium is scattered with focal destruction areas, and many dead cells are found within the endothelial layer (figs. 6, 7) or floating in the aqueous humour.

Active regeneration processes, already present at 24 h., overcome, and 15 to 20 days after the cell inoculation, the endothelium is morphologically normal.

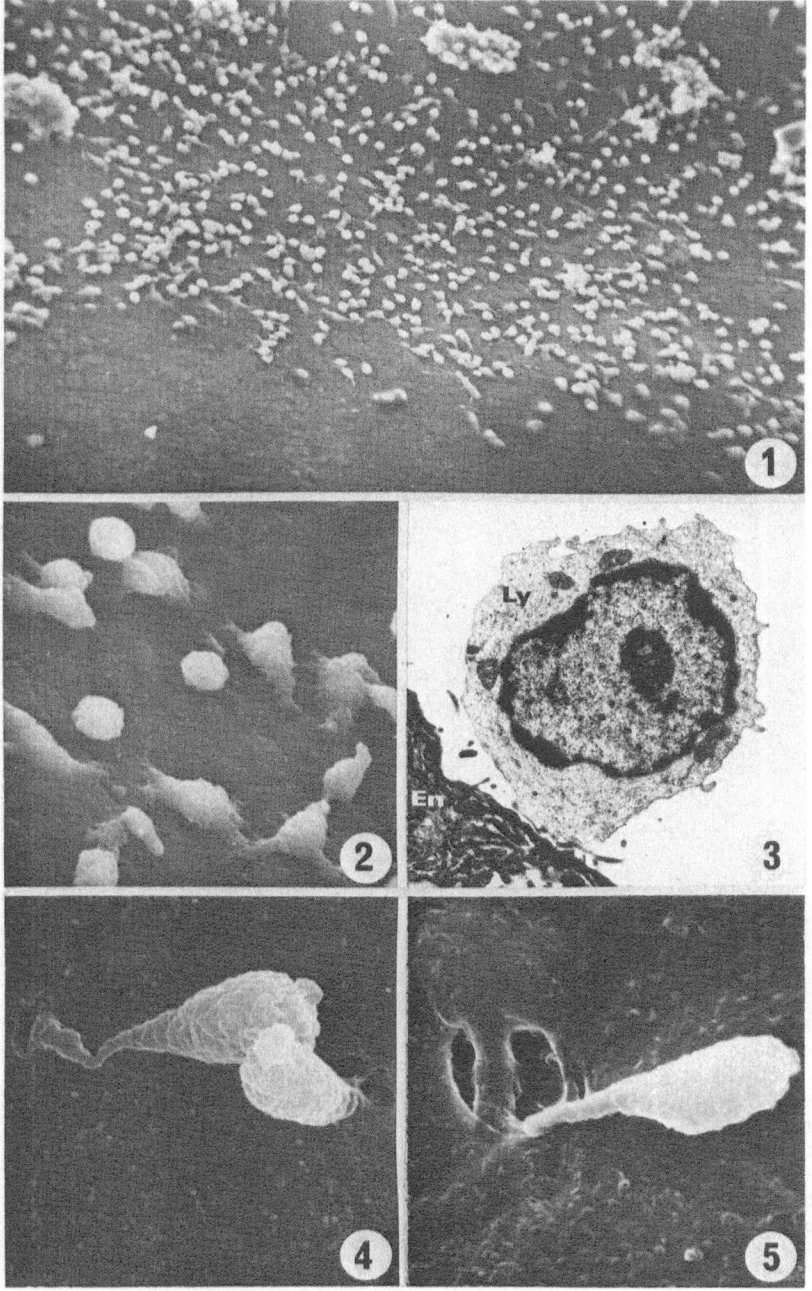

Fig. 1. 1d. after the cell inoculation into the anterior chamber, sensitized lymphocytes sediment and set on the corneal endothelium. x 175. Photo. Dr. G. Renard.

Fig. 2. 2d. Lymphocytes anchor themselves to the endothelium with fine long processes (small and large lymphocytes) or with large pseudopods (large lymphocytes). x 950. Photo Dr. G. Renard.

Fig. 3. 2d. A small typical lymphocyte (Ly) fixed to an endothelial cell (En). Note the relations between effector and target villi. x 10000.

Figs. 4–5. 2d. Typical views of 'hand-mirror' shaped lymphocytes attached to (fig. 4) and infiltrating between (fig. 5) endothelial cells owing to their uropod. x 3500. Photo Dr. G. Renard.

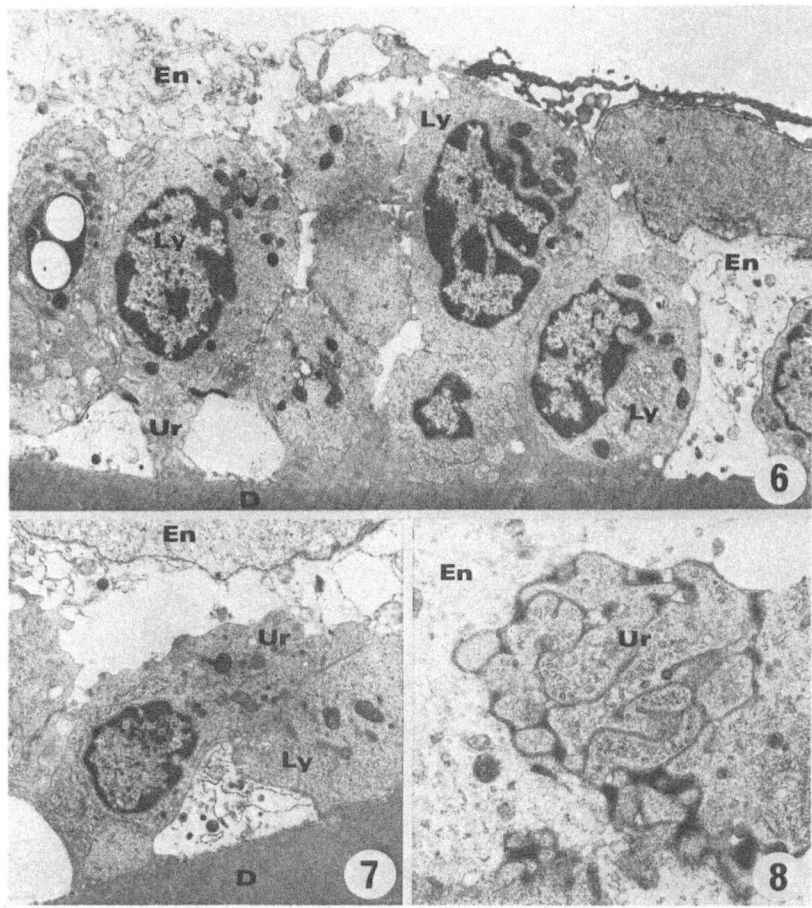

Fig. 6. 3d. Numerous lymphocytes (Ly) infiltrated in the endothelial layer (En). A lymphocyte is attached to Descement's membrane (D) by its uropod (Ur). The endothelium is more than 10 μm thick, and a dead cell is present at the upper left (En). x 7000.

Fig. 7. 3d. A lymphocyte with a short posterior uropod (Ur), neighbouring another lymphocyte (Ly) and a dead endothelial cell (En). Note the cytoplasmic organelles in the uropod, and the small anterior pseudopod close to the Descemet's membrane (D). x 7900.

Fig. 8. 3d. A uropod tip (Ur) forcing the lateral face of an endothelial cell (En). Note the clustered ribosomes in the uropod. Target membranes are intact or tangentially sectionned. x 21300.

DISCUSSION

It is interesting to compare this *in vivo* morphologic model of cytotoxicity with others, *in vitro*. As a matter of fact, the selectivity of the lymphoid suspension filtration on a nylon wool column, proved by the immuno-fluorescence test, allows us to consider this model as mainly T-cell mediated. This is in fact another proof of a local graft-versus-host reaction where T lymphocytes represent the effector cells ((Grebe and Streilein, 1976), which is in agreement with Kaplan's study (Kaplan *et al.*, 1975).

Different *in vitro* morphologic models are used to study the relationships between effector lymphoid cells and target cells. The cytotoxicity can be non specifically induced with plant lectins (Biberfeld, 1971) or with sublytic concentrations of antibodies directed against the target cells (Biberfeld *et al.*, 1973), or it can also be specifically induced by rejection of tumor cells (Able *et al.*, 1970; Kalina and Berke, 1976) or in mixed-lymphocyte-reaction (Barber and Alter, 1978): all these reactions are K- (Biberfeld *et al.*, 1973) or T- (Able *et al.*, 1970; Barber and Alter, 1978; Biberfeld, 1971; Kalina and Berke, 1976) cell mediated.

In both *in vitro* and *in vivo* models, the aspects of the activated lymphocyte are the same, notably concerning volume and form variations, and uropod formation. The uropod is a highly specialized cytoplasmic process, not only involved with movement, but also with a wide variety of interactions with the environment, including other cells (Biberfeld, 1971; MacFarland *et al.*, 1966). It plays an important but unknown role in cell-mediated cytotoxicity (Biberfeld, 1971).

In case of target monolayer (Biberfeld, 1971; Biberfeld *et al.*, 1973), both ocular and *in vitro* reactions are exactly parallel: anchoring and penetration of lymphocytes, and unglueing of monolayer follow the same stages. In the same way, cellular interactions between effector and target cells are identic (Able *et al.*, 1970; Barber and Alter, 1978; Biberfeld, 1971; Biberfeld *et al.*, 1973; Kalina and Berke, 1976). Close contact is a prerequisite for lymphocytes to exert cytotoxicity (Cerottini and Brunner, 1974) and this *in vivo* model is not inconsistent with, nevertheless neither target membrane discontinuities nor intercellular bridges or specialized junctions have been met, as few authors stated (Barber and Alter, 1978; Ferluga and Allison, 1974; Sellin *et al.*, 1971).

A difference between *in vitro* and ocular models is the great regenerative ability of the rabbit corneal endothelium, which heals rapidly and completely wounds caused by lymphocytes.

The graft-versus-host reaction is considered to simulate allograft rejection (Cerottini and Brunner, 1974; Grebe and Streilein, 1976). So this ocular model which can be compared with many *in vitro* models of lymphocyte cytotoxicity, might be used for a better understanding of intimate cellular mechanisms of graft rejection, and particularly of corneal graft rejection.

REFERENCES

Able, M.E., J.C. Lee, & W. Rosenau. Lymphocyte-target cell interaction *in vitro*. Ultrastructural and cinematographic studies. *Amer. J. Pathol.* 60: *421*, (1970).

Barber, T.A., & B.J. Alter. Ultrastructure of effector-target cell interaction in secondary cell-mediated lympholysis. *Scand. J. Immunol.* 7: *57*, (1978).

Biberfeld, P. Cytotoxic interaction of phytohaemagglutinin-stimulated blood lymphocytes with monolayer cells: a study by light and electron microscopy. *Cell. Immonol.* 2: *54*, (1971).

Biberfeld, P. Uropod formation in phytohaemagglutinin (PHA) stimulated lymphocytotoxic interaction between lymphocytes and antibody-coated monolayer cells.

Biberfeld, P., G. Biberfeld, P. Perlmann & G. Holm. Cytological observations on the cytotoxic interactions between lymphocytes and antibody-coated monolayer cells. *Cell. Immunol.* 7: *60*, (1973).

Cerottini, J.-C. & K.T. Brunner. Cell-mediated cytotoxicity, allograft rejection, and tumor immunity. *Adv. Immunol.* 18: *67*, (1974).

Ferluga, J. & A.C. Allison. Observations on the mechanism by which T-lymphocytes exert cytotoxic effects. *Nature* 250: *673*, (1974).

Grebe, S.C. & J.W. Streilein. Graft-versus-Host reactions: a review. *Adv. Immunol.* 22: *119*, (1976).

Inomata, H., G.K. Smelser & F.M. Polack. The fine structural changes in the corneal endothelium during graft rejection. *Invest. Ophthalmol.* 9: *263*, (1970).

Julius, M.H., E. Simpson & L.A. Herzenberg. A rapid method for the isolation of functional thymus-derived murine lymphocytes. *Eur. J. Immunol.* 3: *645*, (1973).

Kalina, M. & G. Berke. Contact regions of cytotoxic T lymphocyte-target cell conjugates. *Cell. Immunol.* 25: *41*, (1976).

Kaplan, H.J., T.R. Stevens & J.W. Streilein. Transplantation immunology of the anterior chamber of the eye. I. An intra-ocular graft-versus-host reaction (Immunogenic anterior uveitis). *J. Immunol.* 115: *800*, (1975).

Khodadoust, A.A., & A.M. Silverstein. Transplantation and rejection of individual cell layers of the cornea. *Invest. Ophthalmol.* 8: *180*, (1969).

Khodadoust, A.A., & A.M. Silverstein. Local graft-versus-host reactions within the anterior chamber of the eye: the formation of corneal endothelial pocks. *Invest. Ophthalmol.* 14: *640*, (1975).

McFarland, W., D.H. Heilman, & J.F. Moorhead. Functional anatomy of the lymphocyte in immunological reactions *in vitro. J. Exp. Med.* 124: *851*, (1966).

Polack, F.M. – Histopathologic and histochemical alterations in the early stages of corneal graft rejection. *J. Exp. Med.* 116: *709*, (1962).

Porter, R. & J. Knight, eds. Corneal Graft Failure. Ciba Foundation Symposium 15, New York, Associated Scientific Publishers, Amsterdam, 1973.

Prendergast, R.A., & R.M. Franklin. Local adoptive immunity in the eye. II. Ocular response following lymph node allograft and specific antigenic challenge. *Invest. Ophthalmol.* 10: *695*, (1971).

Sellin, D., D.F.H. Wallach, & H. Fischer. Intercellular communication in cell-mediated cytotoxicity. Fluorescein transfer between H-2^d target cells and H-2^b lymphocytes *in vitro. Eur. J. Immunol.* 1: *453*, (1971).

Touraine, J.L., F. Touraine, O. de Bouteiller & M. Bonneau. Identification et énumération des lymphocytes T et B chez l'homme en pratique quotidienne. In 'Les techniques de séparation et d'identification des lymphocytes humains'. Séminaire Technologique INSERM, Montpellier, 12–15 Mai 1976. INSERM ed. Paris, 1976, p. 121.

Author's address:
Centre de Recherche d'Ophtalmologie
Fondation Rothschild
29, Rue Manin
75019 Paris
France.

THE CORNEAL ENDOTHELIUM

HERBERT E. KAUFMAN

(New Orleans, U.S.A.)

Clinical specular microscopy has indicated that human cell healing occurs by spreading, there is a limited healing reserve, and premature cell loss is the equivalent of a 'premature aging' that may lead to later decompensation. This instrument has been useful in studying healing and cell damage from surgery, drugs, and special procedures such as intraocular lens insertion. It pointed out extensive cell loss at the time of intraocular lens insertion, and subsequent studies have indicated that at least part of this cell loss may be due to the methacrylate surface of the lens. Laboratory studies suggest that coating that surface can prevent this component of cell loss. The magnitude of benefits to be found from such coating requires further clinical study.

In recent years my concept of the corneal endothelium has totally changed. Many years ago it was thought that the human corneal endothelium was similar to animals. The early experiments of Maumenee and Kornblueth (1948), indicated that the rabbit cornea could be frozen and the endothelium presumably killed, and yet these corneas could regain their clarity within approximately a week. Subsequent studies in the rabbit by Kaufman, Capella, and Robbins (1964), Polack (1963) and others confirmed the fact that rabbit corneal endothelial cells could multiply, but shed little light on the human corneal endothelium.

Flat preparations of large numbers of human corneas (1965) suggested, however, that the number of cells on the cornea decreased with age. They also suggested that once the cornea was injured, healing occurred by spreading but not by cell division. Such conclusions, however, were difficult to confirm until the advent of the specular microscope.

The specular microscope (Fig. 1) was first developed by Maurice (1968) in 1968, and subsequently improved by Laing, Sandstrom, and Leibowitz (1975) and again by Bourne and Kaufman (1976). It permits the detailed observation of the human corneal endothelium in the intact living eye (Fig. 2), and thus opens totally new horizons for a study of this tissue. Patients can be studied at many different ages and the density of the corneal endothelial cells determined. When this is done, it becomes clear that there is a decrease in the number of corneal endothelial cells per unit area with age – despite some biological variability. After injury, even in people as young as 16 years of age, it can be seen that there is a loss of central corneal

51

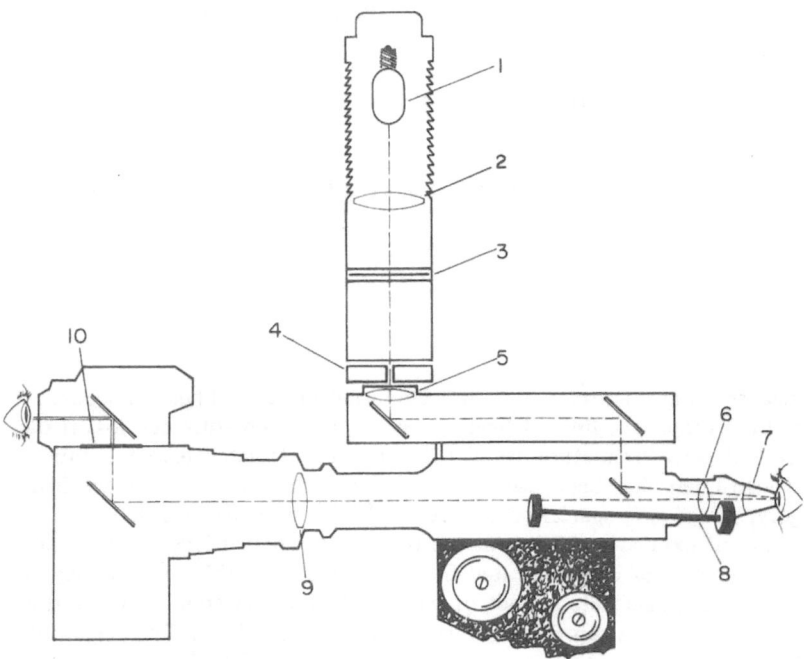

Fig. 1. Scheme of the clinical specular microscope.
1 – Lamp
2 & 5 – Condensing lenss
3 – Xerox flash tube
4 – slit aperture
6 – objective lens
7 – dipping cone lens
8 – focus attachment
9 – eye piece lens
10 – viewing screen

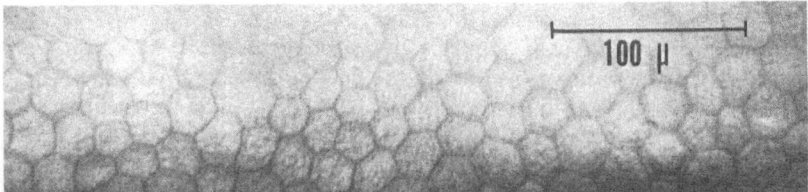

Fig. 2. Normal endothelium as seen by specular microscope.

endothelial cells, and that healing occurs by sliding rather than by cell multiplication with little or no cell regeneration.

These kinds of observations have led to several new concepts which are both scientifically and clinically important in terms of an appreciation of the human corneal endothelium.

52

Healing reserve

Any damage to the corneal endothelium, whether surgical, traumatic, or drug-induced, must be compensated for by spreading of the remaining cells. Although the lower limits of cell numbers have not been defined, it seems clear that there comes a point at which adequate covering of the endothelial surface is no longer possible and corneal edema results. In conditions such as keratoplasty, where there is a wound which must be healed, or in which incidents such as immune reactions may damage some of the cells, it has become generally accepted that the more cells that are transferred to the recipient from the donor, the greater margin of safety because of the 'healing reserve'.

Aging of the cornea and premature aging

The number of endothelial cells decreases with age. In a certain proportion of people this decrease is enough so that corneal decompensation occurs and corneal edema supervenes. We believe that if the cornea is traumatized and cells are prematurely lost from such trauma, the continuing decrease in cells with age may lead to a decompensation and corneal edema many years after the original insult. There are several clinical examples which seem to exemplify this: Spencer and associates (1966) described a group of patients with congenital glaucoma whose pressure had been adequately controlled and who had crystal-clear corneas for approximately 20 years after the initial episode of glaucoma and unevently surgery. Twenty years later, these corneas became edematous − presumably because the initial cell loss from stretching in surgery had been sufficiently great so that continued cell death with time could no longer be tolerated.

Some corneal transplants remain clear for a period of years and yet become edematous and cloudy with no apparent inflammatory incident many years after the initial surgery. We believe that these donor grafts are those with marginal cell populations which can no longer cover the surface of Descemet's membrane as additional cells die with time. In the specimens of such corneas, no abnormality is seen except for corneal edema and inadequate numbers of endothelial cells.

Studies of the corneal endothelium with the specular microscope have both scientific and clinical uses. These include the examination of donor eye tissue before it is used for corneal transplantation. The examination of patients before procedures such as intraocular lens implant is important to be certain that a reasonable number of endothelial cells are present before such surgery which might cause some increase in cell loss. Studies include the evaluation of drugs which may be used in the eye, and it now seems that any drug or any solution inserted into the eye should be checked in man to be certain that it does not cause undue loss of central corneal endothelial cells. Surgical techniques can be checked to determine whether endothelial damage is occurring, and whether modifications can be made to minimize this.

A beautiful example of the possible advantages to man of specular microscopy involves the study of intraocular lenses.

The first study of the effect of intraocular lenses on the human corneal endothelium was done by Bourne and Kaufman (1976) at the University of Florida and indicated substantial endothelial cell loss in a small number of patients. An additional cooperative study was then done by Forstot and associates (1977) from the University of Florida with Jaffe in Miami. This larger study yielded fascinating results. A prospective examination of the patients showed a substantial cell loss which appeared to occur at the time of surgery. This loss seemed to occur regardless of lens type used, and a variety of different types of intraocular lenses resulted in comparable endothelial cell loss. The comparison of intraocular lens insertion with cataract extraction in these two studies revealed an andothelial cell loss from regular intracapsular cataract extraction of 7 to 8 percent, but when aphakic eyes were compared with pseudophakic eyes, there was always a greater loss in the pseudophakic eye, and this loss averaged greater than 40 percent. There was no evidence in this study that the retention of the lens in the eye caused progressive endothelial damage, and these studies indicated that endothelial cell damage was primarily an event occurring at the time of surgery.

This evidence of endothelial cell damage, which was much more extensive than previously believed, and the pinpointing of such damage to the time of surgery focused my attention on possible causes for such an occurrence. The most obvious place to look for such damage was in contact between the methacrylate lens and the corneal endothelium. In both rabbits and man methacrylate lenses which were wet with balanced salt solution and touched to the cornea, caused extensive corneal endothelial damage as judged both by scanning electron microscopy and by nitroblue tetrazolium staining (1977). A careful examination of this damage indicated that its appearance was unique and it appeared as if the methacrylate surface adhered to the central corneal endothelium instantaneously and ripped off the top of the endothelial cells. In fact, examination of a lens which had been in contact with the corneal endothelial cells showed debris on the surface consistent with cell membranes stripped from the endothelial cell. Glass produces similar damage, but covering the glass with a soft contact lens (Bausch & Lomb T lens) eliminates this damage and permits a totally normal endothelium. Instantaneous touch of the unprotected intraocular lens to endothelium produces this cell destruction, but rubbing of the normal human or animal lens on the endothelial surface produces virtually no cell damage.

Because of this I thought I could biophysically alter the methacrylate surface to prevent this component of cell injury. The most effective solution tested was a polyvinyl pyrrolidone (PVP K 29—31, 40 percent, in balanced salt solution). Dipping the lens in this solution permits it to be rubbed against the endothelium without cell loss or cell injury at the time.

As yet I am not certain that all surgeons obtain a comparable cell loss, nor am I certain that this is the only or major mechanism of cell loss in human disease. To acquire such certainty, coated lenses will need to be compared with uncoated lenses from a double-blind controlled series.

In preparation for this, however, I have tested the safety of PVP in rabbit eyes, and find it to be well tolerated. It has been used in human eyes for many years to reform the anterior chamber by some surgeons who do keratoplasty without inflammation or incidence. In two patients with uneventful cataract extractions in whom lenses have been dipped in this PVP solution at the time of surgery, cell loss was 9 and 11 percent, as compared to the 7 to 8 percent cell loss seen in regular cataract extraction, or the average of 40 percent cell loss seen in intraocular lenses. This is certainly not conclusive, but provides further incentive for additional studies.

REFERENCES

Bourne, W.M. & H.E. Kaufman. Specular microscopy of human corneal endothelium. *Am. J. Ophthalmol.* 81: *319*, (1976).

Bourne, W.M. & H.E. Kaufman. Endothelial damage associated with intraocular lenses. *Am. J. Ophthalmol.* 81: *482*, (1976).

Forstot, S.L., W.L. Blackwell & N.S. Jaffe et al. Effect of intraocular lens implantation on the corneal endothelium. *Trans. Am. Acad. Ophthalmol. Otolaryngol.* 83: *195* (1977).

Katz, J.I., H.E. Kaufman & E.P. Goldberg et al. Prevention of endothelial damage from intraocular lens insertion. *Trans. Am. Acad. Ophthalmol. Otolaryngol.* 83: *204*, (1977).

Kaufman, H.E., J.A. Capella & J.E. Robbins. Study of enzyme activity in corneal repair. *Invest Ophthalmol.* 3: *34*, (1964).

Laing, R.A., M.M. Sandstrom & H.M. Leibowitz. In vivo photomicrography of the corneal endothelium. *Arch. Ophthalmol.* 93: *143*, (1975).

Maumenee, A.E., & W. Kornblueth. Regeneration of corneal stromal cells. I. Technique for destruction of corneal corpuscles by application of solidified (frozen) carbon dioxide, *Am. J. Ophthalmol.* 31: *699*, (1948).

Maurice, D.M. Cellular membrane activity in the corneal endothelium of the intact eye. *Experimentia* 24: *1094*, (1968).

Polack, F.M., Isotopic labeling of corneal stromal cells prior to transplantation. *Transplantation* 1: *83*, (1963).

Robbins, J.E., J.A. Capella & H.E. Kaufman. Study of endothelium in keratoplasty and corneal preservation. *Arch. Ophthalmol.* 73: *242*, (1965).

Spencer, W.H., W.J. Ferguson Jr., R.N. Shaffer & M. Fine. Late degenerative changes in the cornea following breaks in Descemet's membrane. *Trans. Am. Acad. Ophthalmol. Otolaryngol.* 70: *973*, (1966).

Author's address:
Louisiana State University
Medical Center
LSU Eye Center
136 South Roman Street
New Orleans, LA 70112
U.S.A.

Docum. Ophthal. Proc. Series, Vol. 20

WIDE-FIELD IN VIVO SPECULAR MICROSCOPY

R. WITMER, FR. BIGAR AND A. THAER

(Zürich/Wetzlar, Switzerland)

The credit of introducing specular microscopy for the study of the corneal endothelium goes to D. Maurice. However, it was Vogt, who showed in 1931 that the corneal endothelium could well be visualized with the conventional slit-lamp. Laing, Sandstrom and Leibowitz on one side, Bourne, Mc Carey and Kaufman on the other side modified the original system for the human in vivo cell evaluation. Several studies have since been published by different groups on the problem of endothelial cell loss after routine cataract operation and after implantation of intraocular artifical lenses. L.W. Hirst, R.C. Snip, W.I. Starck and A.E. Maumenee recently wrote a paper on the same subject and came to the final conclusion, that all the figures published so far should be viewed in the light of the problems of the photography used. The analysis of the data obtained is certainly open to many questions.

With the specular microscopes so far available only a small, strip-like rectangular area of the corneal endothelium can be observed and photographed. On one side of the picture the strong glare of the front surface of the dipping cone and the surface corneal reflex are restricting the image. The other side is limited by the image of the slit-shaped illumination-field diaphragm. The number of cells visible in such a photomicrograph amounts to about 50, one cell row containing between 15–20 cells. The area seen therefore is not more than about 80.000 to 100.00 μ^2 or less than 1/10 of a square millimeter, and often much less. Also, quoted from the paper of Hirst and coworkers, 'many photographs are of poor quality and are rejected at the analytic stage'. But such pictures may well show areas of some endothelial cell damage. In all the papers mentioned the very large standard error of the mean (13–14%) may result from extensive cell variation in cell density, depending on the area of cornea photographed. Hirst and coworkers conclude: 'before the clinical specular microscope is established as a reliable clinical tool, these problems of photography and data analysis require reevaluation'.

My coworker Fr. Bigar, with the very valuable help of A. Thaer of Leitz Wetzlar, have been studying systematically different means to enlarge the observed endothelial area over the last two years. They have shown, that in the donor eye it is easy to obtain photomicrographs of a much larger area of the corneal endothelium with the use of polarized light. The surface reflex

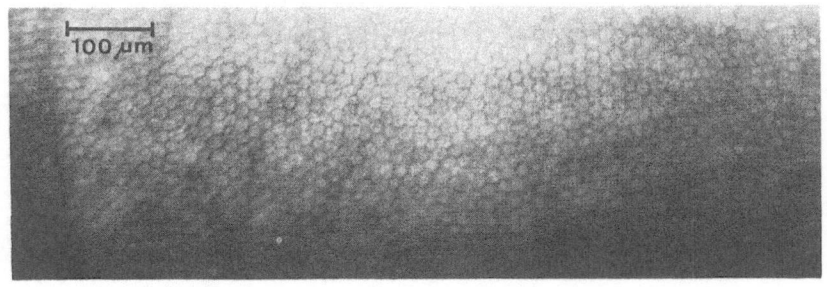

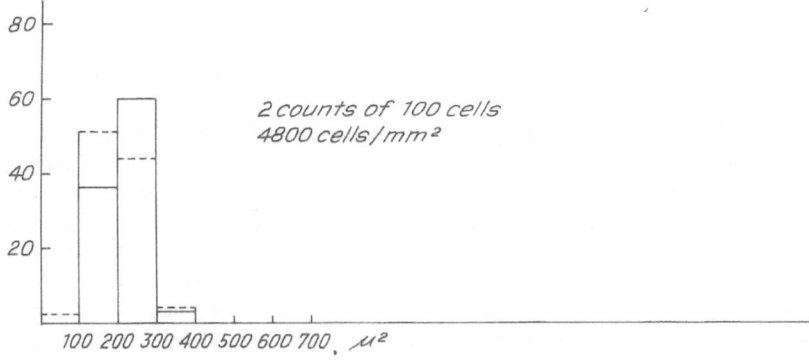

2 counts of 100 cells
4800 cells/mm²

Fig. 1. 10 year old girl with regular endothelial cells. Histogram of endothelial cells.

of the cornea can thus be almost completely eliminated and a total amount of approximately 1500 cells are visible on an area of almost 1 mm². This set-up has been found very convenient for routine evaluation of all donor material used in the eye bank. Only if a regular corneal endothelium of a high cell density is seen, the cornea is excised for storage in a modified McCarey–Kaufman medium. Unfortunately, this technique is up to now not suitable for in vivo observation, since a high amount of the polarized light reflected at the endothelial aqueous humor boundary is extinguished by the analyzer together with the corneal surface reflex. Very long exposure times are therefore needed for photomicrography.

We have been looking for further possibilities to improve specular microscopy. The light reflecting area of the corneal surface has to be displaced laterally by increasing the angle between the incident light beam and the reflected beam for observation. This could be achieved by increasing the numerical aperture of the objective of a vertical illuminator as used in the conventional specular microscopes. The disadvantage of such an optical system, however, is the very small depth of focus.

We have finally chosen another possibility by separating the two beams using two objectives. A joint front lens for both beams is placed as a contact immersion element on the cornea. But non-contact specular microscopy is also possible. This can be very helpful when examining children or patients during the early postoperative period.

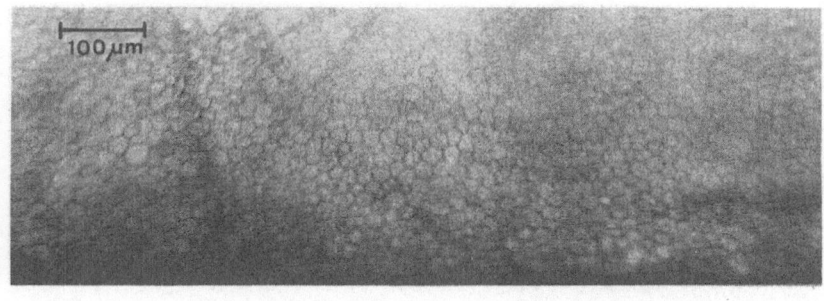

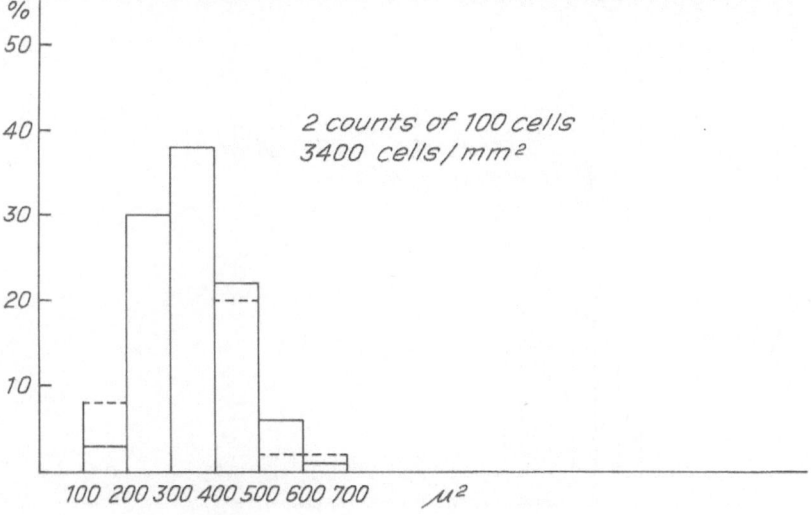

Fig. 2. 34 year old woman. Distribution of endothelial cells.

The analysis of the photomicrographs obtained with this new specular microscope poses the problem of morphometry and counting. In many of the pictures we see several hundred cells. A fully automatic image analysis as seen on a TV screen is not possible because of the constant eye movements and the resulting unsteadiness of the image, as well as the unfavourable contrast conditions.

A semi-automatic analysis, however, is possible by placing the specular photomicrographs on a tracing panel. The contours of the endothelial cells are traced with a special pencil, which converts the data into digital co-ordinate values.

A few examples will show you the possibilities of this system.

A normal 10 year old child shows a very uniform distribution of small endothelial cells (70% between 100 and 200 μ^2) with a very limited variation of size. The number per mm^2 is as high as 4800 cells (Fig. 1).

The 34 year old mother of this child has already a decrease to 3400 cells per mm^2, and the cells vary much more in size. Nearly 40% of the cells have a size between 300 und 400 μ^2 (Fig. 2).

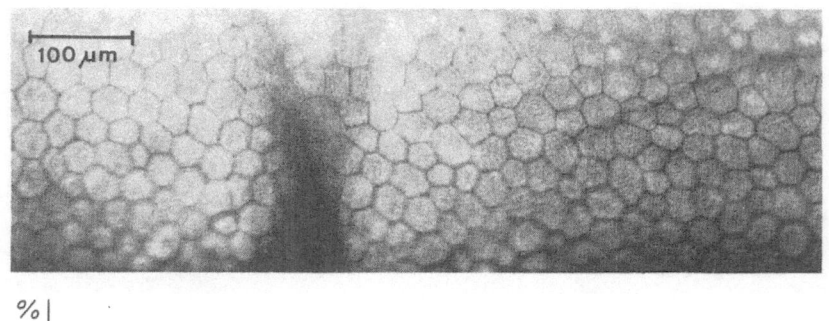

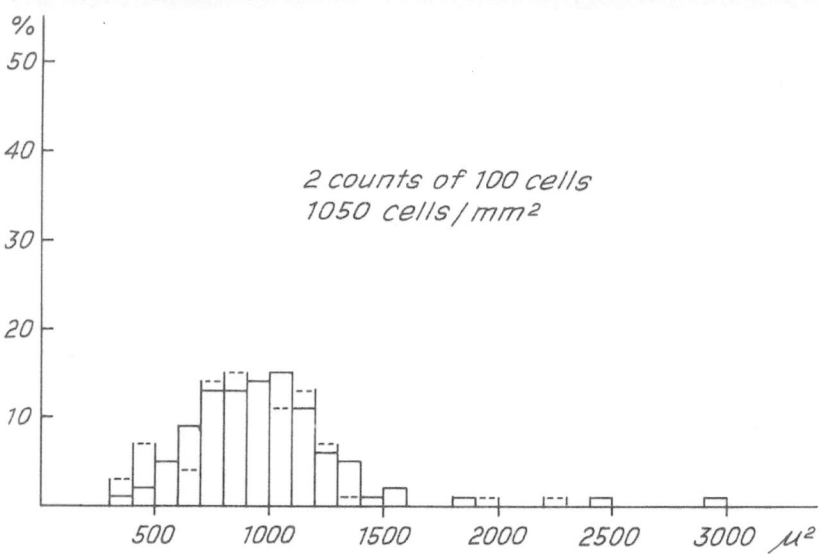

Fig. 3. Homogenously enlarged endothelial cells in a 75 year old aphakic patient. Distribution of endothelial cells.

A 75 year old aphakic patient has a very flat distribution curve of very large cells and only 1050 cells per mm² are left in the central corneal area (Fig. 3).

The next picture is from a 72 year old patient with a typical cornea guttata (Fig. 4). Exact counting of the number of endothelial cells in such a case is difficult, because the cells covering the warts of Descemet's membrane are not visible on the photomicrograph due to the very limited depth of focus of the specular microscope.

CONCLUSION

We can say, that the last word in specular microscopy is certainly not spoken. Our system seems to provide better data for the evaluation of the behaviour of the corneal endothelium in the living human eye than the microscope so far in use. We have confirmed earlier findings, but with more

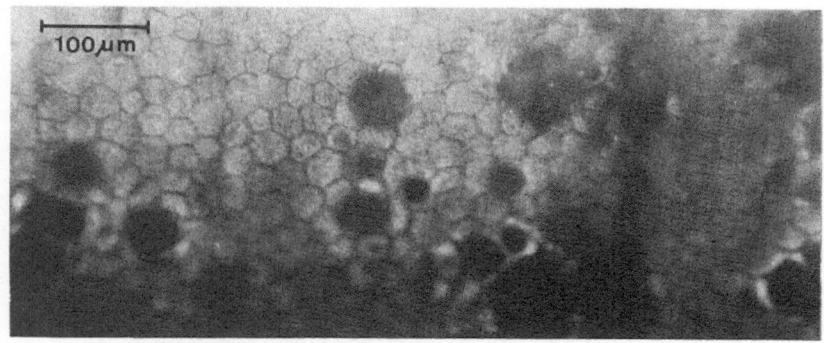

Fig. 4. Cornea guttata in a 72 year old woman.

time and experience a more accurate picture of the corneal endothelium will be obtained.

REFERENCES

Bourne, W.M., B.E. McCarey & H.E. Kaufman. Clinical specular microscopy. *Trans. Am. Acad. Ophthalmol., Otolaryngol.* 81: *743*, (1976).

Hirst, L.W., R.C. Snip, W.I. Stark & A.E. Maumenee. Quantitative corneal endothelial evaluation in intraocular lens implantation and cataract surgery. *Am. J. Ophth.* 84: *775–780*, (1977).

Laing, R.A., M.M. Sandstrom & H.M. Leibowitz. *In vivo* photomicrography of the corneal endothelium. *Arch. Ophthalmol.* 93: *143*, (1975).

Maurice, D.M.. Cellular membrane activities in the corneal endothelium of the intact eye. *Experientia* 24: *1094*, (1968).

Vogt, A. Spaltlampenmikroskopie des lebenden Auges. I, 31, Springer Verlag, Berlin, 1931.

Author's address:
Universitäts Augenklinik
Rämistrasse
8091 Zürich
Switzerland

Docum. Ophthal. Proc. Series, Vol. 20

CLINICAL SPECULAR MICROSCOPY OF THE
CORNEAL ENDOTHELIUM

R.A. LAING, M.M. SANDSTROM AND H.M. LEIBOWITZ

(Boston, Massachusetts, U.S.A.)

Over the past several years, clinical examination of the corneal endothelium has progressed from a cursery examination of its specular reflection using a low power slit-lamp biomicroscope to high magnification specular microscopy. A variety of both contacting and non-contacting methods have been developed for observing the endothelium. Each method has its advantages and disadvantages. For general clinical evaluation and photography of the endothelium, as opposed to special research studies, the Clinical Specular Photomicroscope is the 'method of choice' and will probably remain so for the forseeable future. The first figure shows a photograph of the instrument we used.

Using this instrument, corneal endothelial photography has been demonstrated to be of clinical value for a number of reasons. It has enabled the trauma of surgical procedures and the potential damage due to therapeutic agents to be assessed, thereby facilitating the development of improved techniques and agents. Compared to the slitlamp biomicroscope, it has enabled earlier diagnosis of many types of pathology and has demonstrated changes which are not appreciated by biomicroscopy. Such applications of clinical specular microscopy have been demonstrated not only by us but also by a great many other investigators all over the world.

I will discuss some of the results which we have obtained and the methods which we have used to evaluate endothelial photographs. When we first started taking clinical endothelial photographs in 1973 (1, 2), we felt that the dark and bright areas which we saw on the photographs were not significant and would not be amenable to any type of logical analysis. Because of this we concentrated our efforts on studying the size and shape of endothelial cells since the cell boundaries could be visualized quite well. We felt that such morphological parameters might possibly provide information concerning the status of the endothelium (3).

In our first published study, both eyes of 63 normal subjects ranging in ages from 20 to 83 were photographed. A typical photograph obtained from one of these subjects is shown in figure 2. One notices that the cell boundaries are dark and that there is a granular appearance to the region within the boundary. The cells are quasi-regular in shape and all have nearly the same size. The photographs were analyzed using a digitizer to trace around the cell boundaries of the individual cells. The digitizer was coupled to a

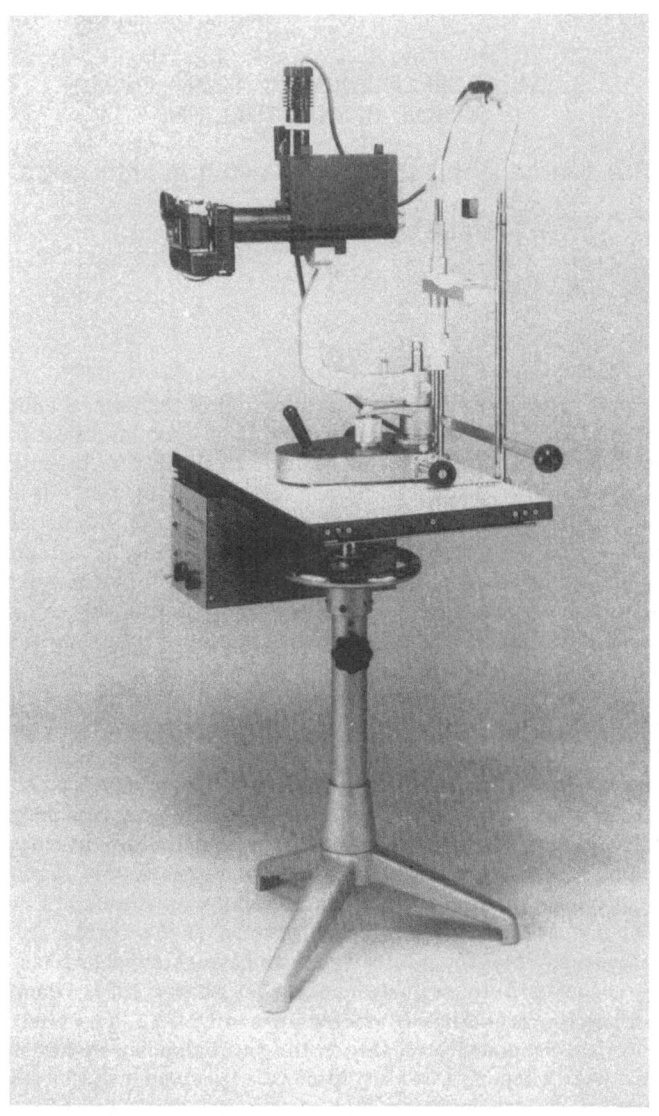

Fig. 1. A photograph of Clinical Specular Photomicroscope.

small desktop computer which calculated the area of each cell as well as its perimeter, its side lengths, its center, and several other parameters associated with cell morphology. When we plotted the average cell area versus age of the subject, we obtained the results shown in figure 3. For the population studied, the average cell area is seen to increase with age. When we compared the difference in cell area between the right and left eyes with age of

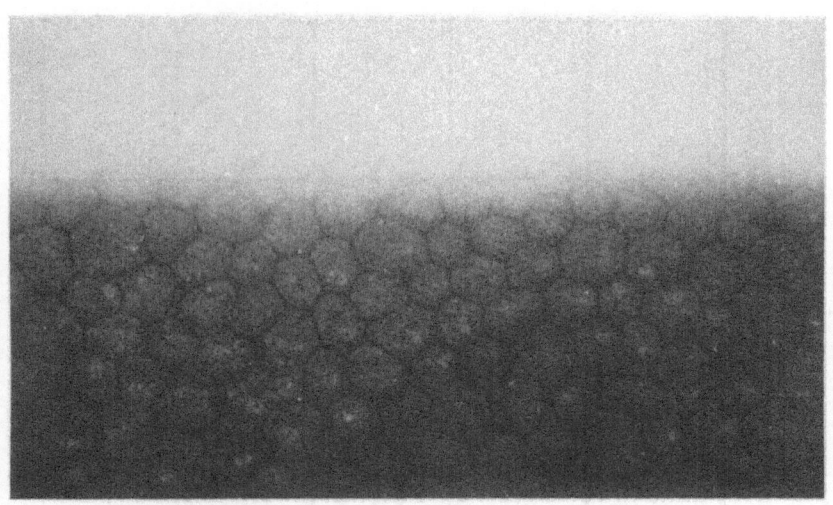

Fig. 2. A typical specular photomicrograph of normal adult eye.

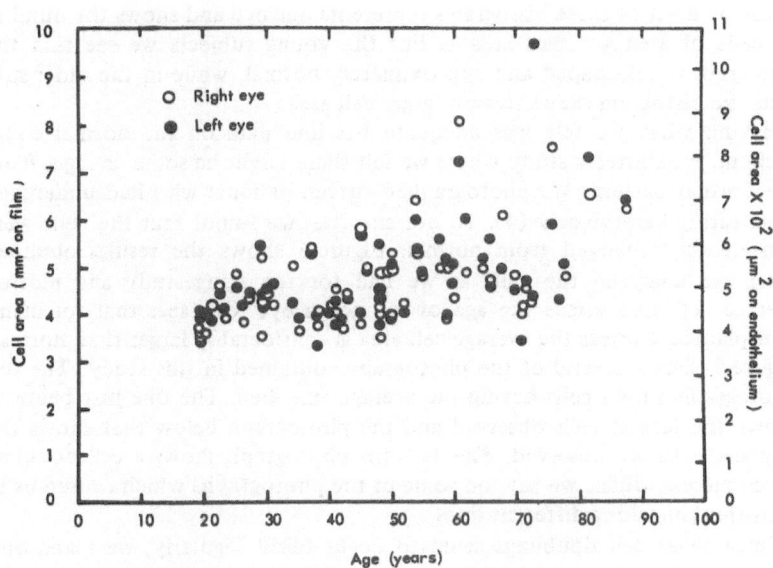

Fig. 3. The average cell area versus age of the subject.

65

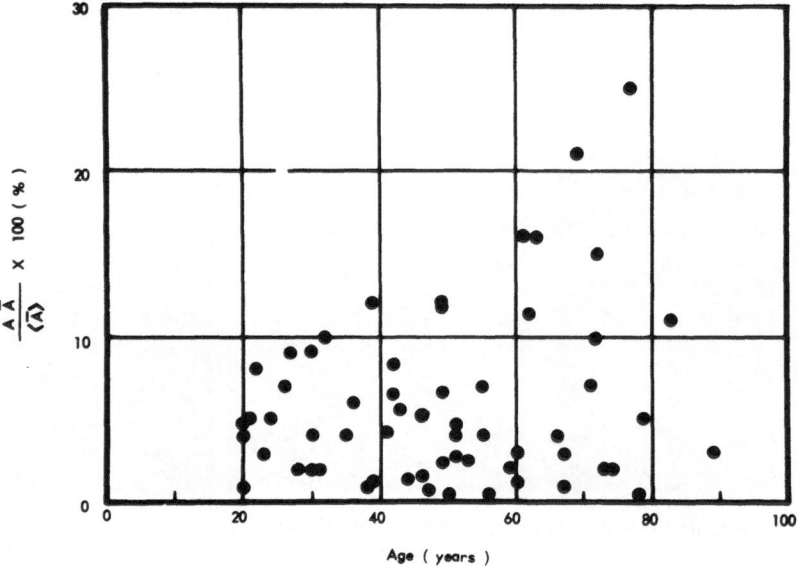

Fig. 4. The difference in cell area between the right and left eyes with age of the subject.

the subject, we obtained the results shown in figure 4. Correlation analysis showed that the right eye-left eye difference did not increase with age although the variation of this difference did. When we calculated the frequency distribution of cell size with age we obtained the results shown in figure 5. Each of these histograms represents one eye and shows the number of cells of area A versus area A. For the young subjects we see that the histogram is bell-shaped and approximately normal, while in the older subjects the histogram skews toward larger cell area.

Having what we felt was adequate baseline data on the normal endothelium, we started a study where we felt there might be some changes from the normal pattern. We photographed fifteen patients who had undergone penetrating keratoplasty (4). To our surprise, we found that the cells were considerably enlarged from normal. Figure 6 shows the results obtained when we analyzed the cells as we had for the aging study and plotted average cell area versus the age of the donor eye. One sees that for many transplanted corneas the average cell area is considerably larger than normal. Figure 7 shows several of the photographs obtained in this study. The top photograph shows cells having the average size seen. The one just below it shows the largest cells observed and the photograph below that shows the smallest cells we observed. The bottom photograph shows a cell doubling phenomenon which we saw on some of the photographs which caused us to start thinking along different lines.

Since these cell doublings seem to occur fairly regularly, we asked ourselves whether there might be other morphological structures which could be resolved by the specular microscope and which might be associated with

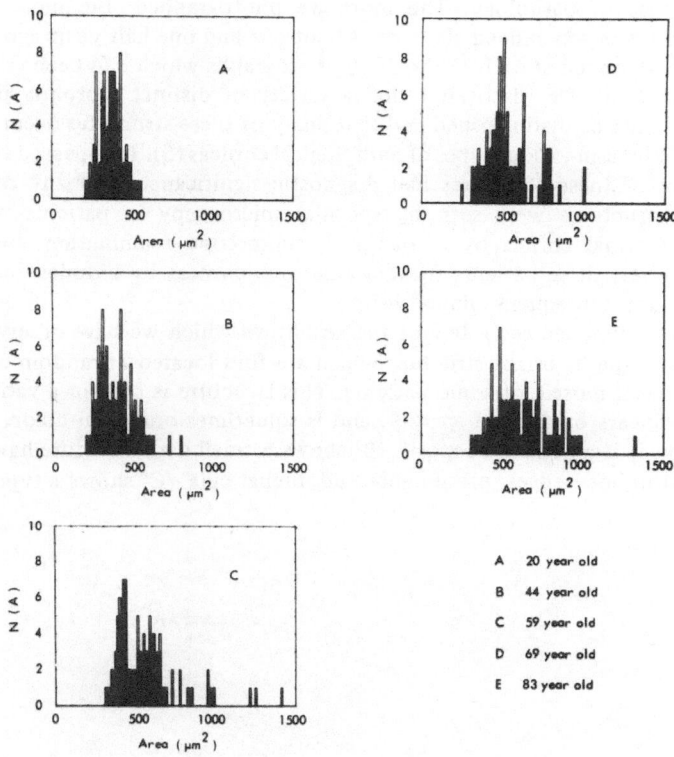

Fig. 5. The frequency distribution of cell size with age.

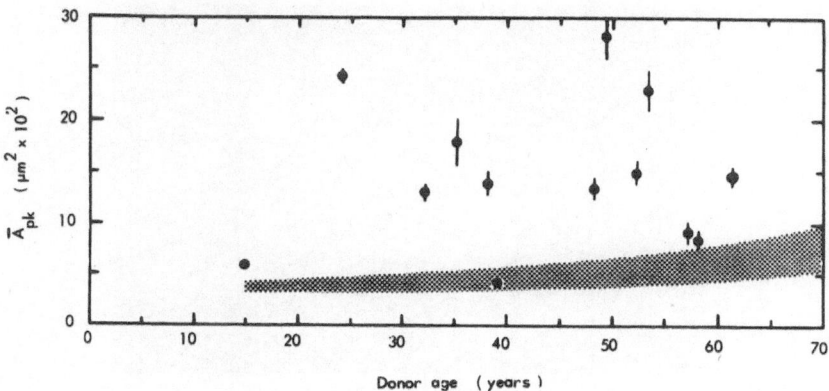

Fig. 6. The average cell area versus the age of the donor eye.

67

specific types of pathology. The more we photographed, the more we realized that this was indeed the case. About one and one half years ago we sat down and looked at each of the 5000 photographs which had been taken up to that time. We discovered that a variety of distinct morphological structures could be distinguished and that many of these structures occurred on a regular basis in various types of pathological corneas (5). It appeared that observation of these structures had diagnostic significance. In many cases abnormal structures were seen by specular microscopy in patients who showed a normal cornea by slit-lamp biomicroscope examination. In all cases, however, these patients showed abnormal corneas by biomicroscope examination in subsequent clinical visits.

On figure 8 you can see a few of the structures which we have observed. 'A' shows a type of bright structure which we find located at random over the endothelial mosaic of some patients. This structure is seen in a variety of sizes, appears bright and sparkly, and is sometimes orange in color. We believe that it is a pigment deposit. 'B' shows a small dark structure having sharp, well defined edges, presumably endothelial cilia. 'C' shows a type of

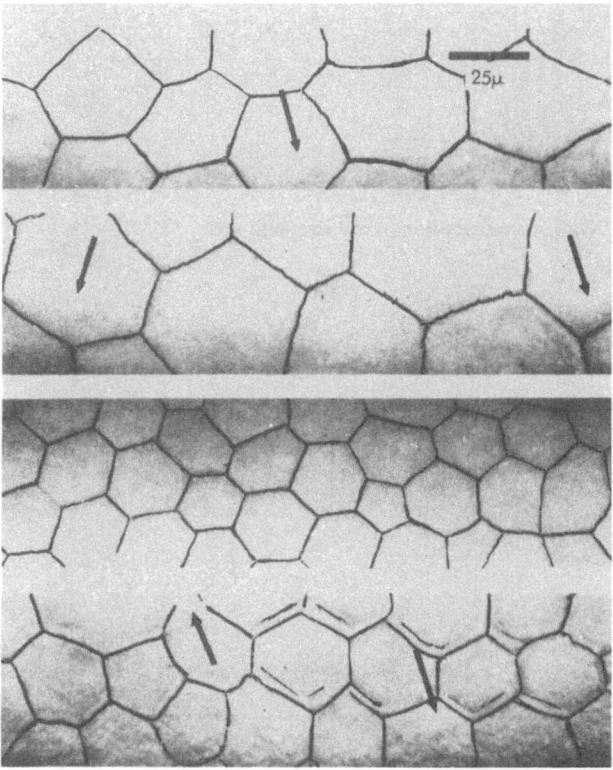

Fig. 7. Several photographs obtained in the penetrating keratoplasty study: 1. average size 2. largest cells 3. smallest cells 4. cell doubling pehnomenon.

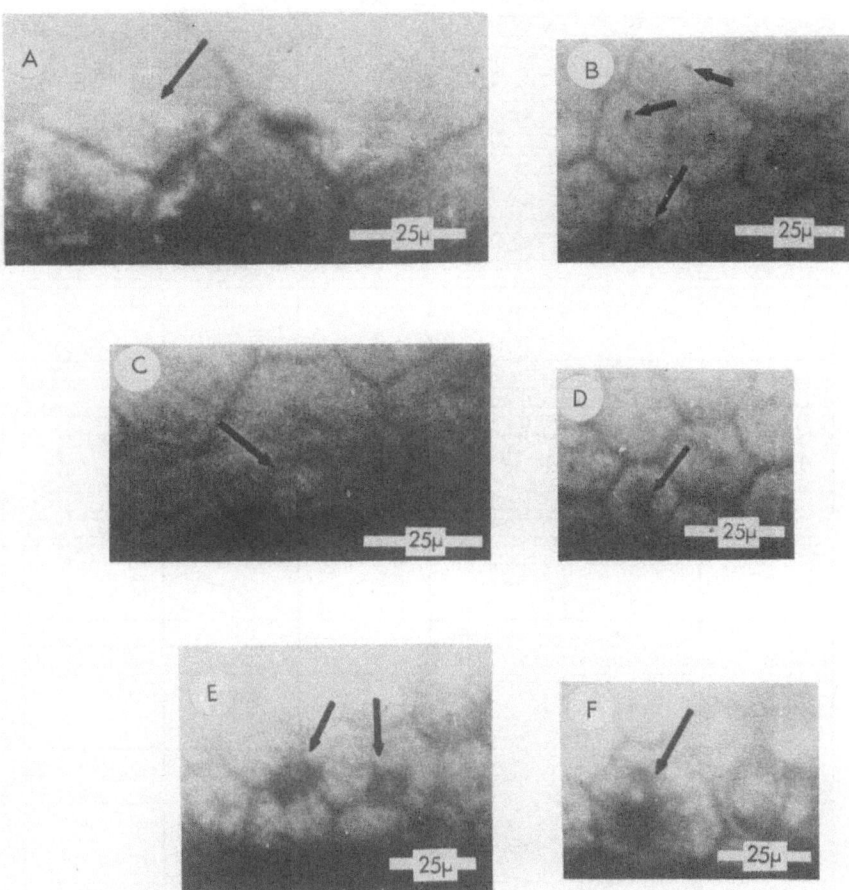

Fig. 8. Miscellaneous structures: A. bright structure; B. dark structure; C. intracellular bright structure which is found in enlarged cells. D. intracellular dark structure which has diffuse edges. E. inflammatory cells. F. dark structure having a central bright spot.

bright structure which is intracellular and found in enlarged cells. Its size is somewhat variable, but in general, the larger the cell, the larger the bright structure, 'D' shows an intracellular dark structure which has diffuse edges. We believe that these are intracellular blebs. 'E' shows several intracellular dark structures which, when seen, tend to be of the same size and are located randomly over the photograph. These are believed to be inflammatory cells. 'F' shows a dark structure having a central bright spot. These structures tend to be in the central or para-central of the cell and can vary in size from smaller to that shown to somewhat larger than the cell. Such structures are always seen in Fuch's dystrophy and are believed to be guttata.

Figure 9 shows a classification chart (6) which shows each of the morphological structures we see on a regular basis. The first row shows the various

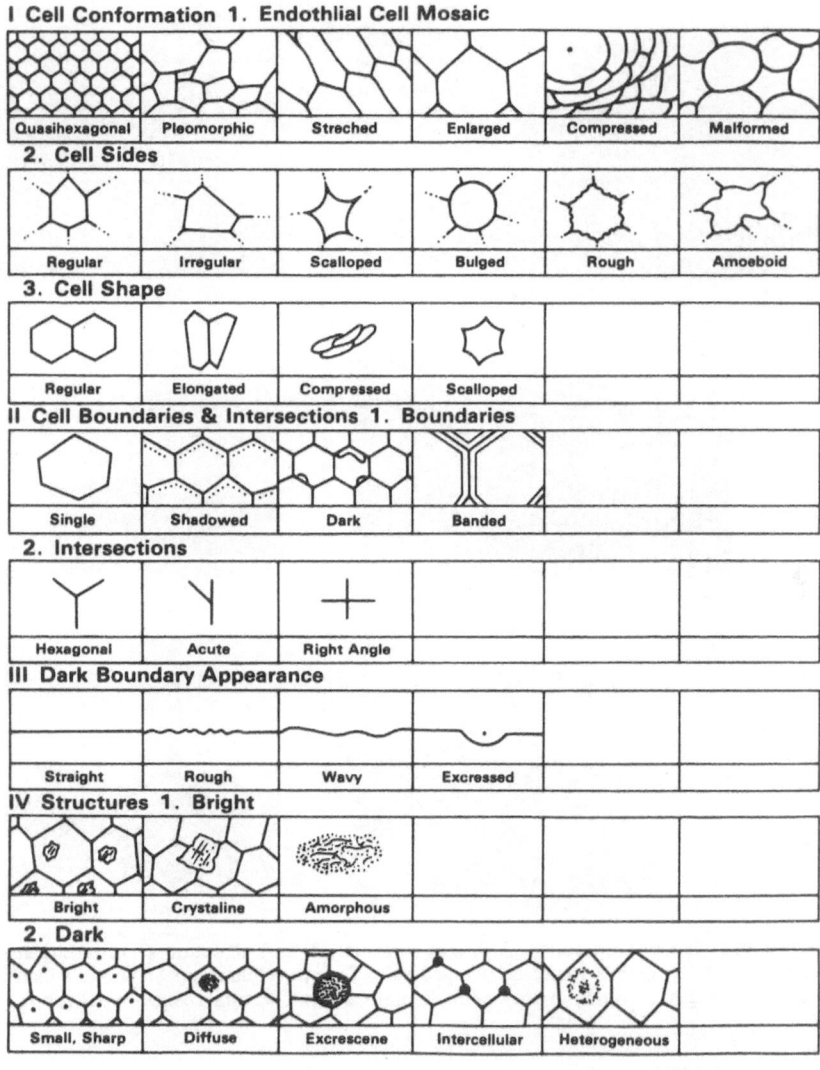

I Cell Conformation 1. Endothlial Cell Mosaic

| Quasihexagonal | Pleomorphic | Streched | Enlarged | Compressed | Malformed |

2. Cell Sides

| Regular | Irregular | Scalloped | Bulged | Rough | Amoeboid |

3. Cell Shape

| Regular | Elongated | Compressed | Scalloped | | |

II Cell Boundaries & Intersections 1. Boundaries

| Single | Shadowed | Dark | Banded | | |

2. Intersections

| Hexagonal | Acute | Right Angle | | | |

III Dark Boundary Appearance

| Straight | Rough | Wavy | Excressed | | |

IV Structures 1. Bright

| Bright | Crystaline | Amorphous | | | |

2. Dark

| Small, Sharp | Diffuse | Excrescene | Intercellular | Heterogeneous | |

© Laing & Sandstrom 1977

Fig. 9. A classification chart which shows each of the morphological structures seen on a regular basis.

types of cell conformation seen. The second row shows various changes in the cell sides. The third, forth and fifth rows show changes in cell shape, in cell boundaries and in cell intersections, respectively. We believe we know what many of these morphological structures represent histopathologically although some are still mysteries. We are currently developing methods for solving these mysteries.

It is interesting to note that a few short years ago it was thought that specular microscopy in vivo would yield little information other than the average cell area or cell count. However, we now know that the Clinical Endothelial Photomicroscope allows us to localize numerous morphological structures which have diagnostic significance. We are close to having both the methods and the knowledge for non-invasive histopathological examination of the human endothelium in vivo thus paving the way for increased accuracy in diagnosis, for better evaluation of treatment, and, in general, for greater benefits in health care delivery to the patient.

REFERENCES

Laing, R.A., Sandstrom, M.M., and Leibowitz, H.M.: In vivo corneal endothelial photomicrography. *ARVO* 74, p. 44(1).

Laing, R.A., Sandstrom, M.M., and Leibowitz, H.M.: In vivo photomicrography of the corneal endothelium. *Arch. Ophthalmol.* 93: *143,* 1975.

Laing, R.A., Sandstrom, M.M., Berrospi, A.R., and Leibowitz, H.M.: Changes in the corneal endothelium as a function of age. *Exp. Eye Res.* 22: *587,* 1976.

Laing, R.A., Sandstrom, M.M., Berrospi, A.R., and Leibowitz, H.M.: Morphological changes in corneal endothelial cells after penetrating keratoplasty. *Am. J. of Ophthalmol.* 82(3): *459,* Sept. 1976.

Laing, R.A., Sandstrom, M.M., and Leibowitz, H.M.: Clinical Specular Microscopy. II. Qualitative evaluation of corneal endothelial photomicrographs. Accepted in *Arch. of Ophthal.*

Laing, R.A., Sandstrom, M.M., and Leibowitz, H.M.: Qualitative evaluation of corneal endothelial photomicrographs. *ARVO* 78, p. 118(4).

Author's address:
Department of Ophthalmology
Boston University School of Medicine
80 East Concord Street
Boston, Massachusetts 02118
U.S.A.

Docum. Ophthal. Proc. Series, Vol. 20

THE ENDOTHELIUM OF THE CORNEAL GRAFT: MORPHOLOGICAL AND FUNCTIONAL ASPECTS

T. SATO, Y. OTA, C. KIMURA, T. TANISHIMA AND S. MISHIMA

(Tokyo, Japan)

INTRODUCTION

Survival of the graft endothelium and maintenance of its functional integrity is the key for successful penetrating keratoplasty (Polack *et al.*, 1964, Salceda, 1967). Studies on the morphological and functional aspects of the endothelial layer of the graft are, therefore, of particular clinical interest. Introduction of the specular microscopy enabled us to photograph the graft endothelium (Maurice, 1968, Bourne *et al.*, 1976) and to perform morphometric analysis of the individual cells (Laing *et al.*, 1976). The integrity of the endothelial cell lining may be studied through determinations of the permeability to fluorescein (Maurice, 1963); the method of Ota *et al.*, (1964) permits such studies in the human eye. Furthermore the active pump mechanism residing in the endothelium maintains constant corneal thickness (Maurice, 1969, Trenberth *et al.*, 1968, Mishima, 1968). Thus corneal thickness would reflect the function of the endothelial layer. This paper summerizes our recent studies on the corneal graft using these three techniques.

MATERIALS AND METHODS

1. Thickness of the corneal grafts

a. Postoperative thickness changes

A total of 34 cases of keratocounus, their age ranging from 10 to 45 years underwent penetrating keratoplasty with 7 mm trephine and 10—0 nylon running sturues (Kimura et al., 1975). Routine postoperative treatment was given, i.e. 0.01 percent betamethasone instillation 3 times a day for two weeks and 0.1 percent betamethasone 3 times a day from the third postoperative week. The steroid instillation was gradually reduced after 10 weeks. Systemic antibiotics and acetazolamide were used. The corneal thickness was measured with a Haarg-Streit pachometer with Mishima-Hedbys' modification (Mishima, 1968).

b. The corneal thickness of the graft at a steady state

The graft thickness was measured in 33 clear grafts after a steady state thickness had been attained, *i.e.* more than 10 months postoperatively (Sato, 1978).

2. The endothelial permeability

The permeability of the graft endothelium to fluorescein was determined using an objective fluorophotometer (Maurice, 1963) by means of a technique of Ota *et al.* (1974). A total of 24 cases of clear graft were studied. The graft thickness was also measured.

3. Morphometry of the endothelial cells

Using a specular micorscope (Topcon Company, Tokyo, Japan) the endothelium of 33 successsful corneal grafts were photographed (Sato, 1978). The photography was carried out at 3 to 4 different places of the graft center. The endothelial cell contour was traced and subjected to analysis using an image analyser (Imagelyser; Hamamatsu T.V., Hamamatsu, Japan) which permitted calculation of the area of individual cells. A total of 150–200 cells were counted for each subject. For a control, a total of 18 normal subjects, 7 males and 11 females and 11 subjects between 10 to 17 years of age and 7 subjects between 62 to 70 years of age, were studied.

RESULTS

1. The thickness of the corneal graft

In all cases, the graft thickness was .greatly increased in the early postoperative period and was subsequently attenuated gradually over a period of 10 to 15 weeks (Fig. 1).

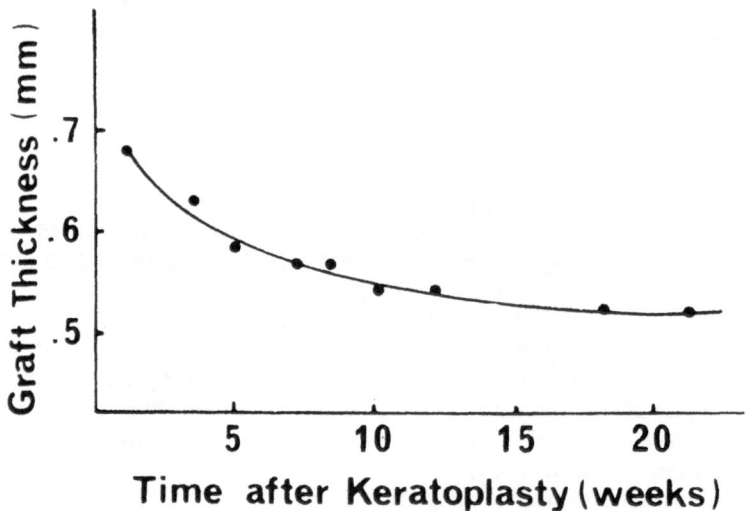

Fig. 1. An example of postoperative changes of the graft thickness. (from Kimura et al., ref. No. 9)

The temporal pattern of the graft thinning could be fitted to an exponential equation which permitted estimation of the graft thickness on the 7th postoperative day. Since there was a great variety in the thickness at this time, factors related to this phenomenon were of interest. Thus, the graft thickness on the 7th postoperative day was correlated with 1) age of donors, 2) intervals from donors' death to enucleation and refrigeration, 3) intervals between enucleation and keratoplasty, and 4) intervals between donors' death and keratoplasty (Kimura, 1975). A significant correlation was found only between the donors age and graft thickness on the 7th postoperative day (Fig. 2). The rate of the graft thinning and the thickness on the 7th postoperative day could also be correlated significantly.

„The corneal thickness at the center of 33 successful grafts averaged 0.539 ± 0.031 (S.D.) mm more than 10 months postoperatively when the thickness was at a steady state. For a control 15 normal corneas were studied and a mean thickness of 0.515 ± 0.025 mm was obtained at the corneal center. The difference between the graft and the normal cornea was statistically significant (Sato, 1978).

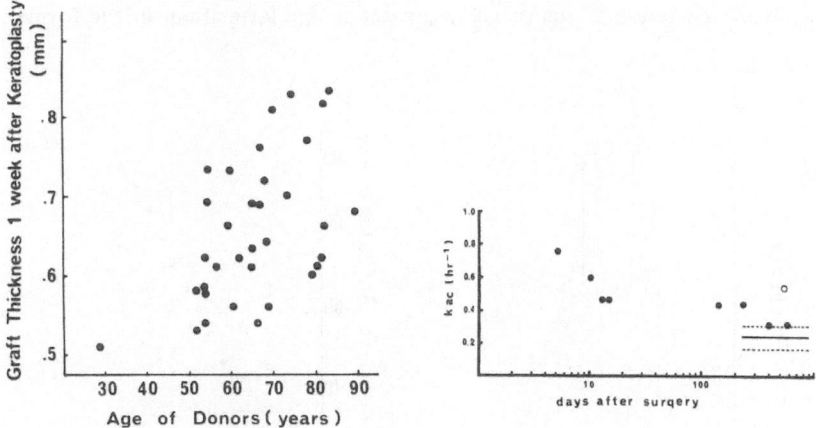

Fig. 2. Correlation between the graft thickness on the 7th postoperative day and the age of donors. (from Kimura et al., ref. No. 9)

Fig. 3. Correlation between the transfer coefficient of the corneal grafts and intervals after surgery. Solid and interrupted lines indicate average and S.D. of the transfer coefficients for normal subjects. The open circle indicates a case where the determination was carried out one month after allograft reaction. (from Ota, ref. No. 19)

2. The endothelial permeability of fluorescein

The permeability of the endothelium to fluorescein was determined in 18 normal corneas and the transfer coefficients averaged $0.228 \pm 0.042 \, \mathrm{hr}^{-1}$ (Ota, 1974). In 9 cases of penetrating keratoplasty, the endothelial permeability were determined at various time intervals after surgery. The transfer coefficient was increased in the early postoperative period but it was reduced in cases with longer postoperative intervals (Fig. 3) (Ota,

75

1975). After one year, the coefficient was close to the normal range. In a case who suffered from allograft reaction showed an increase in the coefficient one month after the reaction had been successfully managed. In 15 cases of the clear graft where the thickness was at a steady state, *i.e.* more than 10 months after surgery, the transfer coefficiet of the endothelium averaged 0.355 ± 0.124 $^{-1}$ .which was signigicantly greater than the normal average (Sato, 1978).

3. *Morphometry of the endothelial cells*

The distribution of the individual cell sizes was studied. In young subjects the distribution conformed with normal distribution (Fig. 4) (Sato, 1978) and the mean cell size of the 11 subjects was $356.3 \pm 45.6 \ \mu m^2$. In the older subjects, the distribution deviated from normal distribution and large cells appeared. The cell size of 7 subjects averaged $436.2 \pm 53.1 \ \mu m^2$ which was significantly greater than that of the young subjects. The standard deviation of the cell sizes was calculated for each individual and it averaged $77.3 \pm 11.7 \ \mu m^2$ in 11 young subjects and $131.1 \pm 27.1 \ \mu m^2$ in 7 old subjects; the standard deviation is significantly greater in the latter than in the former.

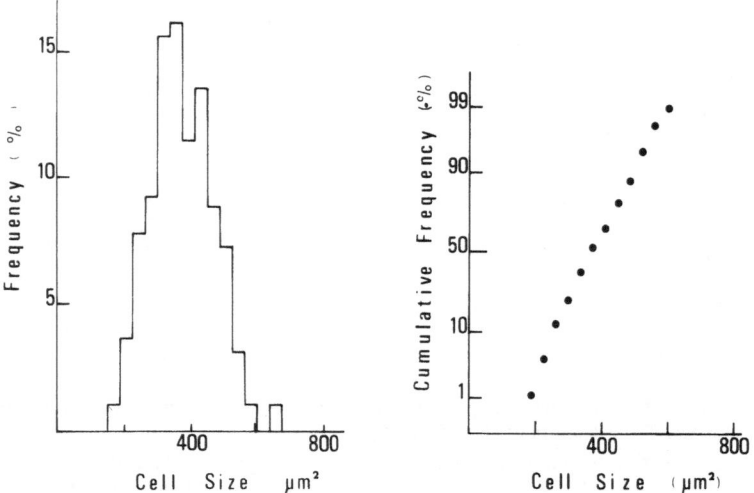

Fig. 4. The histogram and its cumulative plot of the size of the individual endothelial cells of a 15-year-old subject. (from Sato, ref. No. 22)

The endothelial morphometry was conducted in 33 successful grafts 10 months to 6 years after surgery. The individual cell size of the graft was significantly greater than that of the normal subjects (Fig. 5), and the mean cell size was $1131 \pm 461 \ \mu m^2$. The standard deviation of the cell sizes in the individuals averaged $412 \pm 144 \ \mu m^2$, which is significantly greater than those in normal subjects. Eight cases showed a mild rejection episode but the mean cell size did not differ significantly from that of the uneventful cases.

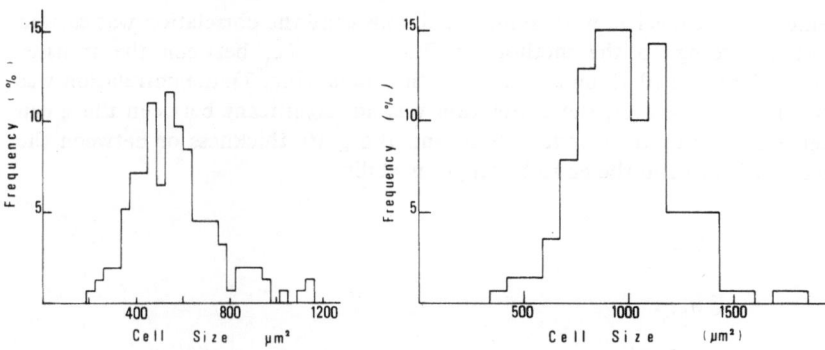

Fig. 5. The histograms of the size of the individual cells in a 68-year-old normal subject (a) and of a corneal graft (b); the donors age was 25 years and recipient was 20 years old, 10 months after keratoplasty. (from Sato, ref. No. 22)

4. Correlation studies

The mean cell size and its standard deviation of the graft endothelium were correlated with 1) age of the donors, 2) the graft thickness at one post-operative week and 3) the steady state graft thickness at the time of the endothelial morphometry (Sato, 1978). However, correlation was not statistically significant. The mean cell size and its standard deviation could, however, be significantly correlated with the intervals after surgery (Fig. 6 a, b). The correlation between the corneal thickness and the postoperative period was not significant. In 15 cases of the graft, 3 measurements; *i.e.* graft thickness, endothelial permeability and endothelial morphometry could be carried out. These cases showed steady state corneal thickness which could be correlated significantly with the endothelial permeability.

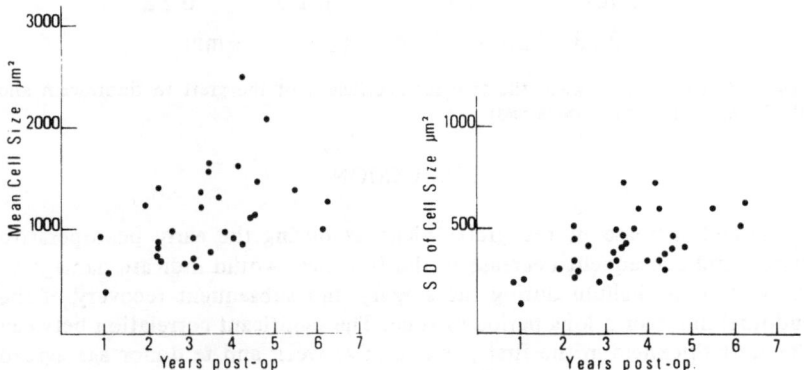

Fig. 6 a, b. Correlation between (a) the mean cell size, (b) the standard deviation of the cell size in the individual graft endothelium and the postoperative period. (from Sato, ref. No. 22)

77

Since these cases had normal intraocular pressure the correlation was carried out according to the method of Ota (1975), *i.e.* between the transfer coefficient and (0.73 mm − the graft thickness) (Fig. 7); the correlation was significant. However, the correlation was not significant between the mean cell size of the graft endothelium and the graft thickness or between the mean cell size and the endothelial permeability.

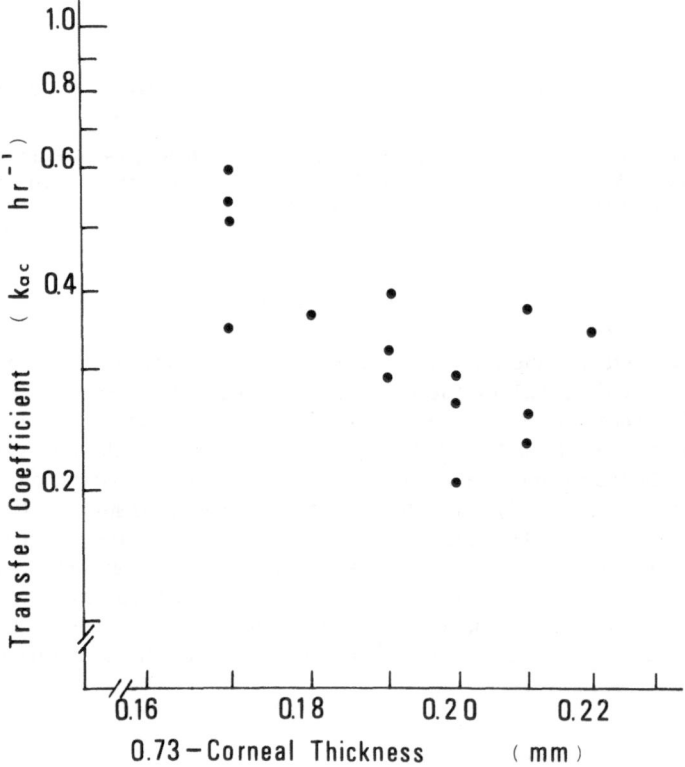

Fig. 7. Correlation between the transfer coefficient of the graft to fluorescein and (0.73 mm − the corneal thickness).

DISCUSSION

A marked increase in the graft thickness during the early postoperative period and subsequent decrease in the thickness would indicate damage to the graft endothelium during the surgery and subsequent recovery of the endothelium over a long period of time. The significant correlation between the graft thickness in the first postoperative week and te donor age agreed with the results of Ehlers (1974) and was thought to point out that the older donors are more vulnerable than the younger donors. A very large size of the graft endothelium shows that the graft endothelium indeed suffered from damage during surgery (Bourne *et al.*, 1976, Laing *et al.*, 1976).

78

In the normal subjects the corneal endothelium of the aged subject was reported to have less cells than in young subjects (Kaufmann *et al.*, 1966, Bourne *et al.*, 1976, Laing *et al.*, 1976). The cell loss is thought to be covered by movement of the neighbouring cells without cell proliferation and probably for this reason the cell size not only increases but also the pleomorphism of the cells is augmented (Von Horn *et al.*, 1975, Sherrard, 1976, Doughmann *et al.*, 1976, Bourne, 1976, Bourne, 1977, Van Horn *et al.*, 1977). The large cell size and standard deviation in the graft would suggest occurrence of similar healing processes.

The endothelial permeability was greatly enhanced during the early postoperative period and was then reduced over a long period. This reduction in the permeability seemed to occur with the thinning of the graft. One can, therefore, assume that the endothelial lining gradually recovered postoperatively. The permeation of fluorescein is thought to take place through the intercellular spaces and is hindered by the intercellular junctional complexes (Kaye *et al.*, 1968, Mishima *et al.*, 1968, Kaye *et al.*, 1973). During the recovery of the endothelium, it was shown that the junctional complex is formed when the endothelial cells come into contact with each other (Kimura *et al.*, 1975, Hirsch *et al.*, 1976). Decrease in the permeability may well be along with the completion of the intercellular junctions.

Three types of measurements could be carried out in cases with clear grafts long after surgery. The steady state graft thickness was close to normal value but was significantly greater than the normal average; this was also the case in the endothelial permeability. Thus, the clear corneal graft covered with fewer cells than the normal cornea shows a slight deterioration of its function. It was of interest that the graft thickness was significantly correlated with the endothelial permeability but not with the mean size of the endothelial cells. Furthermore the latter 2 factors were not correlated significantly. This would suggest that the endothelial cells showed a fairly good intercellular junctions and that within the range of the present cell size variation the junctional integrity was not dependent on the cell sizes. Furthermore the thickness is more dependent on the permeability rather than the cell sizes.

Of clinical significance was the fact that the mean cell size and its standard deviation increased with the postoperative period. Although the graft thickness appeared to be steady, problem remains as to how the graft endothelium and its function changes over a long period of time. A long term follow up using the present three techniques wound provide us with useful information on the fate of the corneal graft endothelium.

SUMMARY

The morphometry of the endothelium and the determination of the thickness and of the endothelial parmeability were carried out on successful penetrating corneal grafts. The thickness is increased during the early postoperative period and gradually decreases subsequently. Thickness in the early period showed a significant correlation with the donor age. The endothelial permeability is high in the early period and then decreases gradually.

In the clear grafts 10 months to 6 years after surgery, the steady state thickness was slightly higher than the normal average and so was the endothelial permeability. The endothelial cells showed a significantly greater mean cell size and standard deviation than those in the normal aged subjects. The mean cell size showed no significant correlation with the thickness nor with the endothelial permeability, but the latter two factors were correlated significantly. The mean cell size and the standard deviation showed a positive correlation with the interval after surgery.

REFERENCES

Bourne, W.M. Specular microscopy of human corneal endothelium *in vivo. Am. J. Ophthalmol.* 81: *319—323* (1976).

Bourne, W.M. & H.E. Kaufman. The endothelium of clear corneal transplants. *Arch. Ophthalmol.* 94: *1730—1732* (1976).

Bourne, W.M., B.E. McCarey & H.E. Kaufman. Clinical specular microscopy. *Trans. Am. Acad. Ophthalmol. Otolaryngol.* 81: *743:753* (1976).

Ehlers, N. Graft thickness after penetrating keratoplasty. *Acta Ophthalmol.* 52: *893—903* (1974).

Hirsch, M., G. Renard, J.P. Fauré & Y. Pouliquen. Formation of intercellular spaces and junctions in regenerating rabbit corneal endothelium. *Exp. Eye* Res. 23: *385—397* (1976).

Kaufman, H.E., J.A. Capella & J.E. Robins. The human corneal endothelium. *Am. J. Ophthalmol.* 61: *835—841* (1966).

Kaye, G.I., S. Mishima, J.D. Cole & N.W. Kaye. Studies on the cornea. VII. Effects of perfusion with a Ca^{++} — free medium on the corneal endothelium. *Invest. Ophthalmol.* 7: *53—66* (1968).

Kaye, G.I., R.C. Sibley & F.B. Hoefle. Recent studies on the nature and function of the corneal endothelial barrier. *Exp. Eye Res.* 15: *585—613* (1973).

Kimura, C. & T. Tanishima. Thickness of the corneal graft after penetrating keratoplasty. *Jpn. J. Ophthalmol.* 19: *348—353* (1975).

Kimura, C. & T. Tanishima. Electron-microscopic studies on the corneal graft endothelium in rabbits. *Jpn. J. Ophthalmol.* 19: *354—367* (1975).

Laing, R.A. M.M. Sandstrom, A.R. Berrospi & H.M. Leibowitz. Changes in the corneal endothelium as a function of age. *Exp. Eye Res.* 22: *587—594* (1976).

Laing, R.A. M. Sandstrom, A.R. Berrospi & H.M. Leibowitz. Morphological changes in corneal endothelial cells after penetrating keratoplasty. *Am. J. Ophthalmol.* 82: *459—464* (1976).

Maurice, D.M. The cornea and sclera. The Eye, ed. Davson, H., 2nd. Ed. Vol. 1: *489—600*, Academic Press, New York & London (1969).

Maurice, D.M. A new objective fluorophotometer. *Exp. Eye Res.* 2: *33—38* (1963).

Maurice, D.M. Cellular membrance activity in the corneal endothelium of the intact eye. *Experientia* 24: *1094—1094* (1968).

Mishima, S. Corneal thickness. *Surv. Ophthalmol.* 13: *57—96* (1968).

Mishima, S. & S.M. Trenberth. Permeability of the corneal endothelium to non-electolytes. *Invest. Ophthalmol.* 7: *34—43* (1968).

Ota, Y. S. Mishima & D.M. Maurice. Endothelial permeability of the living cornea to fluorescein. *Invest. Ophthalmol.* 13: *945—949* (1974).

Ota, Y. Endothelial permeability to fluorescein in corneal grafts and bullous keratopathy. *Jpn. J. Ophthalmol.* 19: *286—295* (1975).

Polack, F.M. G.K. Smelser & J. Rose. Long-term survival of isotopically labeled stromal and endothelial cells in corneal homografts. *Amer. J. Ophthalmol.* 57: *67—78* (1964).

Salceda, S.R. Endothelial cell survival after keratoplasty in rabbits. *Arch. Ophthalmol.* 78: *745—752* (1967).

Sato, T. Studies on the endothelium of the corneal graft. *Jpn. J. Ophthalmol.* 22: *114-126* (1978).

Sherrard, E.S. The corneal endothelium *in vivo*: its response to mild trauma. *Exp. Eye Res.* 22: *347-357* (1976).

Trenberth, S.M. & S. Mishima. The effect of ouabain on the rabbit corneal endothelium. *Invest. Ophthalmol.* 7: *44-52* (1968).

Van Horn, D.L. D.D. Sendels, S.S. Seideman & D.J. Buco, Regenerative capacity of the corneal endothelium in rabbit and cat. *Invest. Ophthalmol.* 16: *597-613* (1977).

Van Horn, D.L. & R.A. Hyndiuk. Endothelial wound repair in primate ocrnea. *Exp. Eye Res.* 21: *113-124* (1975).

Authors' address:
Department of Ophthalmology
University of Tokyo
School of Medicine
Hongo, Bunkyo-Ku
Tokyo
Japan.

HEALING PROCESS IN THE ALKALI–BURNED
CORNEAL ENDOTHELIUM

SHUSAKU KITANO

(Tokyo, Japan)

When the surface of the cornea is burned with alkali, the endothelial layer is also damaged and the denuded area is left.

The defect will be covered with migration and proliferation of surrounding endothelial cells. The healing process in the alkali-burned corneal endothelium was observed by scanning electron microscopy comparing with the findings of endothelial flat preparation and autoradiography.

EXPERIMENTAL METHOD

The burn was made by appling filter paper, 3 mm square, soaked in 4N NaOH, to the surface of the anesthetized rabbit corneas for 10 seconds.

The corneas were observed daily with a slit lamp staining with fluorescein-sodium.

The eyes were enucleated at intervals of 0, 3, 6, 12 and 24 hours and 3, 7 and 14 days after burn. The specimens were fixed with 4% buffered glutaraldehyde, after fixation, they were dehydrated in graded acetone and isoamyl acetate, then dried by the critical point method. After drying specimens were coated with gold-palladium in vacuum chamber and examined with scanning electron microscopy using magnification of X 200 to X 5,000 at 15kV.

An autoradiographic study was made on two groups (Fig. 1, below).
1. To check the incorporation of tritium thymidine into the endothelial cells at various intervals after burn.
2. To trace the movement of regenerating cells which had been labeled at the 24th hour after burn.

Both of flat preparation by van Sallmann's method and praffin sections were dipped with SAKURA-NR-M2 emulsion and kept in dark for 10–14 days.

FINDINGS

Normal endothelial cells observed with scanning electron microscope showed regular distribution of hexagonal pattern with marginal folds resulting from overlapping of the margin of the adjacent cells.

1 Incorporation.

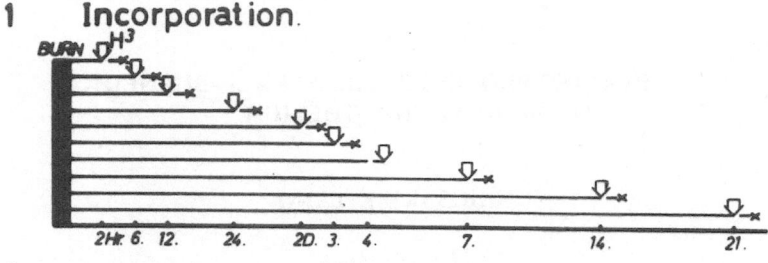

2 Turn over.

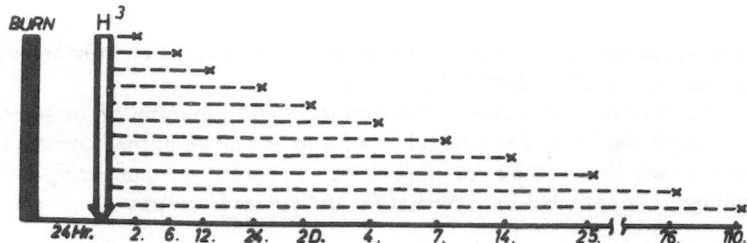

Fig. 1.

Immediately after burn, the endothelium over the entired burned area were completely destroyed and lost normal structual appearance (Fig. 2, below).

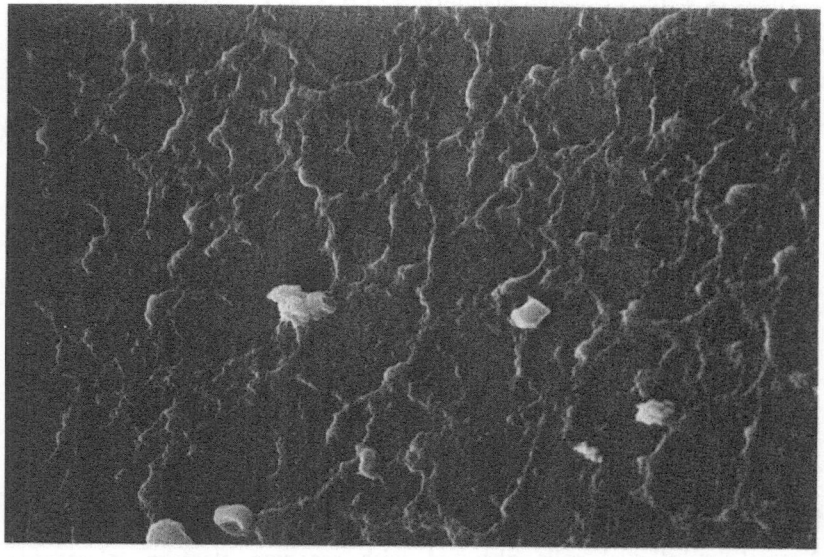

In the marginal region of the wound, various type of the vacuoles were seen intra- and inter-cellularly (Fig. 3, below).

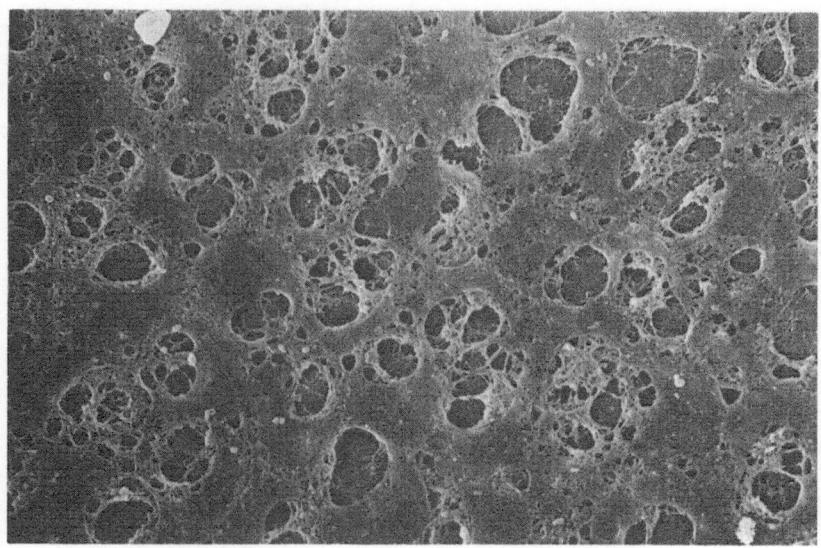

After 3 hours, the degenerated cells were falling off from the Descemet's membrane and there was attachment of fine fibrin on the surface (Fig. 4, below).

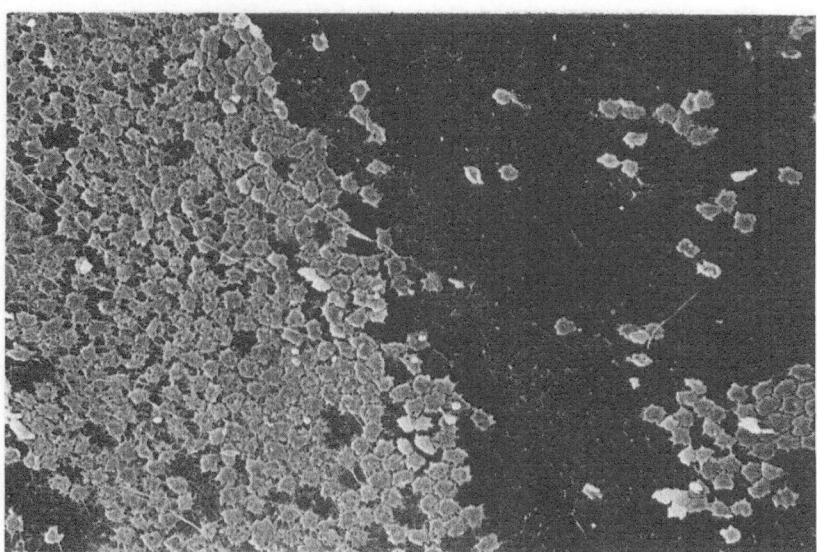

After 6 hours, remained endothelial cells in the margin of the defect became irregular shape and the intercellular space was enlarged. It was thought the first step of the migration of endothelial cells (Fig. 5, below).

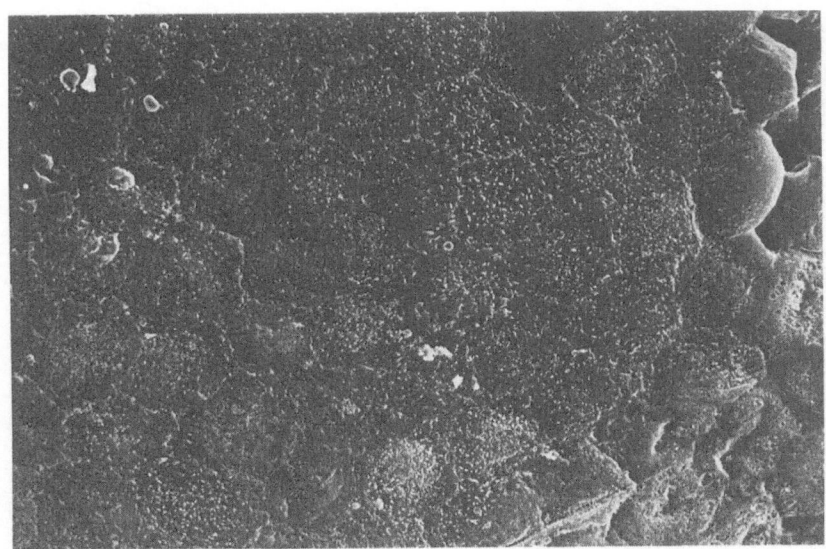

The endothelial cells began to migrate toward the burned area. These cells had oval shape holding a major axis to the center and indistinct marginal folds (Fig. 6, below).

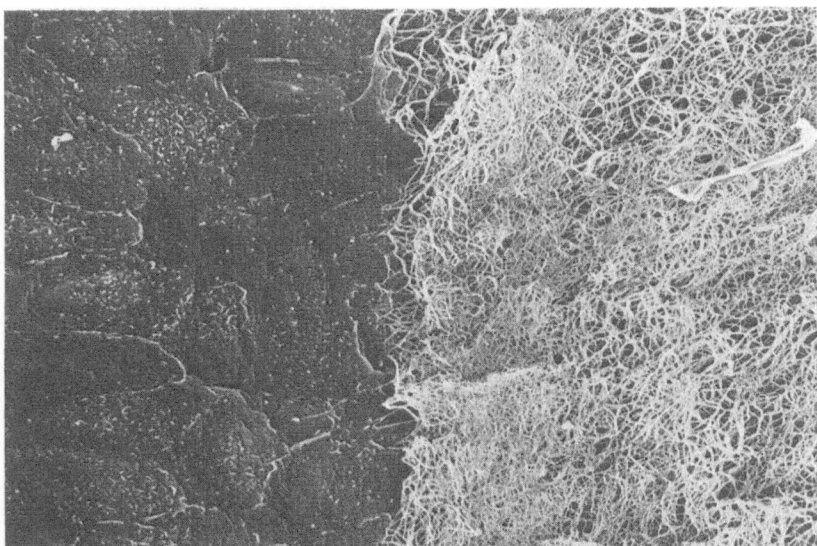

Migrating cells showed frequently quite irregular shape to extend their cytoplasmic processes into and or over the fibrin plug toward the denuded area (Fig. 7, below).

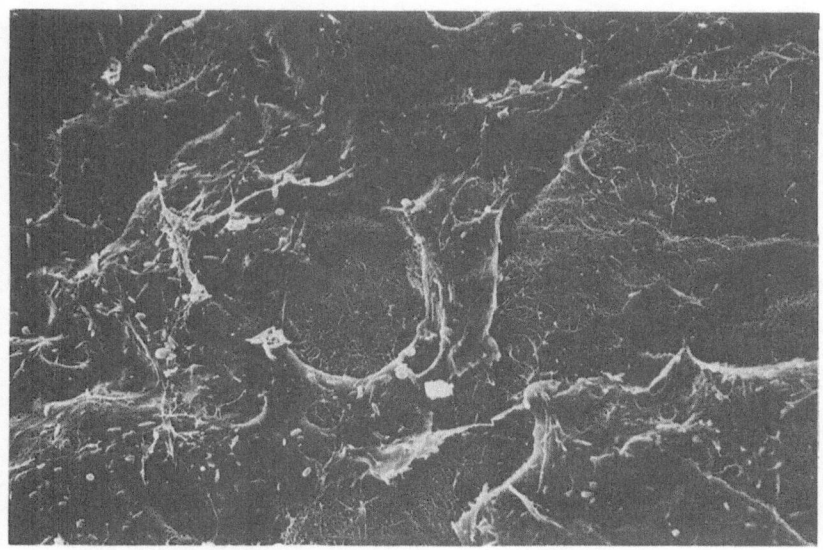

At 24 hr., scanning electron microscopy showed relatively small and thickened round or spindle cells among the migrating cells. It was suggested the these cells were going to mitosis (Fig. 8, below).

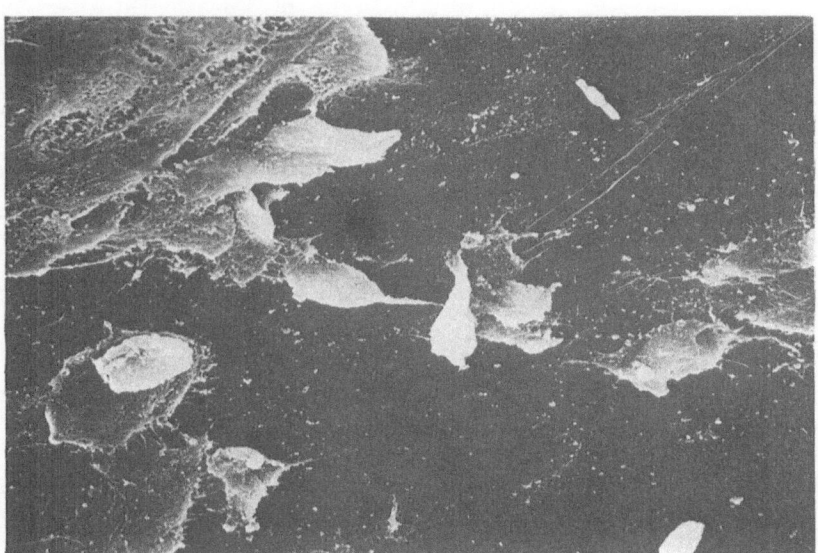

A flat preparation of the endothelium in the same stage, revealed a number of mitotic figure at the margin of the defect (Fig. 9, below).

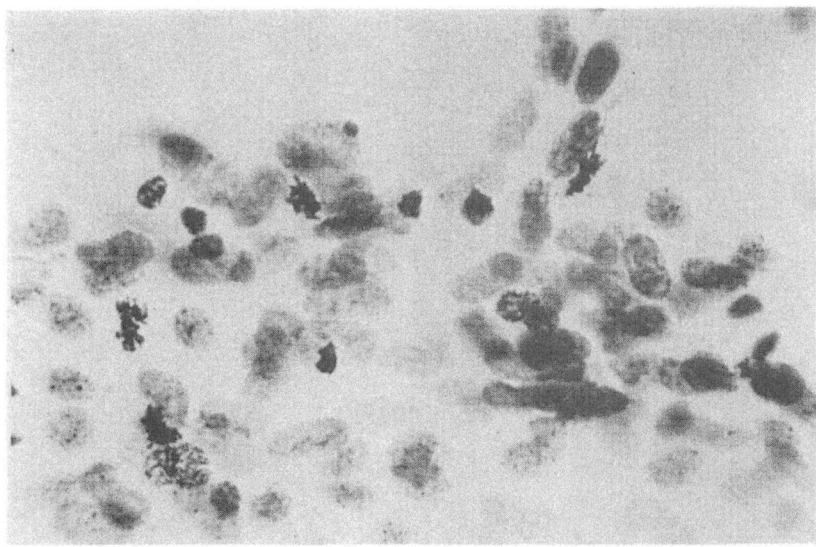

Autoradiography also showed DNA—synthetizing cells labeled with tritium thymidine presented in the limited zone of the surrounding endothelium (Fig. 10, below).

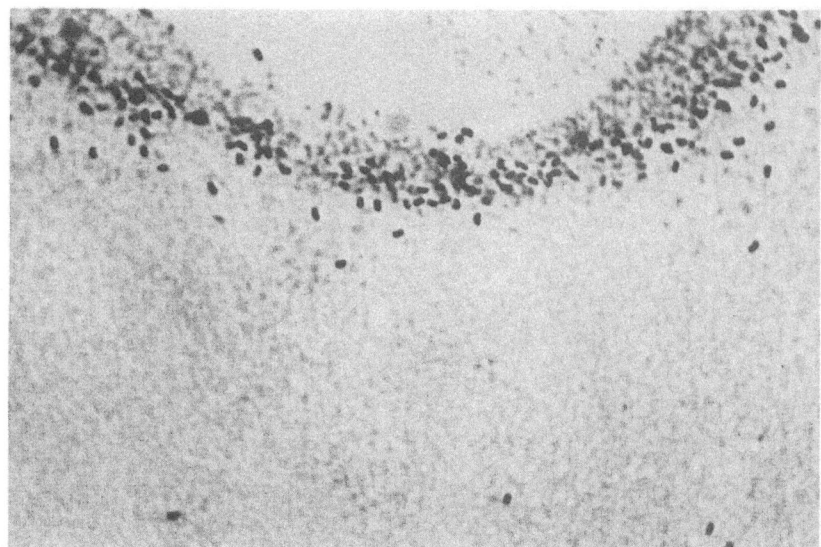

In the paraffin section, tagged cells were shown at the advancing zone of the endothelium indicating that cellular devision was going to occur in these cells (Fig. 11, below).

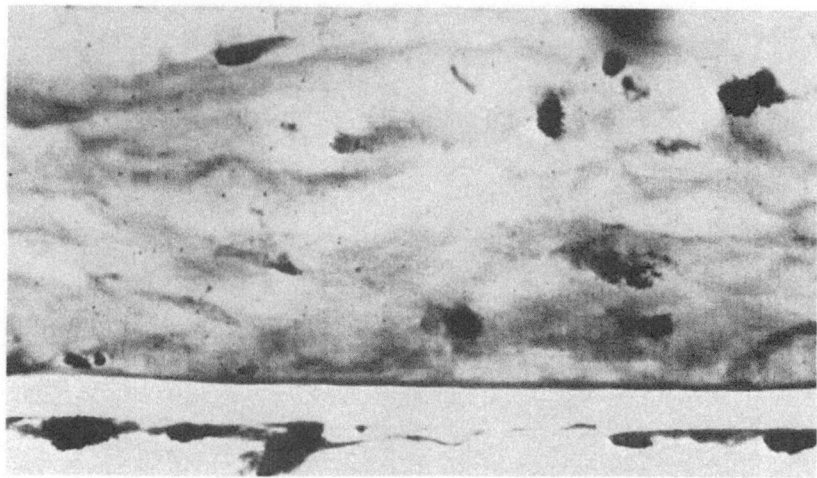

An incorporation of tiritium thymidine into the endothelial layer at the margin of the defect extremely increased between 24 hr. and 48 hr. after burn.

At 3 days, scanning electron microscopy showed the denuded region was covered by a monolayer of large irregular shaped cells migrated from the margin, although degenerating cells and cell debris still existed in the burned area.

In the periphery, there was an aggregation of spindle cells and small round cells where devision took place (Fig. 12, below).

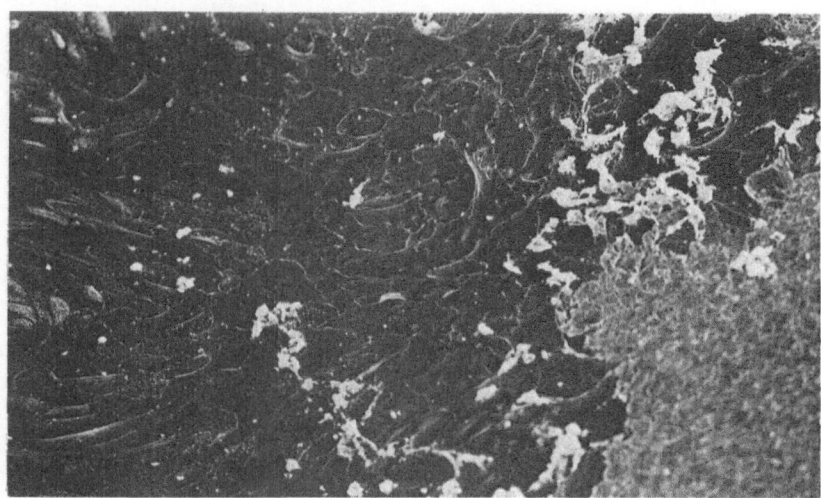

There were a number of mitotic cell between normal endothelial cells and migrated large cells (Fig. 13, below).

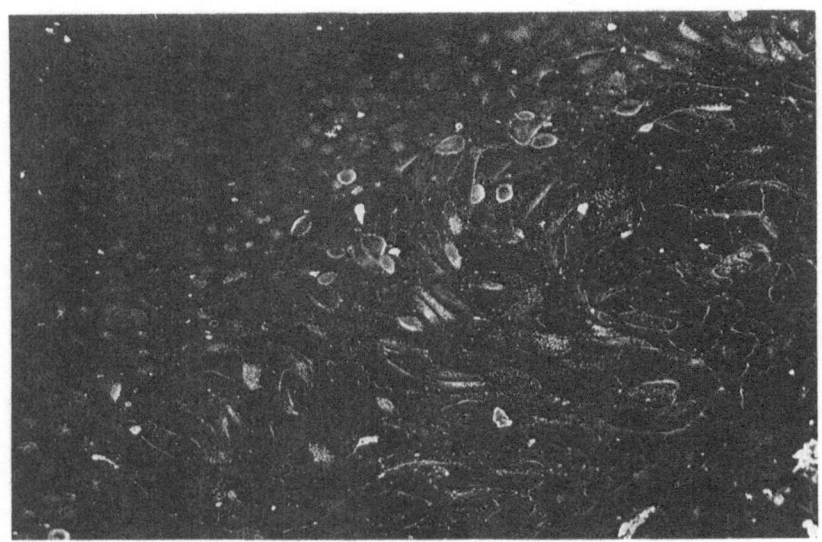

The flat preparation, corresponding to the scanning electron microscopy, revealed irregular shaped migrating cells in the defect, zone of spindle cell aggregation surrounding the denuded area and normal endothelial cells in the periphery (Fig. 14, below).

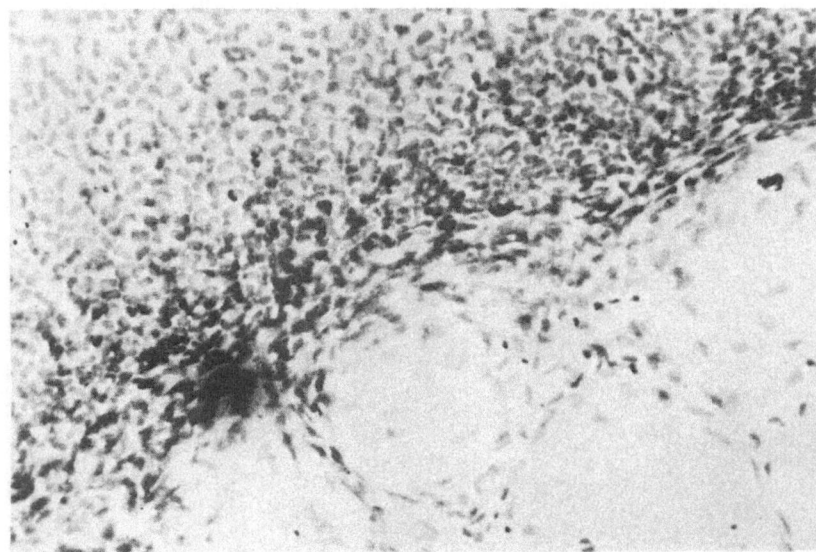

90

The defect of the endothelial layer is covered by the mirgation and mitosis of the marginal cells relatively in a short time. The fact was evidently supported by the findings of autoradiography. At 2 hrs. after intracameral injection of tritium thymidine at the 24th hour after burn, labeled cells were distributed in the marginal region of the wound (Fig. 15, below).

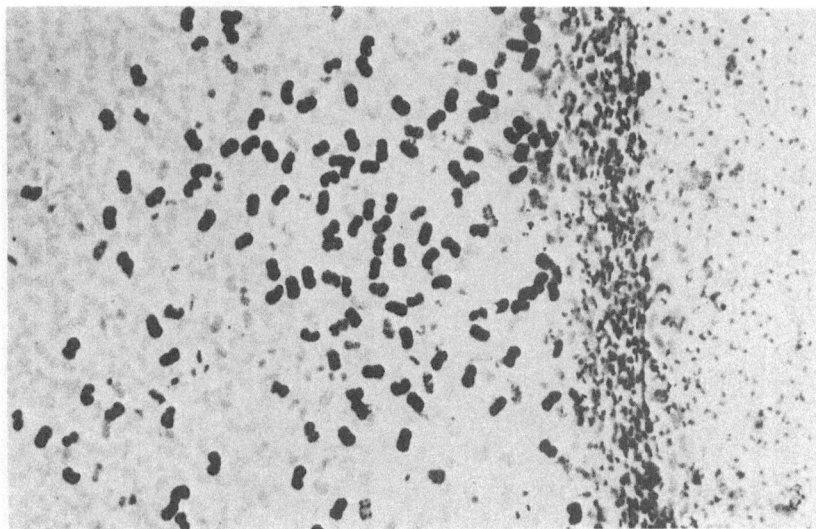

After the lapse of only 10 hrs., almost all of these cells migrated over the wound edge into the denuded area (Fig. 16, below).

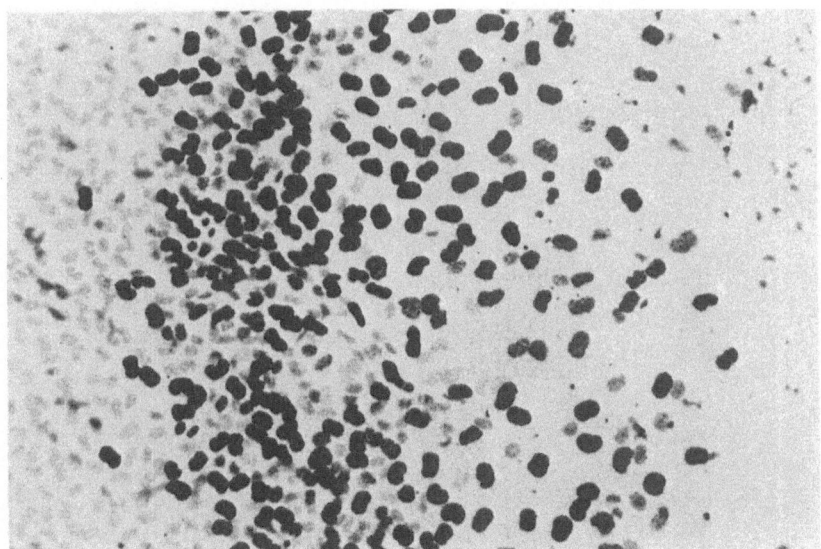

It was noted that migration of the endothelial cells were so rapid. At 48 hrs. after burn, the denuded area was almost covered with migrating cells in which a number of labeled cells were recognized.

On the other hand, there were quite few labeled cells in the marginal region (Fig. 17, below).

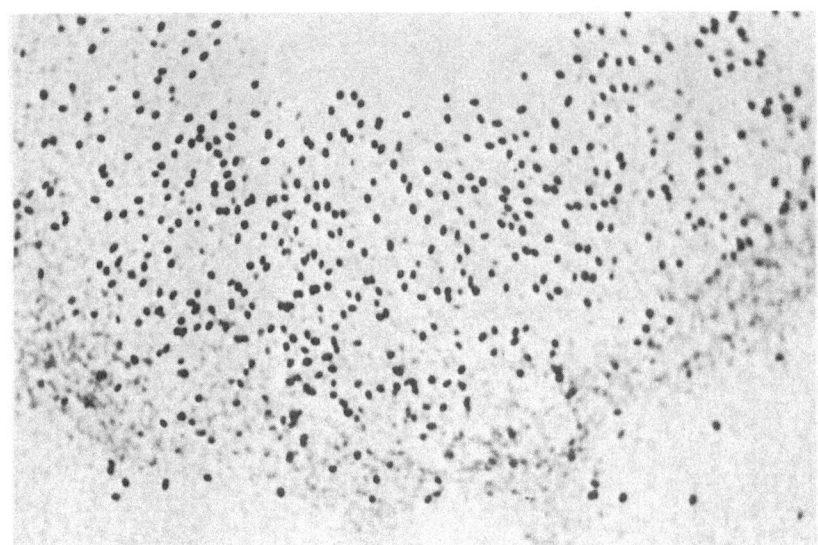

It indicated the mitotic activity of the labeled cells that many daughter cells which had small oval nuclei and light grains were scattered on regenerating endothelium 48 hrs. after labeling (Fig. 18, below).

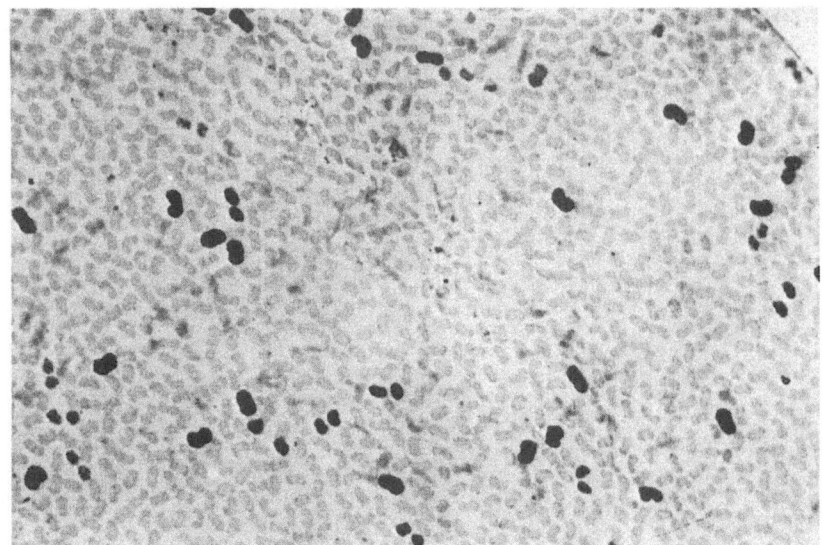

Daughter cells were recognized as small spindle shaped cell having packed microvilli or ruffle on the surface with scanning electron microscopy (Fig. 19, below).

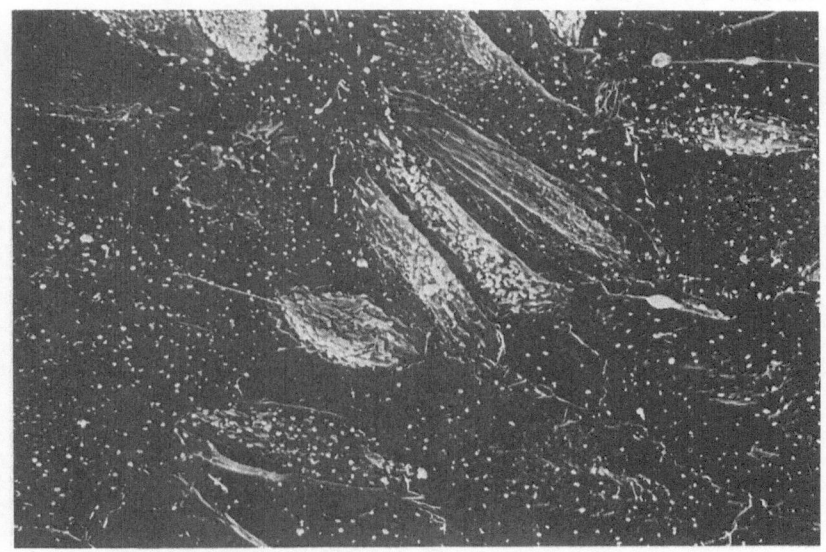

At 14 days after burn, in the marginal region of the wound, oval and spindle shaped cells accumulated to form a multilayer (Fig. 20, below).

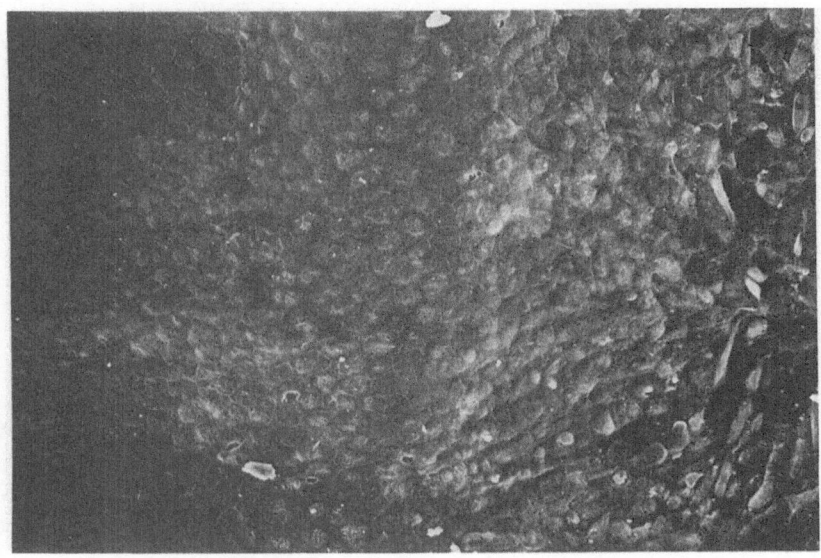

At the same stage, a flat preparation of the endothelium also revealed multi-layered fibroblastic cells with thick stained spindle nuclei (Fig. 21, below), and two or three layers of endothelium were recognize beneath Descemet's membrane in the paraffin section

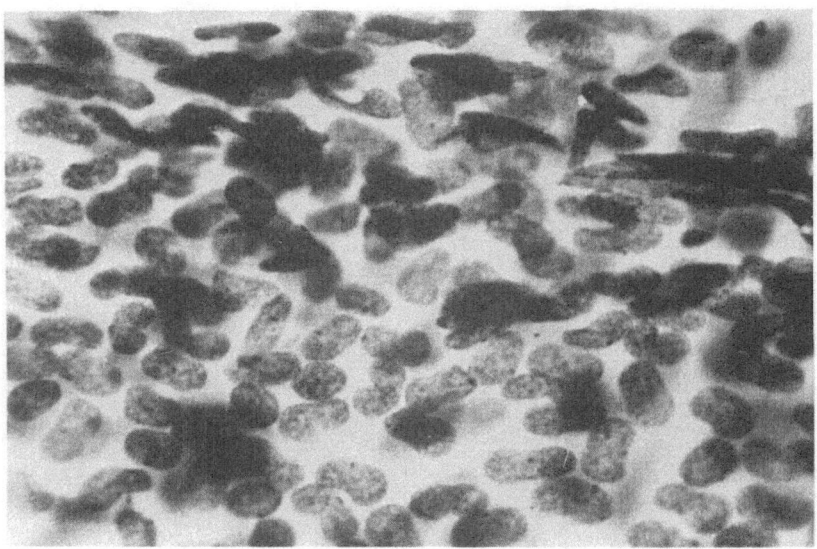

At 3 weeks after burn, scanning electron microscope showed connective tissue was formed along the margin of burned area (Fig. 22, below).

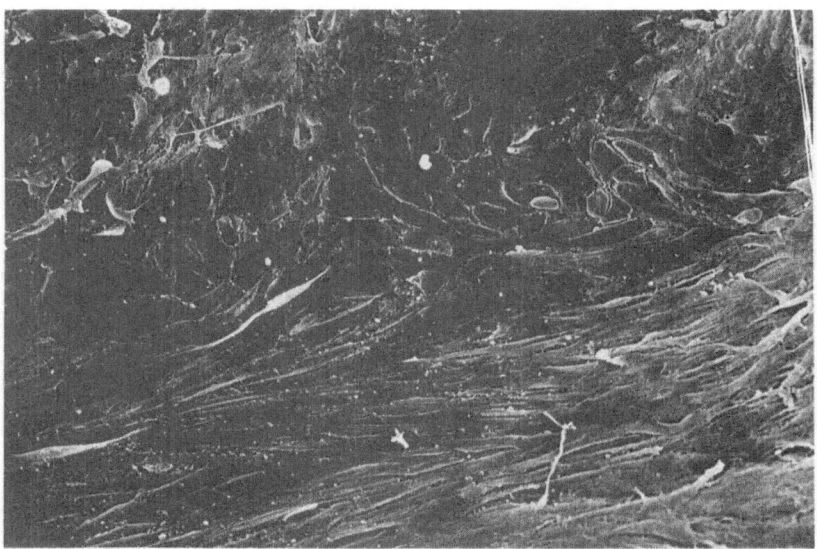

The retension of the labeled endothelial cells in the connective tissue which was formed between stroma and endothelium indicated the over growth of the stimulated edothelium by alkali burn promoted a formation of the retrocorneal membrane (Fig. 23, below).

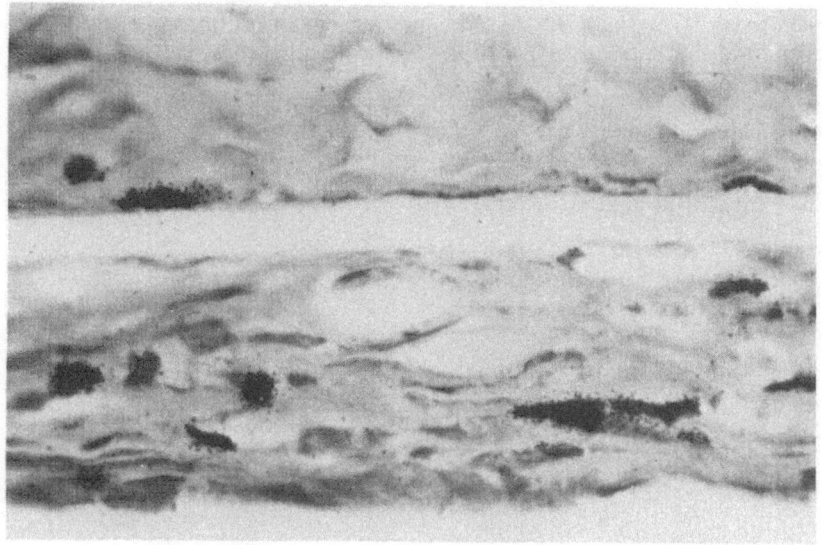

At 2 month after burn, a monolayer of new endothelial cells covered the retrocorneal membrane packed with collagenous fiber.

At this stage, thickness of the cornea returned to normal, the healing of the endothelium was accomplished (Fig. 24, below).

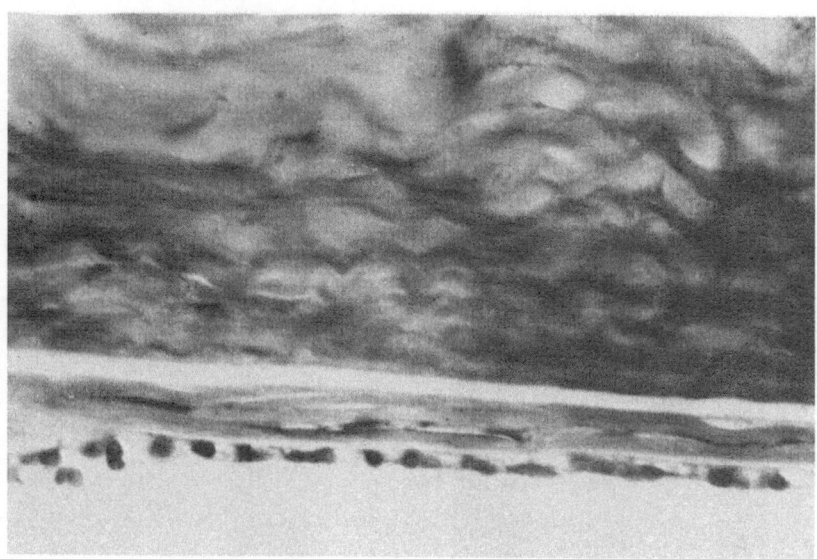

Endothelial cell differentiated form of mesenchymall cell has metaplastic potential to undergo de—defferenciated fibroblast in the process of wound repair.

These fibroblastic cells are capable of synthetizing collagenous fiber and form a new connective tissue, retrocorneal membrane, beneath Descemet's membrane. The cells lining the anterior chamber gradually change in structure and function to that of normal endothelial cells.

Author's address:
Department of Ophthalmology
Nihon University
School of Medicine
30—1 Oyaguchi kamimachi, Itabashi—Ku
Tokyo
Japan

THE ELECTRON MICROSCOPIC STUDY OF FUCHS' DYSTROPHY: THE FIRST PRIMARY CASE IN JAPAN

SHINOBU AKIYA, TAKASHI OHSHIMA AND MACHIKO WADA

(Tokyo, Japan)

INTRODUCTION

Primary Fuchs' dystrophy may be common disease in the world. But, this is rare disease in Japan. Oguchi (1926) has reported one first case based on only clinical findings in 1926.

While there have been several cases thereafter, there has not been any case based on clinical and pathological examinations except for Muramatsu and Hamada's case (1977) in 1977.

The purpose of this paper is to present the certain first case of primary Fuchs' dystrophy to be diagnosed with the findings of a study on clinical and pathological examination in Japan and discuss the pathogenesis of the abnormal Descemet's membrane in Fuchs' dystrophy.

MATERIAL AND METHOD

The material used was corneal button, obtained by perforating keratoplasty. Immediately after operation, the tissue was fixed with 2.5 per cent glutaraldehyde in 0.05 M phosphate buffer (PH 7.4) for 3 hours. Then, one half of the corneal button was dissected and postfixed with 1 per cent OsO_4 in phosphate buffer at PH 7.4 for 2 hours. The corneal button was cut into small pieces while the tissue was in fixative. They were dehydrated with graded alcohol and embedded in Epon 812. After preparing thick (1 to 2 μ) sections stained with toluidine blue for light microscopy, the tissues were trimmed, thinsectioned, and double-stained with uranyl acetate and lead citrate for electron microscopy. A Porter—Blum microtome, and JEM 100B for electron microscopy. Other half of corneal button was embedded in paraffine and used for histochemical studies.

Brief case history of the patient whose corneal button was used in this study is as follows:

This patient was a 28-year-old Japanese woman. She has not had any past history of eye disease. Since Feb. 1976 she had noted blurring of both eyes on arising. Decreasing vision was markedly on right eye. At that time she was in th 9 month of pregnancy. After delivery, vision decreased further.

She came to Keio Hospital's eye clinic on June, 1976. Her visual acuity of the right eye was 0.4 (n.c.) and visual acuity of the left eye was 0.6, corrected acuity was 1.0. By slit lamp examination, epithelial and stromal edema, pigment deposits on the posterior corneal surface and a beaten gold appearance over a wide central area of endothelium were noticed on both eyes, particularly on the right eye.

Intraocular pressure of both eyes was normal. No iritis sign was noted. Her systemic condition was very good except previous slight asthma.

On May, 1977, as patient's vision of the right eye had worsened, perforating keratoplasty was done on the right corneal (Fig. 1).

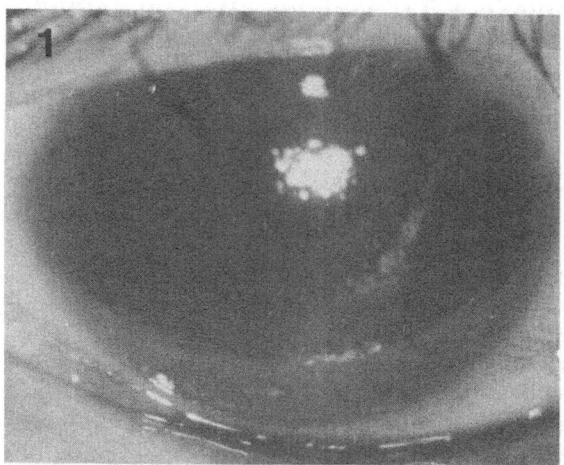

Fig. 1. Pre-operative corneal appearance of the right eye.

Postoperative course was favorable. On May, 1978, patient's visual acuity was 1.5 with contact lens. Corneal edema of the left eye has continued.

RESULTS

Light microscopy:

Many vacuoles were seen in the epitherial layer. Stromal lamellae were separated. Descemet's membrane showed a marked thickening in which several warts involved. The posterior region of Descemet's membrane indicated week stain with eosin. Warts were PAS positive (Fig. 2). The posterior region of Descemet's membrane showed positive staining results for collagen with van Gieson and Mallory's stains.

Furthermore, this region showed positive staining result for mucopolysaccharide with alcian blue stain. No trace of endothelial cells could be found anywhere on the specimen.

Electron microscopy:

Descemet's membrane was about 40 μ thick. The nonbanded region was obscured by presence of the banded pattern (Fig. 3).

The border region was demarcated apparently from the fibrillar region. On the posterior area of Descemet's membrane many warts were observed. At

98

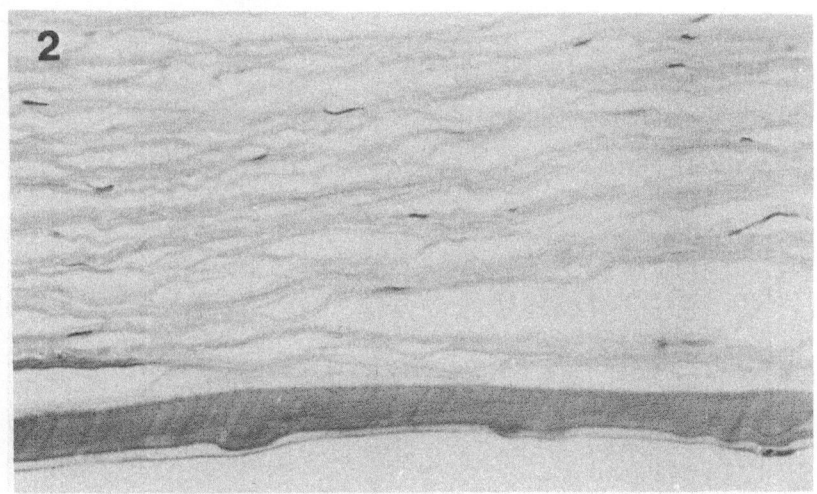

Fig. 2. PAS positive warts of Descemet's membrane.

some places of normal Descemet's membrane there were loosened areas (Figs. 4, 5, 6).

The peripheral part of the wart consisted of the long-spacing bundles, thin fibrils and electron dens fine granules (Fig. 7).

A component of the posterior border region was thin fibrils that sometimes transfer into collagen fibrils on the fibrillar region. However, these findings did not appeared to be more prominent on the region with wart than without wart (Figs. 8, 9, 10).

The long-spacing bundles and thin fibrils with periodicity were seen on the anterior part of the border region (Figs. 11, 12).

When thin fibrils were arranged in close apposition, they showed about 500 Å periodicity, and this sometimes made transition into a banding of 1000 Å, to form long-spacing bundle (Fig. 13).

Some of the long-spacing bundles at the border region of Descemet's membrane had thick double bands (Fig. 14).

The spindle-shaped long-spacing bundles were often surrounded by thin fibrils, electron dense fine granules and almost normal Descemet's membrane pattern (Fig. 15).

The fibrillar region consisted of collagen fibrils and electron dense fine granules (Fig. 16). In the fibrillar region, collagen fibril-electron dense fine granule ratio varied respectively on the places.

On the posterior part of the fibrillar region, electron dense fine granules were apt to be predominant (Figs. 17, 18).

Endothelium was almost missing. But, sometimes, cell nucleous-like structures were observed. High electron dense granules were seen near the ones.

99

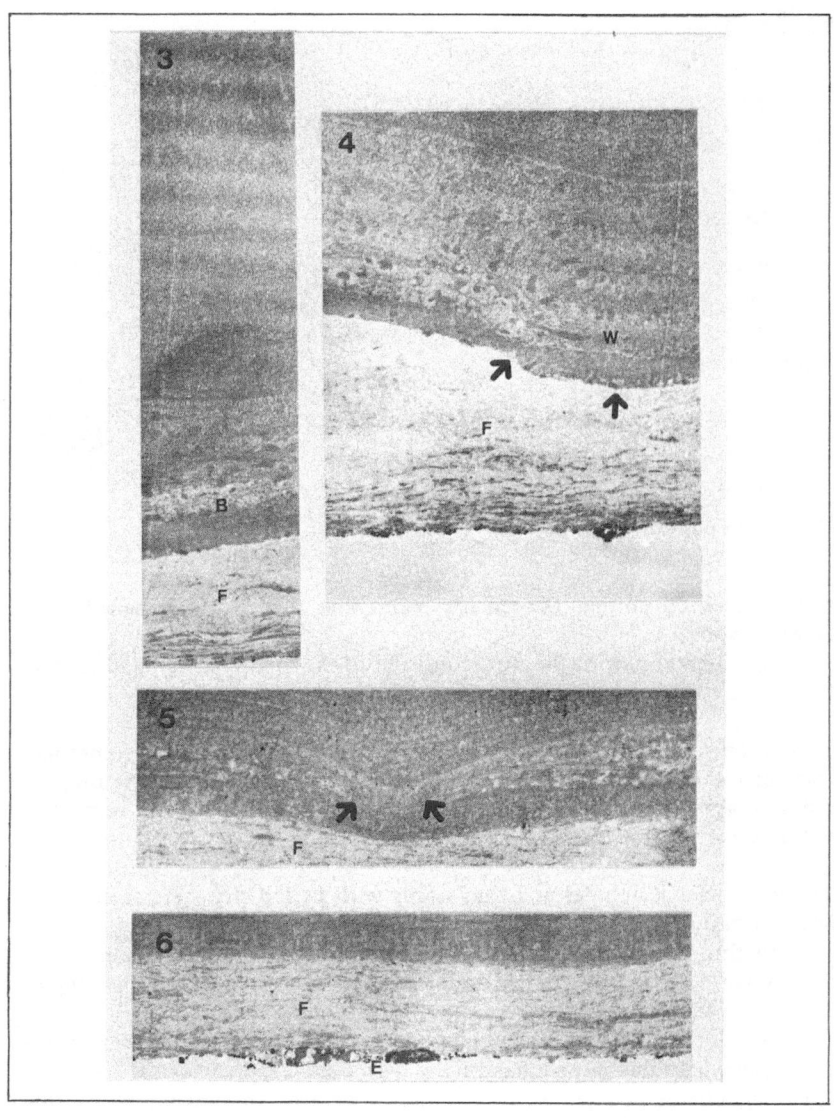

Fig. 3. The marked thickning Descemet's membrane. The non-banded region is obscure by presence of the banded pattern. The fibrillar region is demarcated apparently from the border region. F, fibrillar region; B, border region. (X 3,600.)

Fig. 4. The posterior area of Descemet's membrane showing a wart. Arrows indicate configuration of the wart. F, fibrillar region; W, wart (X 4,200.)

Fig. 5. A wart-like formation in the posterior area of banded region. Arrows indicate configuration of the wart-like formation. The fibrillar region is demarcated distinctly from the border region. F, fibrillar region. (X 3,000.)

Fig. 6. The posterior area of Descemet's membrane without wart. F, fibrillar region; E, abnormal endothelium. (X 3,000.)

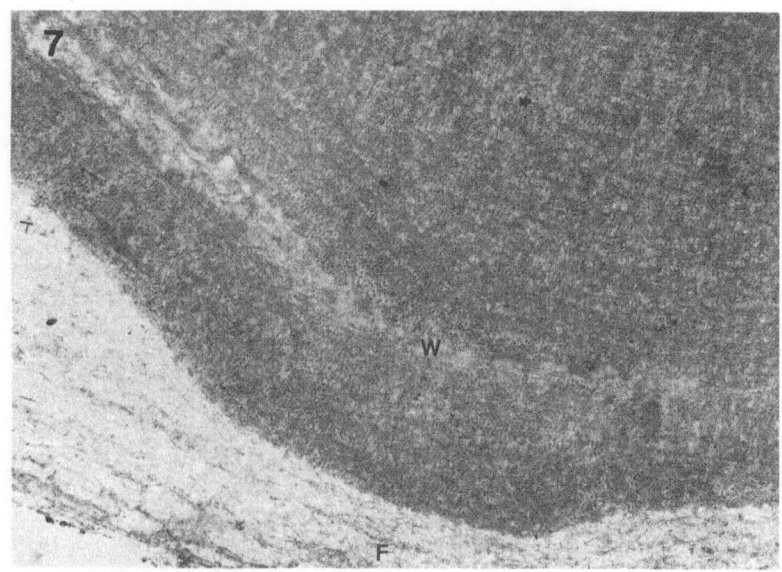

Fig. 7. A wart located in the posterior area of Descemet's membrane. The wart consists of the long-spacing bundles, thin fibrils and electron dense fine granules. W, wart; F, fibrillar region (X 6,000.)

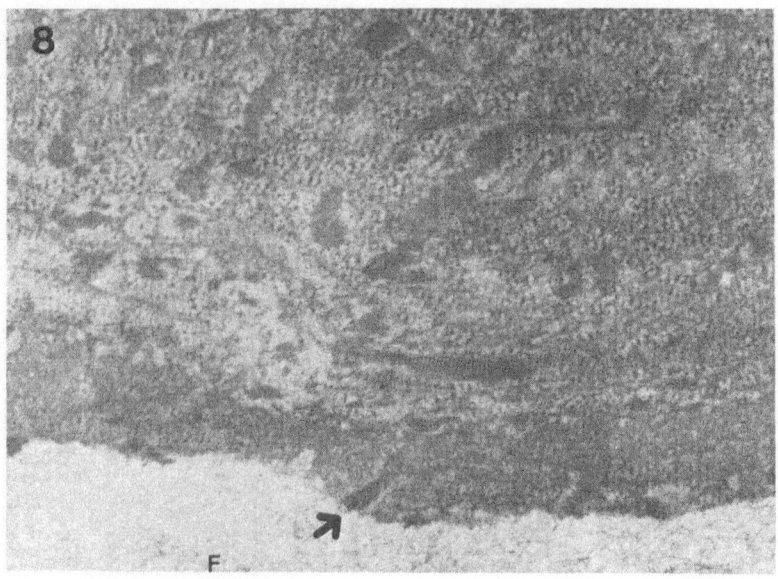

Fig. 8. The peripheral part of the wart. The prominent component of the posterior border region is thin fibrils. These fibrils transfer into collagen fibrils on the fibrillar region (arrow). F, fibrillar region. (X 12,000.)

101

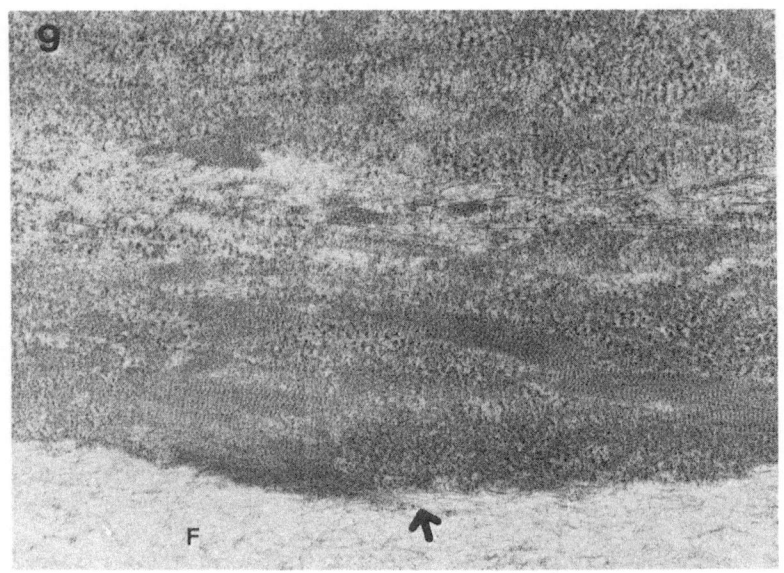

Fig. 9. The border region without wart. Thin fibrils transfer into collagen fibrils on the fibrillar region (arrow). F, fibrillar region. (X 12,000.)

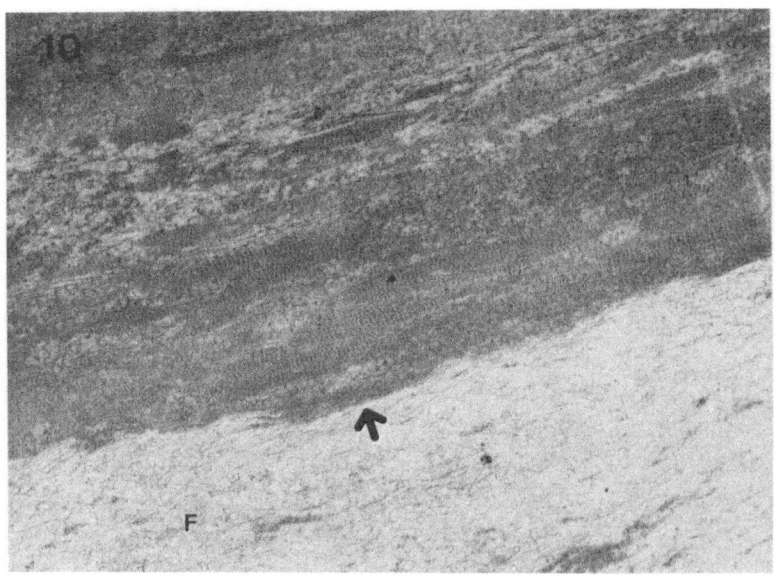

Fig. 10. The border region without wart. The collagen fibrils of the fibrillar region appear to be incorporated into thin fibrils of the border region (arrow). The long-spacing bundles, thin fibrils with periodicity and electron dense fine granules are seen. F, fibrillar region. (X 12,000.)

102

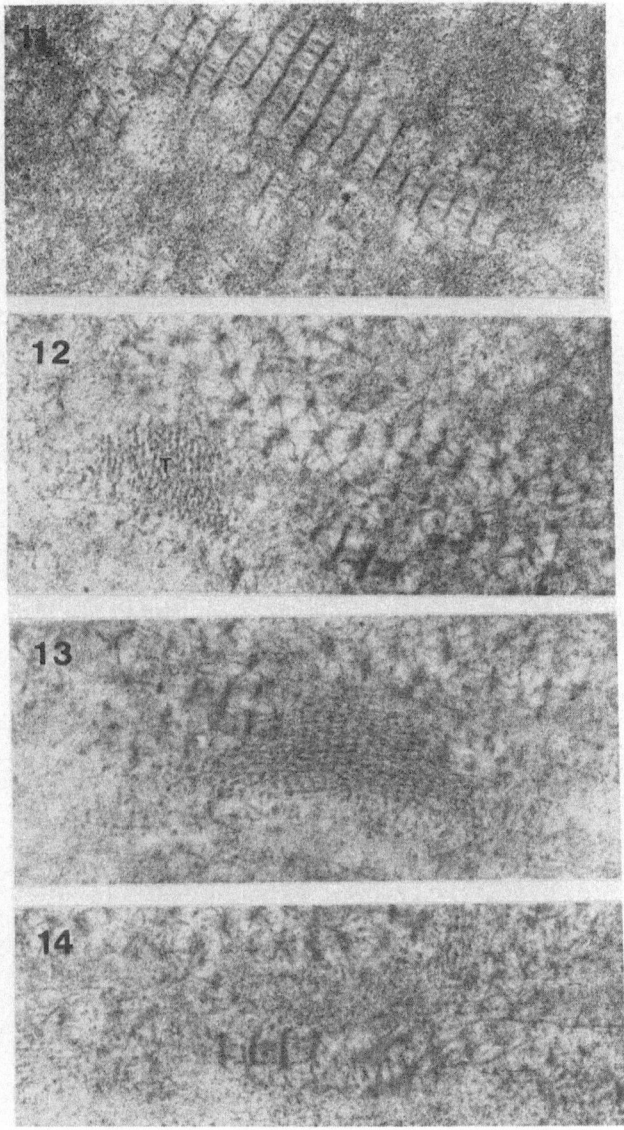

Fig. 11. The long spacing bundles on the border region in high magnification. (X 42,000.)

Fig. 12. The long-spacing bundles and cross section of thin fibrils. T, group of thin fibrils. (X 40,000.)

Fig. 13. When thin fibrils are arranged in close apposition, they show about 500 A periodicity, and this sometimes makes transition into a banding of 1,000 Å, to form long-spacing bundles. (X 40,000.)

Fig. 14. The long-spacing bundle at the border region of Descemet's membrane having thick double bands (arrow). (X 40,000.)

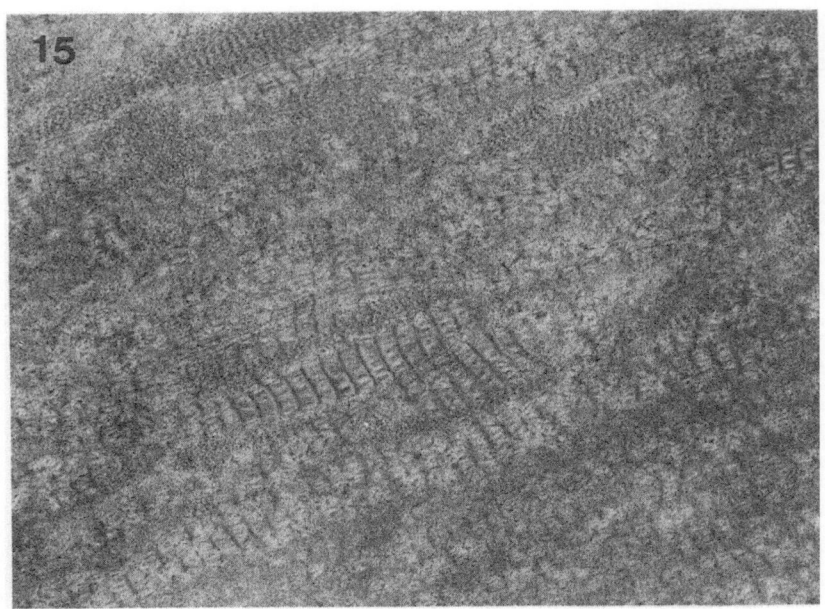

Fig. 15. The spindle-shaped long-spacing bundles surrounded by thin fibrils, electron dense fine granules and normal Descemet's membrane pattern. (X 20,000.)

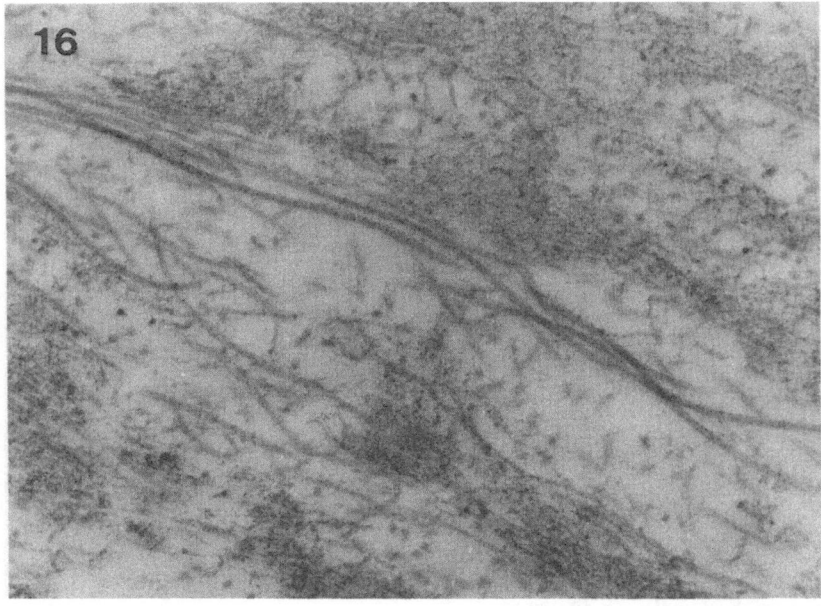

Fig. 16. The fibrillar region of Descemet's membrane. It consists of collagen fibrils and electron dense fine granules. (X 100,000.)

104

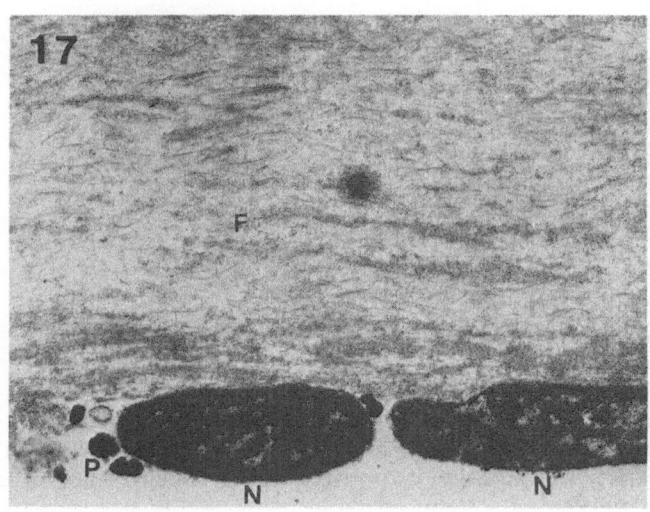

Fig. 17. Endothelial cell nucleus- like structures on the posterior surface of abnormal Descemet's membrane. High electron dense granules are seen near the structure. The electron dense fine granules occupy a large proportion of the posterior area of the fibrillar region. N, endothelial cell nucleus-like structure; P, high electron dense granule; F, fibrillar region. (X 9,600.)

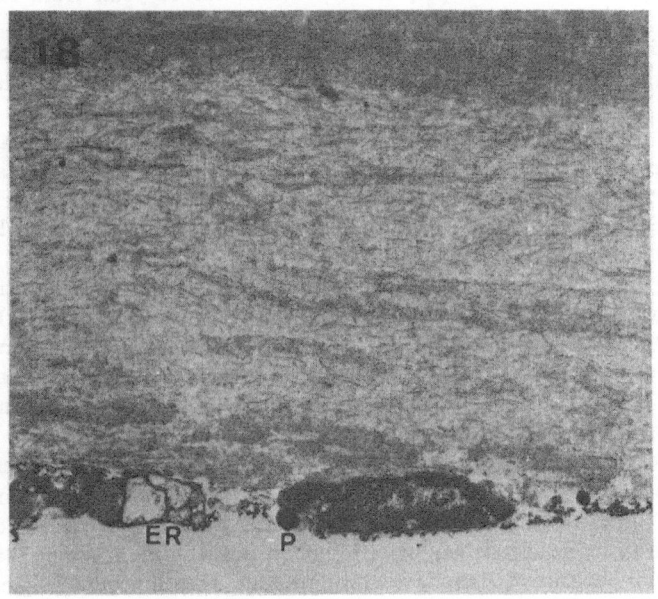

Fig. 18. Abnormal endothelial cells showing enlargement of rough-surfaced endoplasmic reticulum, moderate electron dense material and high electron dense granules in the cytoplasm. ER, rough-surfaced endoplasmic reticulum; P, high electron dense granules. (X 9,600.)

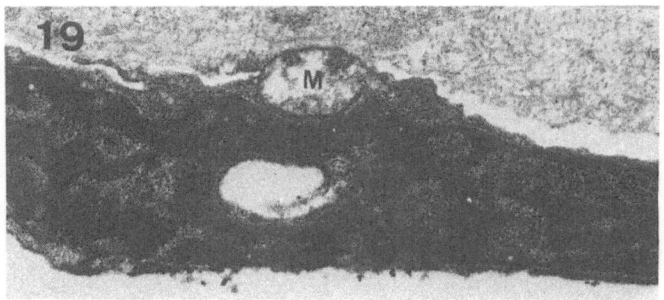

Fig. 19. Abnormal endothelial cell showing vacuolization of mitochondrien. M, mitochondria. (X 20,000.)

Vacuolization of mitochondrien, enlargement of rough-surfaced endoplasmic reticulum, moderate electron dense material and high electron dense granules were seen in the cytoplasm of the residual endothelial cell (Figs. 17, 18, 19).

DISCUSSION

On the basis of the above clinical and pathological findings, this case is able to diagnose primary Fuchs' dystrophy. This patient is the first case among 113,456 patients of Keio Hospital's eye clinic for 10 years from 1968 to 1977.

Electron microscopic findings also showed the same results as the previous reports (Kayes and Halmberg, 1964; Iwamoto and De Voe, 1971; Hamada *et al.*, 1973) in the foreign countries except of a few points.

Fuchs' dystrophy is usually classified primary and secondary. Muramatsu and Hamada's case (1977) that is likely to be Fuchs' dystrophy among previous reported cases in Japan. However, the patient has suffered iritis on the couse of disease. So, our case might be the first case of primary Fuchs' dystrophy in Japan.

About the pathogenesis of abnormal Descemet's membrane formation on Fuchs' dystrophy, a hypothesis has been proposed by Iwamoto (1971).

His hypothesis shows that the endothelial cells undergo transformation into fibroblasts and start producing not only the basement membranelike material but also collagen fibrils and the process of collagen fibril disintegration formes the abnormal Descemet's membrane.

However, the pathogenesis of wart formation can not be elucidated completely with his hypothesis. Although we agree with his hypothesis partially, but, we suppose that the speed and grade of endothelial cell to transform into fibroblast may be different from each others and endothelial cells having abnormal function may produce the abnormal regions of Descemet's membrane involved warts at each time.

Our hypothesis is highly speculative based only on the electron microscopic findings of abnormal Descemet's membrane. Further studies should be examined the case having continuous endothelial cover.

According to the incomplete familiar tree of the patient (Fig. 20), this case may be sporadic. It is very interesting that the corneas of her mother and elder sister who have cornea guttata are clear and normal thick.

Familiar Tree of the Present Case

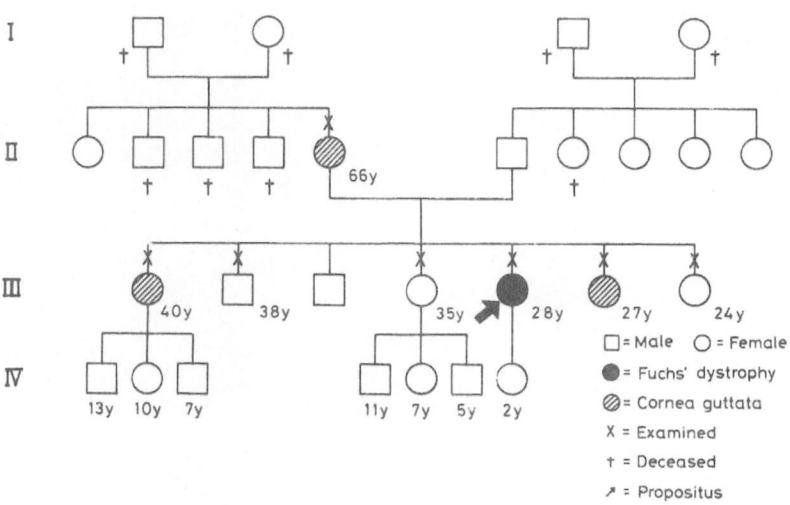

Fig. 20.

It may be right theoretically that the patient has some dispositions to rise cornal edema. We propose that it is important genetically, to know whether the dispositions are governed by hereditary or not.

CONCLUSION

A 28-year-old Japanese woman of primary Fuchs' dystrophy to be diagnosed based on the clinical and morphorogical findings was reported.

This may be the first reliable case of Fuchs's dystrophy in Japan.

For interpretation of the pathogenesis of the abnormal Descemet's membrane, an assumption was made by Iwamoto was corrected a little. Our assumption may be better on comprehension of warts formation than Iwamoto's one.

REFERENCES

Hamada, R., J.P. Giraud & Y. Pouliquen. Electron microscopic study on the Fuchs's dystrophy. *Acta Soc. ophthalm. Jpn.* 77: *531* (1973).

Iwamoto, T. & A.G. DeVoe. Electron microscopic studies on Fuchs' combined dystrophy. I. Posterior portion of the cornea. *Invest. Ophthalm.* 10: *9* (1971).

Kayes, J. & A. Halmberg. The fine structure of the cornea in Fuchs' endothelial dystrophy. *Invest. Ophthalm.* 3: *47* (1964).

Muramatsu, R., R. Hamada, M. Usui & M. Harutake. Scanning electron microscopic studies on the corneal endothelium of three different diseases. (Fuchs' dystrophy, stromal edema of transplanted cornea and alkali burned cornea.) *Folia Ophthalm. Jpn.* 28: *543* (1977).

Oguchi, Ch. A case of Dystrophia epithelialis corneae (Fuchs). *Jpn. Rev. Clinical Ophthalm.* 21: *1* (1926).

Authors' address:
Department of Ophthalmology
School of Medicine
Keio University
Tokyo
Japan

Docum. Ophthal. Proc. Series, Vol. 20

CORNEAL TRANSPLANTATION AND REJECTION

MAX FINE

(San Francisco, California, U.S.A.)

ABSTRACT

With technical problems largely solved and with improved quality of donor material, the immune allograft reaction is becoming the most frequent limitation to corneal transplantation. The over all frequency of the allograft reaction is 15% in the author's experience, varying from about 10% in the most favorable cases to about 35% in the less favorable. Preoperatively vascularized corneas showed a definitely higher incidence of allograft reaction even in the favorable prognostic group. The time of onset of the reaction tended to be earlier and the outcome less favorable in the preoperatively vascularized cases. Regrafted cases also showed a greater frequency of the allograft reaction, almost three times as frequent as in comparable primary grafts. Despite this clear regrafts were obtainable in 64% of all regrafted cases and in 80% of the dystrophy cases.

Corneal transplants may fail from many causes most important of which are poor surgical technique, defective donor tissue, infection, glaucoma, and the immune allograft reaction. As the technical problems of keratoplasty have been progressively solved and as the availability and quality of donor material has improved the role of the allograft rejection as a cause of graft failure has increased in importance to the point that it may soon be considered the ultimate limitation to corneal transplantation. In the most favorable prognostic cases such as keratoconus the success rate is already approaching 100%. With technical improvements the reported incidence of the allograft reaction is decreasing but there is still a wide discrepancy in the incidence reported by various observers. This is true of the most favorable cases undergoing keratoplasty as well as of the least favorable. The allograft reaction in favorable cases such as keratoconus has been variously reported as 11% to 30%. This discrepancy might be explained either on the basis of technique, differences in period of observation, or differences in the criteria for the diagnosis of the allograft reaction. The diagnosis of an immune allograft reaction is not always simple. It was summed up during the Ciba Symposium on corneal graft failure held in 1972 as follows: 'An unequivocal clinical diagnosis of allograft reaction can be made, when, at least 10 days after a first transplantation a previously clear graft in a quiet eye rapidly develops edema with signs of inflammation in the anterior segment including ciliary flush, with cells and usually slight flare in the anterior chamber and when the area of edema in the graft moves across the cornea in the wake of an endothelial line (Khodadoust's rejection line) typically commencing at and moving away from a focus of vascularization in the vicinity of the graft'. It should be added that while the rejection line is essential for a positive diagnosis it is frequently not visible because the cornea is not seen until a late stage of the reaction when it has become obscured by corneal edema or by the debris of the destroyed endothelial cells. The reaction has been held resposible for the majority of failures in the less favorable categories of corneal disease such as the chemical injuries. Maumenee (1973) and Khodadoust (1973) hold that the immune reaction is the most frequent cause of graft failure when gross technical failures have been eliminated. There are on the other hand others (Elliott, 1971; Moore and Aronson, 1971) who feel that there is insufficient evidence for specific donor antigen sensitization in human keratoplasty and that the phenomena observed clinically can be explained equally well by a large group of antigens, microbial, chemical, suture material, etc. Any of these may cause an inflammatory reaction in the recipient with proliferation of mononuclear cells and damage to the endothelium of the graft.

HISTOCOMPATIBILITY

The role of the HL-A histocompatibility antigens in the human allograft reaction has as yet not been clarified. Given the remote likelihood of obtaining a good match of histocompatibility antigens in random donor selection, it is difficult to explain why the great majority of patients receiving corneal allografts do not show a rejection reaction and why the success rate is as high as it is. It has been difficult to demonstrate a direct correlation between HL-A incompatibility and the fate of the graft (Allansmith et al., 1974). Those who have urged such a correlation have in general found their supportive observations limited to grafts transplanted into heavily vascularized corneas of poor prognosis in which greater HL-A incompatibility appeared to be associated with a higher risk of rejection. The suggestion has been made that it is in this latter group of poor prognosis cases that prospective HL-A matching, with all its difficulties and complexities, might be most rewarding (Gibbs et al., 1973; Ehlers and Kissmeyer, 0000; Stark et al., 1973).

CORNEAL VASCULARIZATION

The absence of blood vessels in the cornea has been accepted as an important factor in its relative privilege as a site for an allograft. It has been well documented, however, that the allograft reaction does occur in corneas that are completely avascular (Fine and Stein, 1973). It has been suggested that in such cases the reaction is mediated across the anterior chamber. On the other hand not all heavily vascularized corneas reject an HL-A incompatible donor. For example in a study of corneas scarred by herpes simplex keratitis with moderate to severe stromal vascularization pre-operatively, 20 to 25% showed signs of the allograft reaction (Fine and Cignetti, 1977).

Another type of vascularization worthy of attention but often misinterpreted is early post-operative vascularization following keratoplasty. Many surgeons fear the spread of vessels through the peripheral cornea towards the graft as evidence of an impending rejection and have instituted intensive treatment with corticosteroids to suppress such vascularization. Many times this has resulted in poor wound healing and in certain instances in corneal melting. In the technique of graft fixation with multiple interrupted sutures in which the knots are not buried, whether the sutures are of fine silk or monofilament nylon, most cases will show vessels reaching the cicatrix if some sutures are left in places as long as ten weeks. This is true even in preoperatively avascular corneas but is particularly true in cases in which there has been vascularization of the cornea at some time in the past such as in cases of luetic interstitial keratitis of herpes simplex keratitis, even though no vessels containing blood are present at the time of the keratoplasty. The incidence of the allograft reaction has not, in my experience, been increased by the appearance of these vessels in the recipient cornea during the early post-operative period. Usually such vessels reach the line of union between donor and spread circumferentially in the cicatrix without entering the graft. It is only when the graft is already edematous, whether from an allograft reaction, from poor wound apposition, or from stitch infection that the vessels will invade the graft. In most cases the vessels entering the previously clear cornea will reach the cicatrix through a suture track and at this time the wound will be sufficiently firm so that the suture may be removed and the stimulus for the vascularization at that point is withdrawn. Usually topical instillation of drops containing 1% prednisilone or .1% dexamethasone together with an antibiotic, administered three times a day will be sufficient to suppress the inflammation accompanying this type of vascularization. In many instances where vessels reach the line of union from all quadrants it is possible to remove all the sutures as early as two to three weeks following keratoplasty, since the wound is already firm. Provided the graft is healthy, removal of the sutures will usually be followed by regression of the vessels. I have become so convinced of the innocuous nature of this neovascularization of the peripheral cornea following keratoplasty that in many cases with thin corneas, or other causes of poor cicatrization, I have encouraged the growth of vessels to the border of the graft in order to insure firm wound healing. In some situations in which there has been poor healing of the graft because of previous excessive irradiation it has been possible to obtain better healing and a clear graft by purposely placing the graft so that the border is at the vascular limbus. The allograft reaction has not seemed to be more frequent or more severe in such cases than in other cases of similar prognostic status.

REGRAFTS AND MULTIPLE GRAFTS

Another question related to graft rejection that is yet to be answered definitively is the matter of to what degree multiple grafting in the same eye or grafting to both eyes of the same patient influence a rejection reaction. It has for example been reported that even in the most favorable prognostic group of keratoconus cases a graft performed in the second eye increases greatly the possibility of the rejection reaction. Other observers have not been able to confirm this although most experienced corneal surgeons can cite isolated cases in which an allograft reaction in a second eye was follow-ed soon thereafter by an allograft reaction in the fellow eye, operated months previously.

In approximately 400 bilateral keratoplasties in cases of keratoconus and Fuchs' dystrophy I have observed this event only five times. A typical instance was a young woman age 19 who had a successful penetrating keratoplasty for keratoconus of the left eye in 1955. Four month later a similar keratoplasty was done in the right eye. Two months after this the recent graft became clouded by a typical allograft reaction in the avascular cornea. Treatment was begun with topical corticosteroids with a good response but two weeks later the graft of the left eye (which had had the original graft) became clouded by a similar graft reaction. Both eyes cleared completely with topical corticosteroid therapy and have remained clear for 23 years. This brings up the possibility, however remote, that the two donors to the same recipient shared common histocompatibility antigens to which the recipient had been sensitized.

As might be expected from the immunologic nature of the allograft reaction the frequency of the reaction tends to increase with successive grafts to the same eye. The over all incidence of the reaction in a series of twelve hundred successive primary grafts was 13% (follow up one year or longer). This series was heavily weighted with dystrophy cases (keratoconus 30%, Fuchs' dystrophy 15%) and these cases which are more uniform with fewer variables than traumatic or inflammatory cases were reviewed. The incidence of the allograft reaction in this dystrophy group is shown in Table I. The small number of preoperatively vascularized cases showed the

Table 1. Incidence of allograft reaction in primary grafts for dystrophies

	number	number with reaction	% with reaction
Avascular	583	60	10.2
Vascular	23	8	34.7

allograft reaction three times as frequently as the large group without vessels. When the same type of cases underwent regrafting the frequency of the reaction increased from 10.2% to 27.4% ($P < 0.01$) (Table 2).

Table 2. Incidence of allograft reaction in primary avascular grafts and avascular regrafts.

Dystrophy cases	number	number with reaction	% with reaction
Primary grafts	583	60	10.2
Regrafts	51	14	27.4

The outcome of the allograft reaction following treatment with local corti-costeroids was significantly poorer in regrafted cases than in primary grafts (Table 3).

Table 3. Outcome of allograft reaction in primary grafts and regrafts

Results	primary graft		regraft	
	no.	%	no.	%
Clear	79	60.3	16	43.2
Not clear	52	39.7	21	56.8

Table 4 summarizes the outcome of 137 regrafts performed over a five year period. There is an indication that in the good prognosis cases a regraft has almost as good a chance of remaining clear, in spite of the greater frequency of the allograft reaction.

Table 4. Results of corneal regrafts 1971–1976

	Diagnosis	number	no. clear	(%)
1.	Aphakic bullous keratopathy	42	32	(76%)
2.	Keratoconus	29	23	(79%)
3.	Fuchs' dystrophy	18	9	(50%)
4.	Herpes simplex	13	7	(54%)
5.	Chemical injury	11	2	(18%)
6.	Familial dystrophy	10	8	(80%)
7.	Interstitial keratitis	7	5	(71%)
8.	Mechanical injury	4	1	(25%)
9.	Others	3	1	(33%)
	total	137	88	(64%)

SUMMARY

Although confirmatory laboratory tests of the corneal allograft reaction are not available, a positive diagnosis of graft rejection may be made clinically. The specific antigens involved in the allograft reaction and the pathways of the reaction have not been firmly established. This does not, however, prevent the control of the reaction and the reversal of its effects if prompt and vigorous treatment with local corticosteroids is begun at the earliest sign of the reaction. At the present time selection of donors on the basis of HL-A compatibility does not appear to be promising.

REFERENCES

Allansmith, M.R., M. Fine & R. Payne. Histocompatability Typing and Corneal Transplantation. *Trans. Am. Acad. Ophthalmol. Otolaryngol.* 78: *445*, (1974).

Ehlers, N. & F. Kissmeyer-Nielsen. Influence of Histocompatibility on the Fate Of The Corneal Transplant. pp. 307 In Corneal Graft Failure, Ciba Foundation Symposium 15, Associated Scientific Publishers, Amsterdam, 1973.

Elliott, J.H. Immune FactorIn Corneal Graft Rejection. *Invest. Ophthalmol.* 10: *216*, (1971).

Fine, M. & F.E. Cignetti. Penetrating Keratoplasty in Herpes Simplex Keratitis. *Arch. Ophthalmol.* 95: *613*, (1977).

Fine, M. & M. Stein. The Role of Corneal Vascularization In Human Corneal Graft Reactions. pp. 193 In Corneal Graft Failure, Ciba Foundation Symposium 15, Associated Scientific Publishers, Amsterdam, 1973.

Gibbs, D.D., J.R. Batchelor & T.A. Casey. The Influence of HL-A Compatability on the Fate of Corneal Grafts in Corneal Graft Failure, Ciba Foundation 15 Associated Scientific Publishers Amsterdam, 1973.

Khodadoust, A.A. The Allograft Rejection Reaction: The Leading Cause Of Late Failure Of Clinical Corneal Grafts, in Corneal Graft Failure, Ciba Foundation Symposium 15. Associated Scientific Publishers, Amsterdam, 1973.

Maumenee, A.E. Clinical Patterns of Graft Failure in Corneal Graft Failure, Ciba Foundation Symposium 15. Associated Scientific Publishers, Amsterdam, 1973.

Moore, T.E., Jr. & S.B. Aronson. The Corneal Graft: A Multiple Variable Analysis Of The Penetrating Keratoplasty. *Am. J. Ophthalmol.* 72: *205*, (1971).

Stark, W.J., G. Opelz, D. Newsome et al. Sensitization to human lymphocyte antigens by corneal transplantation. *Invest. Ophthalmol.* 12: *639*, (1973).

Author's address:
Max Fine, M.D.
2233 Post Street
San Francisco, CA 94115 U.S.A.

THE FATE OF CORNEAL REGRAFTS
AFTER PREVIOUS REJECTION REACTIONS

ALI A. KHODADOUST AND ABBAS ABIZADEH

(Shiraz, Iran)

The prognosis for a clear corneal regraft is usually considered hopeless. However, it is not clear whether it is a poor recipient bed, technical difficulties, or the immune reaction which is the most important determining factor in the outcome of these grafts.

The clinico-pathological patterns of the allograft rejection reaction in each of the three cellular layers of cornea with experimental corneal transplantations have been defined under a variety of conditions (Khodadoust and Silverstein, 1969 and 1972). These observations enabled us to make a definite clinical diagnosis of the allograft rejection reaction. The incidence of rejection could be correlated to the degree of host corneal vascularization; once the host is sensitized, practically all vascularized grafts succumb to the rejection process.

Subsequent observations on a clinical series of penetrating grafts showed specific patterns of rejection reaction similar to those of experimental animals (Khodadoust, 1973). The incidence of rejection could also be correlated to the degree of host corneal vascularization.

To evaluate the role of previous sensitization in the fate of clinical corneal regrafts, we have selected a series of regraft patients in whom the previous graft had failed, specifically because of allograft rejection reaction. The purpose of this communication is to report the results of follow-up observations on the fate of these regrafts in terms of incidence and clinical picture of the rejection reaction.

PATIENTS AND METHODS

The records of all 63 regrafts done on 45 patients at the Department of Ophthalmology, Pahlavi University, Shiraz, Iran, between 1975–1977, were reviewed. Excluding the non-immunologic causes of previous graft failures, we selected 50 regrafts done in 32 patients in whom conclusive clinical diagnosis of allograft rejection reaction had been made as the principal cause of previous graft failure.

Most of the initial transplants and all of the regrafts were done by the same surgeon, at the same department, and with the same technique. The source of donor material and technique of anesthesia and surgery were identical to those reported earlier (Khodadoust, 1973). The size of the regraft was almost always the same as the initial transplant.

Of 50 regrafts done in 32 patients, there were 32 instances of second graft, 15 instances of third graft, and 3 instances of fourth graft. The indications for the initial surgery, in order of frequency, were: quiet corneal scar (of smallpox, trauma, or trachoma) 46.8%; recurrent herpetic keratitis 25%; keratoconus 12.5%; infected ulcers and keratitis 12.5%; and chemical burns 3.2%.

The indication for regrafts in this selected series was corneal graft failure due to specific allograft rejection reaction. The age of patients ranged from 17 to 80 years. There were 24 males and 8 females. Two of the patients were aphakic, and in 4 other cases the second graft was combined with uneventful intracapsular cataract extraction. The donor epithelium was removed mechanically in all cases before transplantation.

No systemic immunosuppressive agents were used prior to regrafts. Systemic corticosteroid (60–80 mg prednisolone in divided doses every other day was used in all cases with second or third grafts from the second postoperative day, and then tapered off as soon as all reaction in the anterior chamber and limbal congestion had disappeared. Topical steroid (Dexamethason) with antibiotic was started 6 times a day one week postoperatively and tapered off to one drop at bedtime 4–5 weeks later.

Sutures were removed 6 weeks to 6 months or more after surgery, depending on the loosening of suture loops.

RESULTS

All the recipient corneas were moderately to severely vascularized. To evaluate the prognostic significance of previous sensitization in allograft rejection reaction, we will separate the results of this study into three groups: second, third, and fourth graft.

1. The second graft. This group included 32 eyes of 32 patients. The time interval between initial graft and rejection ranged from 4 weeks to 6 years, and the time interval between rejection of the first graft and the second transplant ranged from 2 weeks to 18 months. This depended on the severity of the allograft rejection reaction and the condition of the patient's second eye. In severe rejection reactions leading to necrosis, descemetocele, or impending perforation, regrafting had to be done earlier, whereas in endothelial rejection reaction alone, with a useful working second eye, we generally postponed the regraft for a period of 6 months or more. This approach was based on our unpublished observations on several cases in which the host endothelium had regenerated after endothelial rejection and the graft had regained its transparency within 6–8 months.

During the average follow-up of one year, 21 of these 32 regrafts succumbed to the allograft rejection reaction. In these, the time interval between transplantation and rejection ranged from 2 weeks to 2 years. Eleven grafts remained clear during the same period of time.

The clinical pattern of the rejection reaction in the majority of cases was similar to that described earlier in primary graft rejection reaction. However, they seemed to have a more rapid course as compared to the first graft

116

rejection. In some instances, with early onset of the rejection process the reaction had a fulminating course. There was rapid onset of intense keratic precipitate all over the graft endothelium, followed by folds in Descemet's membrane and diffuse edema of the graft. Heavy cellular infiltration of stroma, mimicking the clinical picture of corneal abscess, was followed by necrosis, descemetocele, and perforation. In none of these fulminating cases could the course of the rejection process be altered or stopped with a combination of systematic, subconjunctival, and topical corticosteroid therapy.

In 6 of the 21 cases with milder allograft rejection reactions, the process could be stopped by steroid therapy. In the other 15 cases, either the patient appeared too late, or steroid therapy failed to control the process. These cases had to be regrafted.

2. The third graft. In this group there were 15 eyes of 15 patients. The time interval between rejection of the second and the third graft ranged from 10 days to 2 years, with an average of 4 months.

During an average follow-up of 9 months, 12 of these 15 grafts succumbed to an allograft rejection reaction and 3 grafts remained clear. The time interval between transplantation and rejection ranged from 4 days to 12 months, with an average of 2 months.

The pattern of the rejection process was similar to that of the second graft rejection. In 2 instances, there was rapid loss of endothelial cells with minimum cell infiltration on the 4th to 5th postoperative day. This was associated with failure in wound healing and necrosis of the graft. Both eyes became phthisical after conjunctival flap procedures. In only one case could the process of rejection reaction be stopped with systemic and topical corticosteroid therapy; this graft remained clear during the 4 months of follow-up. In the other 3 cases, the eyes were regrafted for the fourth time.

3. The fourth graft. In this group there were three eyes of three patients, one eye aphakic and theother two phakic. The time intervals between rejection of the third graft and retransplantation were 1, 3, and 12 months. In the first case, the graft rejected 10 days after operation. The other two cases were maintained on systemic steroids and cytoxan starting on days 2 and 3 postoperatively, and both grafts were clear 5 months and 1 year after surgery.

DISCUSSION

This communication presents the results of a study to determine the effect on subsequent regrafts of host sensitization to transplantation antigens during the course of earlier rejection of corneal grafts. While neither the donors nor recipients were tissue-typed to determine histoincompatibility relationships, the chance occurrence of a given antigen on a regraft corneal button, against which the host had become sensitized during the course of an earlier rejection reaction, might put the new graft at greater risk of rejection. An earlier study (Khodadoust, 1973) established the precise incidence of the allograft rejection reaction in a large series of grafts with different degrees of vascularization. Thus, a study of the incidence of rejection of corneal regrafts performed with the same technique and by the same surgeon offers the opportunity of assessing the effect of prior rejection processes on the success of regraft procedures.

The following evidence suggests that prior sensitization to the histocompatibility antigens of even unrelated corneal donors markedly influences the incidence and pattern of subsequent corneal graft rejection reactions:

1. Whereas the rate of allograft rejection reactions in comparably vascularized recipient beds is estimated at less than 50% following a first graft, specific rejection occurs in 68% of all second grafts and in 80% of third grafts. Not enough fourth grafts were done to provide statistically significant data.

2. Once the rejection process has started in the regraft, the reaction proceeds more rapidly as compared with the rejection of first grafts.

3. The time of onset of the rejection reaction in regrafts occurs earlier than in initial grafts, so that onset of rejection was seen in some instances within a week to 10 days after operation in the regraft as compared with a minimum interval of three weeks in initial grafts.

4. Specific graft rejection in regrafts had more of a tendency to follow a fulminating course than was true in initial grafts.

In addition to the above, there is yet another hint that sensitization against the tissues of one donor may lead to the rejection of the tissues of a second donor. Among a group of patients with unrelated bilateral corneal grafts, we have on our records two patients who had clear corneal grafts in one eye for 4—5 years, at which time the second eye received a corneal graft from an unrelated donor. A few days after the initiation of rejection in the recently grafted second eye, the originally successful grafts succumbed to severe allograft rejection reactions, although in both instances there was only mild to moderate vascularization present. In neither case could the rejection process be altered by steroid therapy.

These observations suggest that one or more of the antigenic constituents of one donor may be shared by the tissues of another donor, but not by the recipient, so that sensitization against the antigens of one graft may put the second at greater risk of rejection. While we do not have a clear statistical evaluation of the probability of such antigen-sharing, rough approximations such as are outlined in Table 1 support the assumption that prior exposure to and sensitization by histocompatibility antigens put a graft recipient at greater risk for rejection. This is, of course, the same reason that a history of blood transfusions is important for kidney and other organ transplant recipients.

It is possible, of course, that the phenomenon that we have described above is unrelated to histocompatibility antigen cross-reactions, but rather may be ascribed to increasing deterioration of the quality of the recipient graft bed which might accompany each subsequent rejection process. While this cannot be ruled out absolutely, it is our clinical impression, based upon a very large series of observations on recipient eyes in all extremes of vascularization and other damage, that the regraft eyes in the study did not differ appreciably on average from those receiving inital grafts.

We are not aware of similar reports in the literature on the outcome of

Table 1. Approximations of histoincompatibility probabilities

Given that there are 20 alleles at locus A:

The *average* probability of having any given allele = .05 + .05 = .1
The *average* probability of having any given 2 alleles = $(.05)^2$ = .0025
The *average* probability of a second person having either of the 2 given alleles = $(.1 + .1)-(.005)^2$ = .1975

Given that there are 30 alleles at locus B:

The *average* probability of having any given allele = .033 + .033 = .066
The *average* probability of having any given 2 alleles = $(.033)^2$ = .0011
The *average* probability of a second person having either of the 2 given B locus alleles = $(.066 + .066)-(.033)^2$ = .131

The HLA−B 5 cross-reacting group occurs in 70% of the Iranian population.

The probability of a corneal recipient being negative for B5 Creg = .30
The probability of incompatibility = $(.3 \times .7)$ = .21
The probability of a negative recipient and 2 positive donors = $(.3 \times .7^2)$ = .147

The *average* probability of 2 persons sharing any A or B = $(.1975 + .131)-(.1975 \times .131)$ = .3026
The *average* probability that a recipient shares no antigen with 2 donors who share one or more antigens with each other = $.3026 (1 - .3026)^2$ = .1476

corneal regrafts in a group of patients who had previously rejected their corneal graft. The largest series of regrafts described were reported by Cowden and coworkers (1974). In their series of 51 regrafts, they reported they reported 64% clear grafts, but all of their cases were in aphakic eyes. These workers did not mention the degree of vascularization at the time of grafting, nor was it clear what proportion of their patients had lost their original graft due to specific allograft rejection reactions.

The response of the rejection process to steroid therapy was quite variable in the present group of patients. Because of the rapid course of the rejection process in the majority of cases, by the time they were referred to the clinic there was often complete loss of endothelial cells, and steroids could not reverse the process. However, clinical observations on those cases referred at early stages of rejection suggested that this group is generally more resistant to steroid therapy than was our experience with initial grafts.

In the patients with a fourth graft, one succumbed to the rejection process while on steroids, although the other two patients maintained clear grafts on a combination of steroids and cytoxan. Although the number of such patients is small and no solid conclusion can be drawn, this observation would seem to justify the use of such immunosuppressive agents for grafts in heavily vascularized corneas or for regrafts with a specially poor prognosis, as has been advocated by others (Polack, 1965; Leibowits and Elliott, 1966; D'Amico and Castroviejo, 1969; Hughes and Kallmeyer, 1967).

CONCLUSION

We do not recommend bilateral corneal grafts in patients in whom one or both corneas are vascularized, due to the high incidence of allograft rejection reaction in patients with highly vascularized corneal beds. In such cases, appropriate selection of suitable donors by tissue-typing would appear to be strongly indicated.

REFERENCES

Cowden, J., H.E. Kaufman & F.M. Polack. The prognosis of keratoplasty after previous graft failures. *Am. J. Ophthal.* 78: *523*, (1974).

D'Amico, R.A. & R. Castroviejo. Suppression of the immune response in keratoplasty. *Am. J. Ophthal.* 68: *829*, (1969).

Hughes, W.F. & J. Kallmeyer. Etiology and treatment of the corneal homograft reaction including azathioprine (Imuran). *S. Afr. Med. J.* 41: *548*, (1967).

Khodadoust, A.A. The allograft rejection reaction: the leading cause of late failure of clinical corneal grafts. *In* Corneal Graft Failure. A Ciba Foundation Symposium. Elsevier, Amsterdam. 151, (1973).

Khodadoust, A.A. & A.M. Silverstein. Transplantation and rejection of individual cell layers of the cornea. *Invest. Ophthal.* 8: *180*, (1969).

Khodadoust, A.A. & A.M. Silverstein. The survival and rejection of epithelium in experimental corneal transplants. *Invest. Ophthal.* 8: *169*, (1969).

Khodadoust, A.A. & A.M. Silverstein. Studies on the nature of the privilege enjoyed by corneal allografts. *Invest. Ophthal.* 11: *137*, (1972).

Leibowitz, H.M. & J.H. Elliott. Chemotherapeuric immunosuppression of the corneal graft reaction. I. Systemic antimetabolotes. *Arch. Ophthal.* 75: *826*, (1966).

Polack, F.M. Inhibition of immune corneal graft rejection by azathioprine (Imuran). *Arch. Ophthal.* 74: *683*, (1965).

Author's address:
Department of Ophthalmology
Pahlavi University Medical School
Shiraz
Iran.

KERATOPLASTY AND TRANSPLANTATION ANTIGENS*

WALTER J. STARK, HUGH R. TAYLOR, AND WILMA B. BIAS

(Baltimore, Maryland, U.S.A.)

INTRODUCTION

When the recipient corneal bed is avascular, allograft rejection occurs in about 10% of keratoplasty cases (Khodadoust, 1973; Stark *et al.*, 1972; Chandler and Kaufman, 1974). If the preoperative recipient cornea is heavily vascularized, however, the incidence of immunogenic graft failure can range as high as 65% of cases (Khodadoust, 1973; Batchelor *et al.*, 1976).

In cases of allograft rejection after keratoplasty, the precise role of donor-recipient histocompatibility (HLA) antigens is not fully known. Some authors have found a significant correlation between the number of matching donor and recipient HLA antigens and the graft results in high-risk cases of vascularized corneas (Batchelor *et al.*, 1976; Vannas *et al.*, 1976), but other studies have not shown a similar correlation (Allansmith *et al.*, 1974).

The HLA antigen system is the major transplantation antigen system in man as demonstrated by analysis of familial renal transplantation results (Opelz *et al.*, 1977; Mickey *et al.*, 1971). Due to the complexity of the HLA antigen system, the probability for complete matching of donor and recipient antigens for unrelated, cadaver transplants is low. In renal transplantation, preimmunization of the recipient to HLA antigens of the donor increases the risk of rejection (Terasaki *et al.*, 1971; Opelz and Terasaki, 1971; Opelz *et al.*, 1973; Opelz *et al.*, 1972; Terasaki *et al.*, 1968). However, for keratoplasty, the effect of recipient preimmunization has not been fully evaluated.

It is known that patients can become immunized and develop lympho-cytotoxic antibodies by exposure to foreign HLA antigens from previous transplants, including corneal transplants as we have reported (Stark *et al.*, 1973), blood transfusions (Opelz and Terasaki, 1971), or pregnancy (Dausset, 1954). Preimmunization of the recipient to antigens of the donor may be detected by preoperative cross-match testing between the recipient's serum and the donor's lymphocytes (Terasaki *et al.*, 1968; Kissmeyer-Nielsen *et al.*, 1966).

* This work was supported in part by the National Eye Institute, Bethesda, Maryland, Grant EY01302

The purpose of this paper is to present our results of penetrating kerato-plasty in 84 potentially preimmunized recipients with severe preoperative corneal vascularization. The donor corneas that were used for these cases were selected on the basis of obtaining a negative donor-recipient cross-match test before surgery. No attempt was made to match donor and recipient HLA antigens specifically.

MATERIALS AND METHODS

Eighty-four penetrating keratoplasties were performed between November 1973 and November 1977. Patients selected for this study had significant vascularization of the corneal stroma in at least three quadrants, extending into the visual axis. Of the 84 patients studied, 64 (76%) had previously had at least one corneal transplant failure in that same eye. These 64 patients had an average of 1.9 previous graft failures, with a range of from 1 to 6 previous graft failures in that eye. The remaining 20 patients had previously been exposed to foreign HLA antigens by keratoplasty in the other eye or by blood transfusion or pregnancy. Of the 84 patients 50 were female and 34 were male. The age of recipients ranged from 13 years to 80 years (mean, 60 years). The original diagnosis before the first graft in the study eyes was as follows: vascularized corneal scars, 31 eyes; corneal edema, 17 eyes; corneal dystrophies, 10 eyes; alkali burns, 8 eyes; and vascularized corneas of unknown etiology, 14 eyes.

Preoperatively, sera from all waiting keratoplasty patients were cross-matched individually against lymphocytes of all the potential corneal donors. A specific donor cornea for an individual recipient was selected on the basis of a negative cross-match reaction with the donor's lymphocytes. If a positive cross-match was obtained, the cornea was not used for that recipient, because a positive cross-match indicates that the recipient has antibodies that are specific for one or more antigens of that donor. In addition, HLA typing of both donor and recipient was obtained but no attempt was made to match donor and recipient antigens specifically.

Donor material for these 84 cases was stored in McCarey-Kaufman medium (McCarey and Kaufman, 1974) until used for keratoplasty. Surgery was performed within 60 hours of the donor's death. All grafts were sutured with 10−0 monofilament nylon suture (Stark et al., 1972). Of the 84 grafts, 70 were 7.5 mm in diameter, 10 were 8.0 mm in diameter, and 4 were 7.0 mm in diameter. Forty-four grafts were performed on phakic eyes and 19 of these were combined with lens removal. The remaining 40 grafts were performed on aphakic eyes.

The diagnosis of immune graft rejection was made only if the graft remained clear for at least 2 weeks after surgery and then developed edema or clouding associated with keratic precipitates on the graft endothelium or a rejection line. Non-immune causes of graft failure included grafts that clouded within 2 weeks of surgery or graft clouding associated with infection, trauma, glaucoma or persistent epithelial defects with exposure keratitis.

124

NUMBER OF PATIENTS				
Total	Allograft Rejection	Non-Immune Graft Failure	Total Clear	Mean Follow-up (Range-Months)
84	13(15%)	6(7%)	65(77%)	14.3(3—45)

Table 1. Outcome of keratoplasty, potentially pre-immunized recipients with dense corneal vascularization. Negative donor-recipient cross-match.

RESULTS
Negative Donor-Recipient Cross-Match Pairs

Postoperatively 65 of the 84 corneal grafts (77%) are clear, with an average follow-up of 14.3 months (range 3 to 45 months). Fifteen percent of the grafts (13 of 84) have failed by immune allograft rejection, and 7% have failed from causes other than rejection (Table 1). Ninety-two percent of grafts failures from rejection (12 of 13) occurred within 6 months of surgery, with the average time for occurrence of rejection being 3.6 months. Twenty-two of the 84 patients (26%) had evidence of an immune event, either rejection or a reversible allograft reaction. Nine of the 22 immune events (41%) could be reversed with corticosteroids, and 13 (59%) of the cases progressed to graft clouding (Table 2).

Total Number of Grafts	Total Number of Immune Events (Rejection or Reaction)	Allograft Reaction (Graft Clear)	Percentage Reversed
84	22(26%)	9	41%

Table 2. Immune reactions in potentially pre-immunized recipients with dense corneal vascularization.

In these 84 keratoplasty cases with dense corneal vascularization, our incidence of graft rejection, which was 15%, is less than that reported in similar high-risk cases. Khodadoust (1973) has reported graft failure from rejection in 65% of cases with dense corneal vascularization, and Batchelor and co-workers (1976) reported 60% of such cases with graft failure from rejection. Although there may have been differences between their series and ours in factors such as the quality of donor material, or patient follow-up availability, these factors are unlikely to account for all of the large

125

Number of HLA Antigens Matched	Number of Patients	Allograft Rejection	Nonimmune Graft Failure	Clear Graft
0	51	7(14%)	5(10%)	39(76%)
1	35	6(17%)	1(3%)	28(80%)
2	11	0	0	11(100%)
3	5	2(40%)	0	3(60%)
4	1	0	0	1(100%)
TOTAL	103	15(15%)	6(6%)	82(80%)

Table 3. Donor-recipient HLA antigen matches and graft outcome.

difference in incidence of rejection failures between those series and ours. A major cause of the lower incidence of rejection in our series is probably our use of negatively cross-matched donor material. These findings for kerato-plasty are in agreement with the results in other tissue and organ trans-plantation systems (Terasaki *et al.*, 1968; Kissmeyer-Nielsen *et al.*, 1966).

Retrospective Donor-Recipient HLA Antigen Matching

The donor and recipient HLA typing results were known for the 84 cases that received negative cross-matched grafts. There were 19 additional cases for whom the donor and recipient HLA types were known. These additional cases likewise had dense corneal vascularization but the cross-match test had not been performed. The donor-recipient HLA antigen matching was analyzed retrospectively for these 103 cases.

The occurrence of graft rejection was compared with the number of matching donor and recipient antigens as shown in Table 3. When the donor and recipient shared no matching antigens, rejection failures occurred in 14% of the cases (7 of 51). When one matching antigen was shared, rejection developed in 18% of cases (6 of 34). In 11 cases in which the donor and recipient shared two matching antigens, we had no graft failures from rejection. However, rejection accounted for failure in 2 of 5 cases (40%) in which three matching antigens were shared. We have only one case in which the donor and recipient shared four matching antigens, and this graft is clear.

Thus, the incidence of graft failure from rejection does not correlate clearly and consistently with the number of matching HLA antigens shared between the donor and recipient. Also, the incidence of immune events and the reversibility of allograft reaction did not appear to correlate with the number of antigens shared (Table 4).

126

Number of HLA Antigens Matched	Number of Patients	Total Number of Immune Events (Reaction or Rejection)	Allograft Reaction (Graft Clear)	Percent Reversed
0	51	14(27%)	7	50%
1	35	9(26%)	3	33%
2	11	1(9%)	1	100%
3	5	2(40%)	0	0
4	1	0	0	–
TOTAL	103	26(25%)	11	42%

Table 4. Donor-recipient HLA antigen match and graft outcome.

Batchelor and co-workers (1976) have the largest series published to date regarding donor-recipient HLA antigen matching and the graft outcome. In 73 keratoplasty recipients with dense corneal vascularization, they showed a reduction in graft failure from rejection as the donor and recipients shared increasingly more matched antigens. Our work does not confirm this in similar high-risk cases (Fig. 1). However, the majority of our cases received

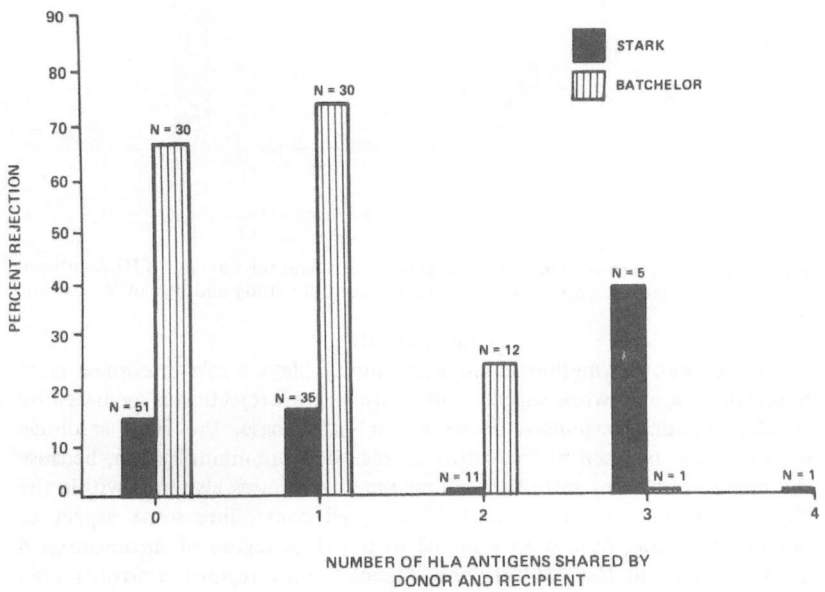

Fig. 1. The incidence of rejection after keratoplasty in recipients who have shared zero, one, two, three or four HLA antigens with their donor. Comparison between this study and that of Batchelor and co-workers.

corneas from negatively cross-matched donors. Batchelor did not report having used cross-match testing for donor selection, although the probability of negative cross-matches will obviously be higher with donor-recipient pairs that are well-matched for specific antigens. Vannas and co-workers (1976) prospectively matched donor and recipient antigens and obtained a negative donor-recipient cross-match test in 18 keratoplasty cases with all degrees of corneal vascularization. Their cases showed a lower incidence of rejection as the number of matched donor-recipient antigens increases (Fig. 2). However, Vannas and co-workers' series included cases with any degree of corneal vascularization, and their recipients may not have had as high a risk of graft rejection as those included in our series and those reported by Batchelor and co-workers (1976).

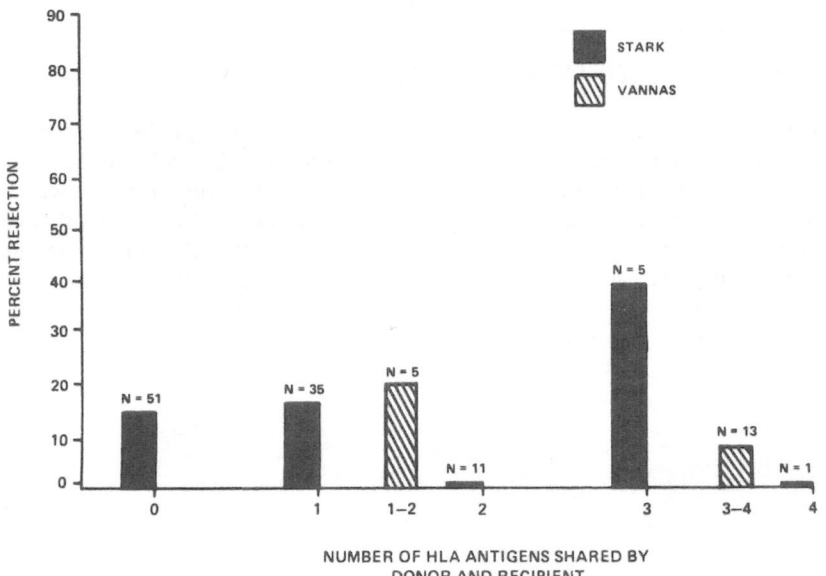

Fig. 2. The incidence of rejection after keratoplasty and the number of HLA antigens shared by recipient and donor. Comparison between this study and that of Vannas and co-workers.

DISCUSSION

It is not known whether humoral immunity plays a role in corneal graft rejection. Previous work suggests that corneal graft rejection is mediated by cellular immune responses. However, in either case, the HLA serologic reactions can be used as indicators of recipient preimmunization, because the major gene loci controlling cell-mediated responses also map within the HLA complex. Thus far, about 10 loci, all controlling some aspect of immune function, have been assigned to the HLA region of chromosome 6 in man (Bias and Hsu, 1977). The D locus (or sub-region) controls mixed lymphocyte responsiveness, and is an in-vitro indicator of cellular immune responsiveness. The entire HLA complex occupies a very small segment of the chromosomal length, allowing one to characterize a given haplotype (the gene complex on one chromosome of the pair) by the serologic specificities it contains.

Our results show a lower incidence of corneal graft failure from rejection when cross-match testing was used for donor selection than did other series involving similar high-risk cases with dense corneal vascularization (Khodadoust, 1973; Batchelor *et al.*, 1976). We conclude that this difference is due primarily to our use of preoperative donor-recipient cross-match testing as a means for donor selection. By so doing, we are able to avoid giving a donor cornea to a recipient who happens to be presensitized to that cornea's antigens (Newsome *et al.*, 1974).

Although we found no consistent correlation between the number of matching HLA antigens shared between the donor and recipient and graft outcome, the role of antigen matching may still deserve further evaluation. However, if further attempts at donor-recipient HLA antigen matching are to be made they must be combined with preoperative cross-match testing, because even if all but one of the known donor-recipient antigens are favorably matched, the recipient still might be preimmunized to the one unmatched donor antigen, or perhaps to donor HLA antigens that are not yet known. Although perfect donor-recipient HLA matching for corneal transplantation may be beneficial, it is not at this time practical because of the complexity of the HLA system (WHO Committee, 1978). Our study, however, demonstrates that the use of cross-matching to avoid donors with transplantation antigens to which the recipient is immunized is feasible and apparently beneficial.

We therefore propose that all potential corneal transplant recipients with vascularized corneal beds be screened for lymphocytotoxic antibodies when there is a history of exposure to foreign HLA antigens through pregnancy, blood transfusion, or previous corneal transplant. Preoperative cross-match testing should be performed to avoid using a cornea from a donor that has any of the same HLA antigens to which the recipient may have been preimmunized. Our preliminary data indicate that, by following these principles and methods, graft prognosis in high-risk keratoplasty cases can be significantly improved.

SUMMARY

The outcome of keratoplasty in 84 high-risk cases is presented. All cases had densely vascularized corneas and a history of prior exposure to HLA antigens by pregnancy, blood transfusion, or previous transplantation. Donors were selected on the basis of a negative cross-match to avoid donor antigens to which the recipient was preimmunized. The overall rate of graft failure from rejection was 15%. A retrospective analysis of donor-recipient HLA matching in 103 high-risk cases showed no consistent correlation between the number of antigens shared and graft outcome. These findings would indicate that a negative cross-match is of prime importance in donor selection for keratoplasty in high-risk cases.

129

REFERENCES

Allansmith, M.R. M. Fine & R. Payne. Histocompatibility typing and corneal transplantation. *Tr. Am. Acad. Ophthalmol. Otolaryngol.* 78: *445*, (1974).

Batchelor, J.R., T.A. Casey, D.C. Gibbs, D.F. Lloyd, A. Werb, S.S. Prasad & A. James. HLA matching and corneal grafting. *Lancet* 1: *551*, (1976).

Bias, W.B. & S.H. Hsu. HLA, the major histocompatibility system in man: An overview. *Acta Anthropogenetica* 1: *15*, (1977).

Chandler, J.W. & H.E. Kaufman. Graft reactions after keratoplasty for keratoconus. *Am. J. Ophthalmol.* 77: *543*, (1974).

Dausset, J. Leuco-agglutinins. IV. Leuco-agglutinins and blood transfusion. *Vox Sang.* 4: *190*, (1954).

Khodadoust, A.A. The allograft rejection reaction: the leading cause of late failure of clinical corneal grafts. In: Corneal Graft Failure, Ciba Foundation Symposium, Elsevier, Amsterdam, 1973, p. 151.

Kissmeyer-Nielsen, F., S. Olsen, V. Posborg-Petersen & O. Fjeldborg. Hyperacute rejection of kidney allografts associated with pre-existing humoral antibodies against donor cells. *Lancet* 2: *662*, (1966).

McCarey, B.E. & H.E. Kaufman. Improved corneal storage. *Invest. Ophth.* 13: *165*, (1974).

Mickey, R.M., M. Kreisler, E.D. Albert, N.,Tanaka & P.I. Terasaki. Analysis of HL-A incompatibility in human renal transplants. *Tissue Antigens* 2: *57*, (1971).

Newsome, D.A., M. Takasugi, K.R. Kenyon, W.J. Stark & G. Opelz. Human corneal cells in vitro: morphology and histocompatibility (HL-A) antigens of pure cell populations. *Invest. Ophth.* 13: *23*, (1974).

Opelz, G., R.M. Mickey & P.I. Terasaki. Identification of unresponsive kidney-transplant recipients. *Lancet* 1: *868*, (1972).

Opelz, G., M.R. Mickey & P.I. Terasaki. Calculations on long-term graft and patient survival in human kidney transplantation. *Transpl. Proc.* 9: *27*, (1977).

Opelz, G., D.P.S. Sengar, R.M. Mickey & P.I. Terasaki. Effect of blood transfusions on subsequent kidney transplants. *Transpl. Proc.* 5: *253*, (1973).

Opelz, G. & P.I. Terasaki. Histocompatibility matching utilizing responsiveness as a new dimension. *Transpl. Proc.* 4: *433*, (1971).

Polack, F.M. & C.E. Gonzales. The response of the lymphoid tissue to corneal heterografts. *Arch. Ophthalmol.* 80: *321*, (1968).

Stark, W.J., G. Opelz, D. Newsome, R. Brown, R. Yankee & P.I. Terasaki. Sensitization to human lymphocyte antigens by corneal transplantation. *Invest. Ophthal.* 12: *639*, (1973).

Stark, W.J. D. Paton, A.E. Maumenee & P.E. Michelson. The results of 102 penetrating keratoplasties using 10-0 monofilament nylon suture. *Ophth. Surg.* 3: *11*, (1972).

Terasaki, P.I., M. Kreisler & R.M. Mickey. Presensitization and kidney transplant failures. *Postgrad. Med. J.* 47: *89*, (1971).

Terasaki, P.I., D.L. Thrasher & T.H. Hauber. Serotyping for homotransplantation. XIII. Immediate kidney transplant rejection and associated antibodies. In Advance in Transplantation. Edited by J. Dausset, J. Hamburger, G. Mathe. Baltimore, Williams and Wilkins, 1968, p. 225.

Vannas, S., K. Karjalainen, P. Ruusuvaara & A. Tiilikainen. HLA-compatible donor cornea for prevention of allograft reaction. *Graefe Arch. Ophthal.* 198: *217*, (1976).

World Health Organization Committee: Nomenclature for factors of the HLA system 1977. *Tissue Antigens* 11: *81*, (1978).

Author's address:
The Wilmer Institute
The Johns Hopkins Hospital
600 N. Wolfe St.
Baltimore, Maryland 21205
U.S.A.

HLA – B 12 AND HLA – B 27 ANTIGENS AND SUSCEPTIBILITY TO THE CORNEAL ALLOGRAFT REACTION

SALME VANNAS, ANJA TIILIKAINEN, ANTTI VANNAS
AND KARI KARJALAINEN

(Helsinki, Finland)

INTRODUCTION

In our earlier series of patients with avascular keratoconus the risk of a corneal allograft reaction (AR) appeared to be highest among recipients bearing histocompatibility antigens HLA-B 12 and/or HLA-B 27 (Vannas *et al.*, 1977). This led us to the working hypothesis that recipients bearing these antigens are generally susceptible to factors or agents promoting AR. In the present investigation we have tested this hypothesis further, paying special attention to the significance of vascularization of the corneal bed.

PATIENTS AND METHODS

Our corneal graft recipients included 36 with HLA-B 12 and/or B 27 antigen. For each of these subjects the two nearest control recipients were chosen. In the control groups 8 patients had received the antigen HLA-B 12 or B 27 in the graft, and they were excluded. Thus the whole series comprised 100 grafts. Corrosive eye injuries were not included in this study. The corneal lesions that led to transplantation are listed in Table 1.

Table 1. Recipient series

Diagnosis	Number of cases
Keratoconus	52
Fuchs' combined dystrophy	5
Salzmann's nodular dystrophy	3
Other dystrophies	5
Phlyctenular keratitis	7
Parenchymatous keratitis	8
Herpetic keratitis	7
Other inflammations	3
Injuries	5
Regraftings	2
Others	3
Total	100

Forty-three of the recipient corneal beds were vascularized. In each case corneal vessels were documented by fluorescein angiography, but the corneas were not grouped according to the extent of vascularization.

The ages of the patients ranged from 6 to 81, with a mean of 41.8 years; 58 patients were male. The observation period varied from 4 months to 8 years and was equal in both groups. In all recipients and, whenever possible, in donors HLA histocompatibility antigens were determined by the lymphocytotoxicity test with a panel of well-defined antisera (Amos *et al.*). Cross-match tests were made, too. The best possible donor was selected for each patient, considering A and B loci as well as ABO blood groups. If there were only 0–1 foreign antigens the graft was regarded as well-matched.

Possibilities for obtaining compatible grafts were greatly improved by corneal cryopreservation (Capella *et al.*, 1965), started at our clinic in 1973,

Table 2. Type of grafts

Cryopreservation	53
M-K medium time storage	16
Fresh or moist chamber	31
	100

and M-K medium time storage (McCarey and Kaufman, 1974), introduced in 1975. Our corneal graft material (Table 2) included 53 cryopreserved corneas. The longest preservation time was more than 3 1/2 years, and the graft still had a regular endothelium (Fig. 1). Photograph taken after keratoplasty.

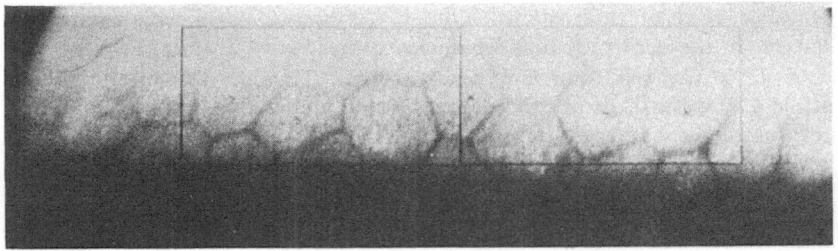

Fig. 1. Specular micrograph of the endothelium of the graft. Before the transplantation this graft was cryopreserved over 3 yrs. Endothelial cell density 1 yr. postoperatively was 1 475 mm^2. Magn. x 100.

Operative technique

The grafts vary in diameter from 7–8 mm. They were mostly sutured with a 10–0 monofilament, either with interrupted stitches or with a running suture. In the earliest patients the suture material was 9–0 virgin silk. Single stitches were removed after 4 to 6 weeks and running sutures after 6 to 8 months.

Postoperatively the patients were given corticosteroids both locally and also orally in a low dosage. In highly vascular cases immunosuppressive therapy (Imurel) was given, too.

AR occurred in 14 of the 100 patients at intervals ranging from 4 weeks to 4 years after the operation (Fig. 2).

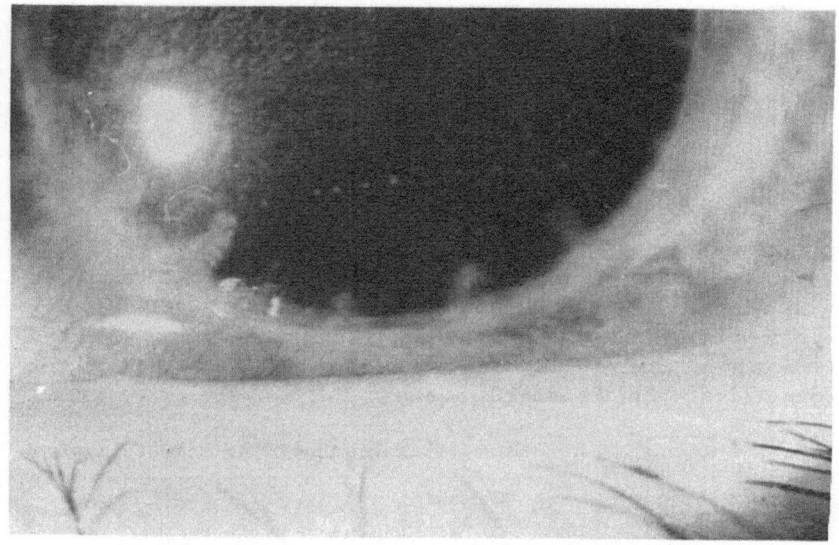

Fig. 2. Allograft reaction with characteristic Khodadoust line 14 months after the transplantation was triggered by a common cold infection. HLA-typing of the recipient: Aw 19, A 28, B 12 and of the graft: Aw 19, A 10, Bw 40, B 18.

Table 3. Frequency of AR in the HLA-B 12/B 27 group in relation to histoincompatibility matches

No. of HLA mismatches	HLA-B 12/B 27 series			Control series		
	No. of cases	AR + No.	%	No. of cases	AR + No.	%
0 ⎫ 1 ⎭	12	0	0	31	1*	3
2	12	5	42	16	0	0
3 ⎫ 4 ⎭	6	4	67	3	0	0
Not known	6	4	67	14	0	0
Totals	36	13	36	64	1	2

* had vascularized cornea and broad anterior synechia

RESULTS

Frequency of AR in HLA-B 12/B 27 carriers and controls

In our HLA-B 12/B 27 group (Table 3) AR developed in 13 of the 36 patients (36%), as compared with 1 of the 64 patients of the control group

(2%). The difference is statistically highly significant.

In the HLA-B 12/B 27 group the frequency of AR increased in parallel with the histoincompatibility; of the 6 patients with untyped grafts 4 developed AR. By contrast, among the controls only one patient developed AR; in this patient histoincompatibility could not be demonstrated. Interestingly, of the 14 controls with untyped grafts not a single developed AR. Thus, the control group failed to demonstrate an unfavourable influence of histoincompatibility.

Frequency of AR in relation to vascularization of recipient corneal bed

a. The whole series

AR developed in 14% of recipients with vascular corneal beds and in 14% with avascular beds, too (Table 4). The equal frequency may be partly explained by the fact that the grafts for vascular recipient beds were more cautiously selected; 44% of the vascular cases had well-matched grafts compared to 32% of the avascular cases.

Table 4. Frequency of AR in relation to vascularization of the recipient corneal bed.

AR	Vascular No. of cases	%	Avascular No. of cases	%
AR+	6	14	8	14
AR −	37	86	49	86
Totals	43	43	57	57

A well-matched and cross-match-negative graft was regarded highly necessary for the two regraftings. Both of these cases had vascularised corneal bed due to previous AR, in one of them associated with vessels of an old parenchymatous keratitis. Their recovery was fine and these well-matched grafts have remained clear.

b. The HLA-B 12/B 27 group and vascularization

Among the vascular and avascular cases of the HLA-B 12/B 27 group AR developed in 31% and 40%, respectively (Table 5). Neither this nor the control group gave conclusive evidence as to whether vascularization contri-

Table 5. Relation between AR and vascularization of the recipient corneal bed in the HLA-B 12/B 27 and control groups

AR	HLA-B 12/B 27 group Vascular No.	%	Avascular No.	%	Control group Vascular No.	%	Avascular No.	%
AR +	5	31	8	40	1	4	0	0
AR −	11	69	12	60	26	96	37	100
Totals	16	100	20	100	27	100	37	100

buted to AR. AR was especially frequent in patients with the B 12 and/or B 27 antigen, whether the recipient beds were vascular of avascular. However AR did not develop in all of such cases and vascularization was not a decisive prognostic factor even in the B 12/B 27 group.

Influence of matched or mismatched HLA-B 12 and/or B 27 antigens on the development of AR

No AR (Table 6) occurred in the 16 cases in which the recipient and the graft had matching HLA B 12 or B 27 antigens, despite some other incompatibilities. But AR developed in 9 of the 14 cases with mismatched HLA-B 12 and/or B 27 antigens, and in 4 of 6 further cases in which the graft was not tissue-typed.

Table 6. Incidence of AR when recipient had HLA-B 12 and/or B 27 antigens

Recipient/graft	AR +	AR −	Total	Incidence of AR
	No.	No.		%
HLA-match of B 12/B 12				
B 27/B 27	0	16	16	0
HLA-mismatch of B 12/BX*				
B 27/BY*	9	5	14	64
HLA-match: not known	4	2	6	67
Totals	13	23	36	36

* BX: some other B antigen than 12
* BY: some other B antigen than 27

Importance of HLA B 12/B 27 and other mismatches in development of AR

Of the 16 cases of matched B 12 or B 27 grafts (Table 7) only 3 grafts were fully compatible, 8 had 1 and 5 grafts 2 incompatible antigens, but no patient developed AR. In the cases of mismatched B 12/B 27 grafts incompatible antigens were more numerous than in those where the graft was

Table 7. Relation of HLA-B 12/B 27 and other mismatches to the development of AR

Total No. of HLA mismatches	Matched for B 12 and/or B 27			Mismatched for B 12/B 27			
	AR + No.	AR − No.	AR + %	AR + No.	AR − No.	Total	AR + %
0 }							
1 }	0	11	0	0	2	2	0
2	0	5	0	4	1	5	80
3 }							
4 }	0	0	0	5	2	7	71
Total	0	16	0	9	5	14	64

matched to B 12/B 27; the frequency of AR seemed to increase with histoincompatibility. Though the number of cases is small we had also the possibility to compare two equally large subgroups with 2 HLA-mismatches: AR developed in 4 of 5 when the graft was mismatched to B 12/B 27 antigens but in none of the cases, when it was matched (P 0.02).

DISCUSSION

As our results show, patients with B 12 and/or B 27 antigens have a higher frequency of AR, whether the recipient corneal bed is avascular or vascular. The frequency of AR in the avascular cases of this series was lower than in our earlier study (Vannas *et al.*, 1977). The slight difference may depend on the increased number of well-matched grafts with matching HLA-B 12/B 27 antigens, grafts with 3–4 mismatches having been avoided.

In the control group (without HLA-B 12 or B 27 antigens) no AR developed in avascular recipient corneas. Vascularization of the recipient cornea was not associated with AR, except in one complicated case. In this case, however, AR probably resulted from the unfavourable influence of anterior synechia, although the effects of other immunological factors, such as HLA-D antigens and antigens of other loci, cannot be excluded.

In our HLA-B 12/B 27 group AR was correlated with histoincompatibility. A mismatch of HLA-B 12 or B 27 was the indicator of risk and seemed especially liable to promote the development of AR. Five of these mismatched patients have not yet developed AR, but this situation may still change with time, because the longest interval from surgery to AR in our series is 4 years. As stated earlier by us (Vannas *et al.*, 1977) AR was often of the late type and in these instances triggered by a somatic infection.

The frequency of HLA-B 12 antigen was 15 per cent in 900 subjects of a healthy Finnish population and that of HLA-B 27 antigen was 14 per cent (Vannas *et al.*, 1977). The coincidence of these two antigens is not common. Conceivably, the extent of the risk group of HLA-B 12/B 27 carriers focuses consideration on these patients. Our data indicate that for recognizing the carriers of HLA-B 12 and/or B 27 antigen HLA-typing of the recipients may be of value. Though compatible grafts were not available it is important to keep these patients under close control, giving immediate therapy for transient infections and graft reactions.

SUMMARY

Our series comprised 100 penetrating corneal transplantations: 36 cases with HLA-B 12 and/or B 27 antigen in the recipient and, as controls, 64 cases without these antigens. The cornea was vascular in 44% of the HLA-B 12/B 27 group and in 40% of the controls.

In the HLA-B 12/B 27 group AR developed in 13 of 36 cases, 36%; but in the control group only in one case (2%). In vascular and avascular cases the incidence on AR was equal.

Among the high-risk cases of the HLA-B 12/B 27 group with definite mismatching of B 12 or B 27 antigens, 9 of the 14 recipients had developed

AR. Six further recipients of this group had untyped grafts, and AR occurred in 4 of the 6, but in none of the 16 cases that were matched for B 12 or B 27 antigens.

The value of a compatible graft, at least to the carriers of HLA-B 12 and/or B 27 antigens is thus confirmed.

REFERENCES

Amos, D.B., H. Bashir, W. Boyle, M. MacQueen & A. Tiilikainen. A simple microcyto-toxicity test. *Transplantation* 7: *220–222*, (1969).

Capella, J.A., H.E. Kaufman & J.E. Robbins. Preservation of viable corneal tissue. *Cryobiology* 2: *116–121*, (1965).

McCarey, B.E., & H.E. Kaufman. Improved corneal storage. *Invest. Ophthalmol.* 13: *165–173*, (1974).

Vannas, S., K. Karjalainen, P. Ruusuvaara & A. Tiilikainen. HLA-compatible donor cornea for prevention of allograft reaction. *Albrecht v. Graefes Arch. klin. exp. Ophthal.* 198: *217–222*, (1976).

Vannas, S., A. Vannas & K. Karjalainen. HLA-Antigene und Allograftreaktion bei Kera-tokonus. *Klin. Mbl. Augenheilk.* 170: *391–396*, (1977).

Vannas, S., A. Vannas & A. Tiilikainen. Corneal transplantation reaction in avascular keratoconus patients due to HLA-associated immune aberration against infection. A hypothesis. *Invest. Ophthalmol. Visual Sci.* 16: *644–646*, (1977).

Author's address:
Prof. Salme Vannas
Department of Ophthalmology
University of Helsinki
SF-00290 Helsinki 29
Finland.

Docum. Ophthal. Proc. Series, Vol. 20

HLA MATCHING AND CORNEAL GRAFT REJECTION

D.C. GIBBS, J.R. BATCHELOR, T.A. CASEY, A. WERB, G. LIAKOS AND C. TAYLOR.

(East Grinstead, U.K.)

INTRODUCTION

For the last six years, wherever possible, we have been HLA typing the donors and recipients of full thickness keratoplasties to try to determine how, if at all, HLA matching affects their fate. This is a report on the first 300 cases with an attempted follow up of 2 years.

DESCRIPTION OF SERIES

The grafts are consecutive and there are no exclusions whatsoever, the only criterion for inclusion is whether HLA typing has been successfully carried

300 FULL THICKNESS GRAFTS

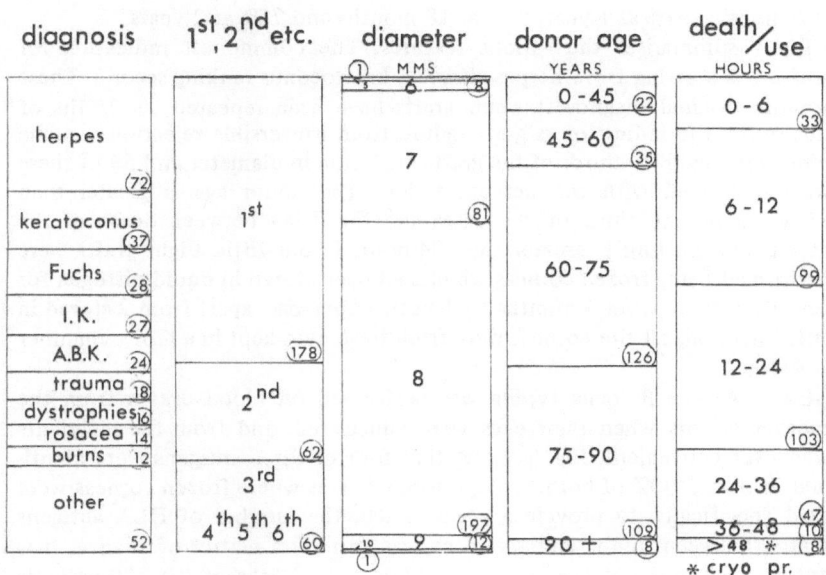

Fig. 1. Description of series.

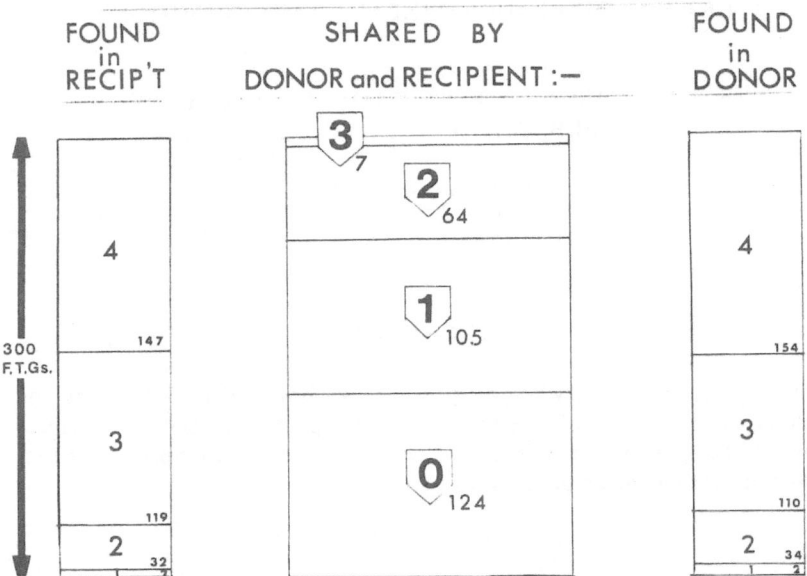

Fig. 2. HLA data.

out. Because 5 patients died, 11 were lost overseas and 47 have not been at risk for the full period, the follow up is not perfect. It is, nevertheless, 97% at 6 months, 91% at 1 year, 84% at 18 months and 78% at 2 years.

Fig. 1 summarises the various features. The commonest indication for grafting is scarring from herpes simplex, keratoconus ranking second. These are the original diagnoses; when grafts have been repeated, as 2/5ths of this series, the indication is graft failure from irreversible rejection or some other mishap. Two-thirds of the grafts are 8 mm in diameter and 53 of these were combined with cataract extraction. The donor age is greater than 75 years in one third of the cases and the delay between death of the donor and grafting is greater than 24 hours in one-fifth. Eight grafts were performed using frozen corneas which had been stored in liquid nitrogen for periods ranging from 4 months to 1 year. Otherwise, apart from 2 stored in M.K. medium, all the corneas were from fresh eyes kept in a moist chamber at 4 deg. C.

HLA – A and B locus typing was performed on blood drawn from the cadaver donors when their eyes were enucleated, and from the recipients whenever convenient. Fig. 2 shows that four or three antigens were identified in nearly 90% of both. Except in the 8 cases where frozen corneas were used specifically to provide a good match, the number of HLA antigens shared between donor and recipient was entirely a matter of chance. It is unfortunate, but not therefore surprising, that 2/5ths of the 300 patients received a total HLA mismatch.

140

RESULTS

The survival of functioning grafts has been calculated by the actuarial method (Barnes, 1965) and because of the usual uncertainties in diagnosing rejection the results are analysed in two ways (Fig. 3). In the first, grafts have been classified as clear or opaque regardless of the reason for failure; and here 63% are clear at 1 year and 53% at 2 years. In the second, cases which failed for reasons other than rejection are excluded, so that all fail-

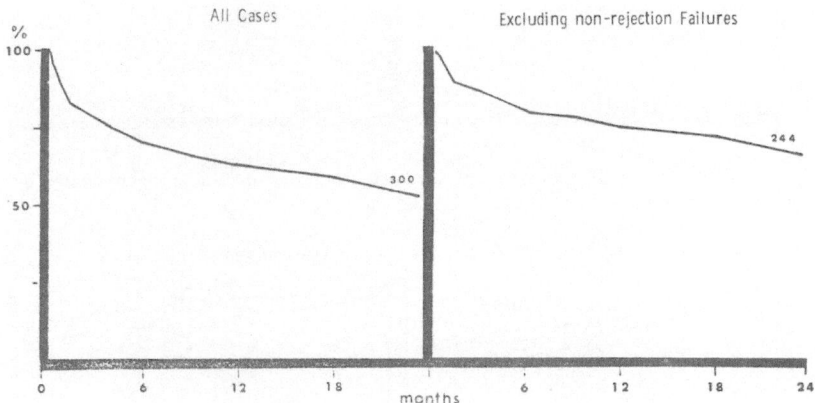

Fig. 3. Duration of graft clarity.

ures are due to irreversible rejection. Here the survival rates are 75% at 1 year and 66% at 2 years. Our criteria for rejection have been described elsewhere (Gibbs *et al.*, 1974), and in the absence of a specific test we have no doubt made mistakes, particularly as rejection may be provoked and go unrecognised in grafts that start to fail for other reasons. Virtually all cases receive topical steroids prophylactically, and rejection episodes occurring despite this are treated with sub-conjunctival Depomedrol and occasionally with systemic steroids as well. To guard against bias, the serological data are not kept in the clinical records and are not known to the ophthalmologists when they are trying to assess the cause of cloudiness.

Let us now see whether the number of HLA antigens shared by donor and recipient – shown on symbols ▽ – affects survival (Fig. 4). Considering all cases, the curves overlap a little and are only approximately in the expected order; but when non-rejection failures are excluded the ranking becomes clear at about 6 weeks. At 18 months the survival rates for cases sharing 3, 2, 1 and no antigens are 100%, 80%, 73% and 65% respectively. However, the number of cases sharing 3 antigens is very small, and the differences are not quite statistically significant.

It is common experience that certain grafts, such as those for keratoconus, nearly always remain clear, so HLA matching can have little or no effect on their outcome. Likewise, cases with epithelial deficiencies and fierce vascularisation such as chemical burns, nearly always fail, and HLA matching may

141

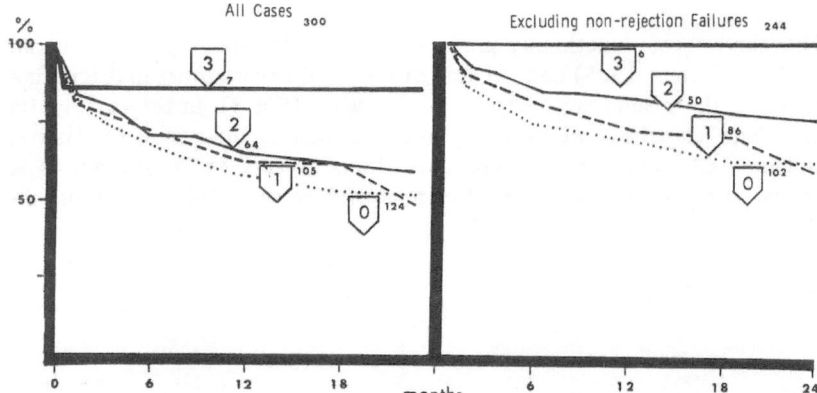

Fig. 4. Duration of graft clarity according to the number of HLA antigens shared by donor and recipient.

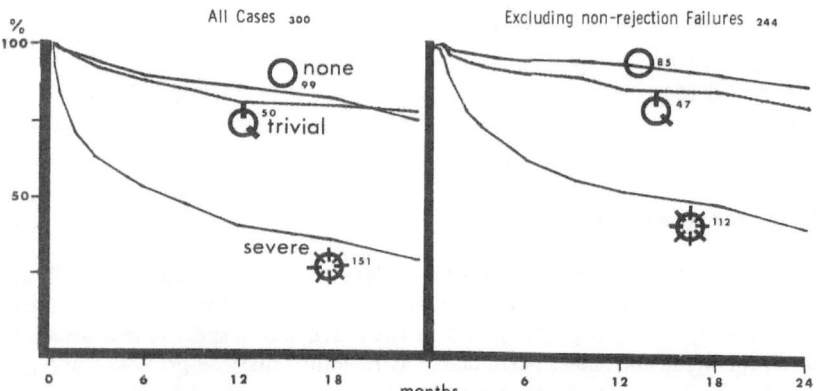

Fig. 5. Duration of graft clarity according to degree of vascularisation of host cornea.

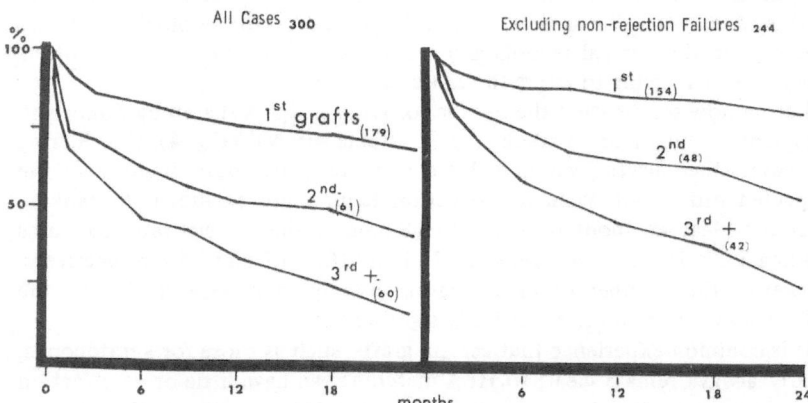

Fig. 6. Duration of clarity according to whether graft is first or subsequent (on same eye).

not be of much help to them either. So it could be misleading to consider the effect of HLA matching on the series as a whole; it would seem more sensible to exclude those cases which are almost bound to succeed plus those that are almost bound to fail, or, at least, to examine them separately. We have done this by subdividing the 300 according to two of the oldest observations in corneal grafting; firstly, that the greater the degree of host vascularisation the less likely is a graft to remain clear; and secondly, that the more often a graft is repeated on the same eye the less likely it is to succeed.

By scrutinising the clinical notes, the photographs and when necessary the histology of the excised disc, we have assessed vascularisation as 'none' ○ when there are no blood vessels, 'trivial' ◔ when merely an occasional vessel is cut by trephine, or 'severe' ✵ . The 'severe' category includes a wide range, but we believe further subdivision is too subjective to be of value. Fig. 5 shows survival curves drawn according to the degree of vascularisation, and the difference in outcome between the trivial and severe groups is around 40% at 1 year and at 2 years, both overall, and when non rejection failures are excluded. Fig. 6 shows the effect of repeat grafts on the same eye. At 1 year the difference between 1st and 3rd-and-subsequent grafts is about 40%, and at 2 years 55% − again both overall and when non-rejection failures are excluded. We have suggested in a previous paper (Gibbs and Casey, 1976) that this worsening outcome is due partly to more blood vessels being attracted by repeat grafts, but unless subtle sub-division of vascularisation is all important, another factor is at work, presumably an immunological one.

Using these two criteria it is now a simple matter to divide the series into three levels of risk (Fig. 7). At low risk are the cases that share the two best features, blood vessels are absent and they are first time grafts. At high risk are the cases that share the two worst features, vascularisation is severe and they have been grafted at least twice before. The remainder fall into the medium risk group. Fig. 8 shows the dramatic difference in the survival rates for these three categories. At 18/12 for example, 85% of the low risk grafts are clear compared with 18% in the high risk group. In fact only 4 of the latter survived for two years, and during the third year two of these failed. When non-rejection failures are excluded the differences are similarly impressive.

We can now examine the effect of HLA matching at each of these three levels of risk. In the 83 low risk cases (Fig. 9) there are only 6 failures from irreversible rejection. One of these shared 2 antigens, two shared 1 antigen and three shared no antigens. There seems nothing to be gained from studying this further. The 169 medium risk cases (Fig. 10) show survival curves that rank clearly according to the number of antigens shared. (Unfortunately one of the cases sharing 3 antigens had a cloudy graft from the start due to primary failure of frozen material.) Overall the differences are not quite significant, but when non-rejection failures are excluded, there is a significant advantage in sharing 3 + 2 antigens compared with sharing 1 + no antigens at 18/12 and at 2 years. Here at 18/12 months the survival rates for cases sharing 3, 2 or fewer antigens are 100%, 83% and 66% respectively.

143

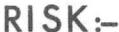

RISK:–

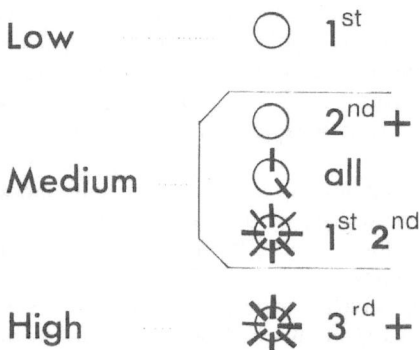

Low .... ○ 1st

Medium .... ○ 2nd +
Q all
※ 1st 2nd

High .... ※ 3rd +

Fig. 7. Levels of risk.

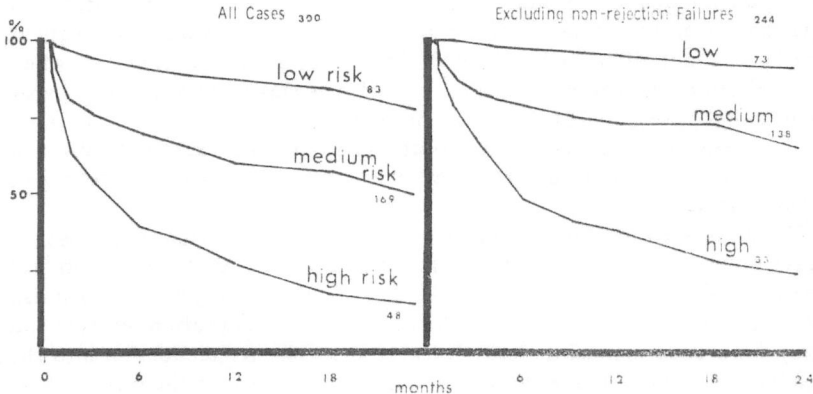

Fig. 8. Duration of graft clarity according to the level of risk.

The 48 high risk cases (Fig. 11) fared very badly except for the 3 sharing 3 antigens. Frozen material was used for these and the two of them which have reached one year remain clear. The cases that shared two antigens fared worst of all, no doubt because a high proportion happened to suffer from epithelial difficulties, several were in fact chemical burns.

As in a previous analysis on a smaller number of patients (Batchelor *et al.*, 1976) HLA matching does not appear to influence the incidence of rejection, but rather the response of rejection episodes to treatment. Considering only the 273 grafts which have been followed up for one year, during this first year the incidence of cases that rejected once or more was around 50% no matter whether 2, 1 or no antigens were shared. However, when 2 antigens were shared, 69% responded to treatment, compared to 57% when 1 antigen was shared and 50% when no antigens were shared. Too few

144

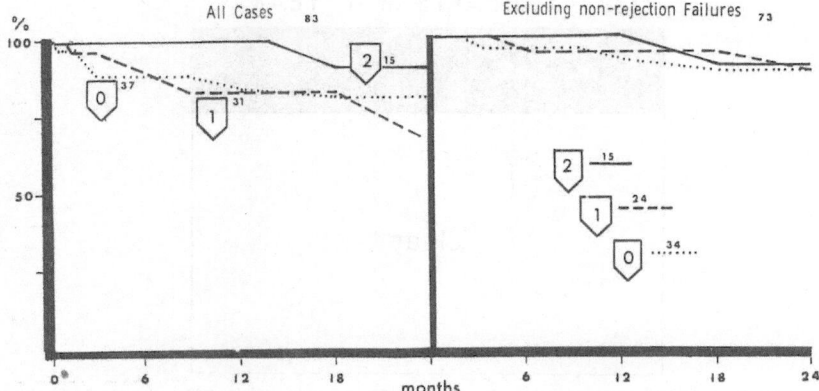

Fig. 9. Duration of clarity of grafts at low risk according to the number of HLA antigens shared.

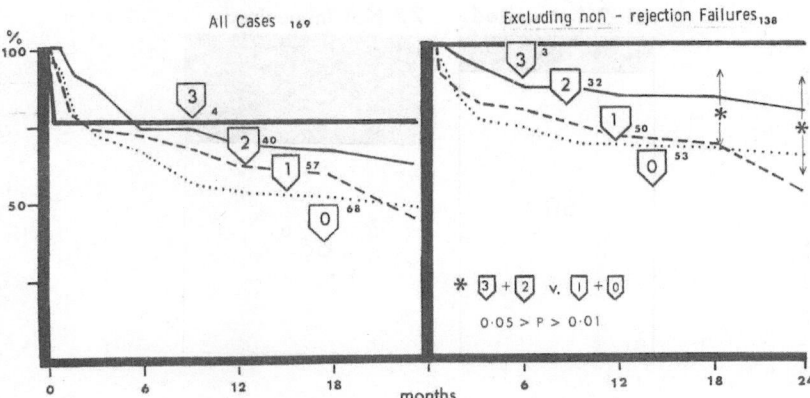

Fig. 10. Duration of clarity of grafts at medium risk according to the number of HLA antigens shared.

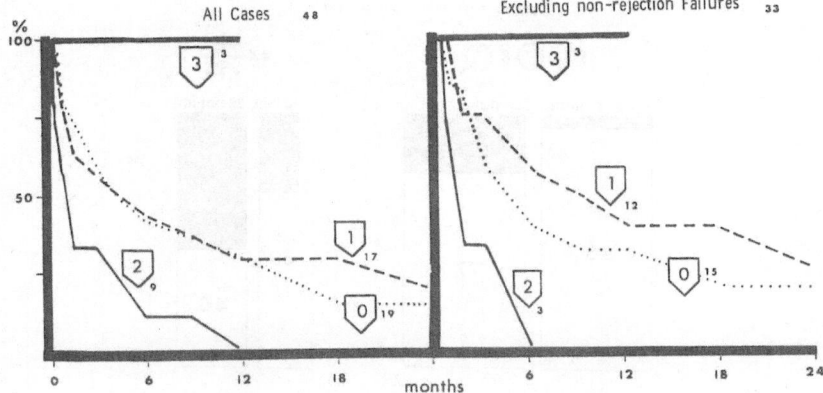

Fig. 11. Duration of clarity of grafts at high risk according to the number of HLA antigens shared.

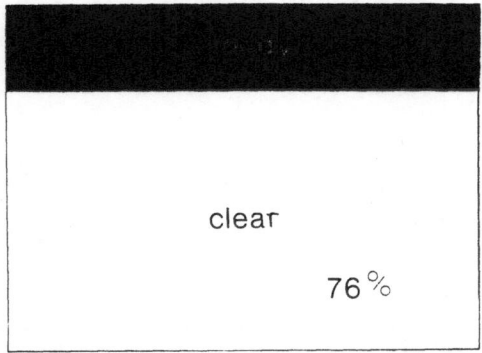

Fig. 12. Patients questioned *re* previous allografts, pregnancies and blood transfusions.

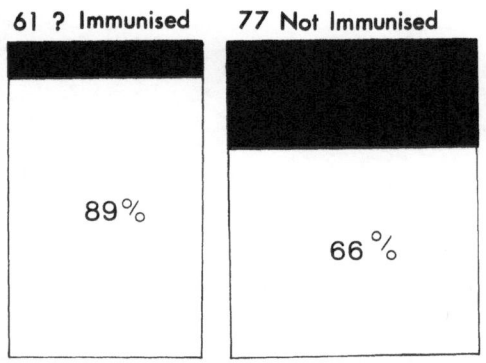

Fig. 13. Division according to immunity.

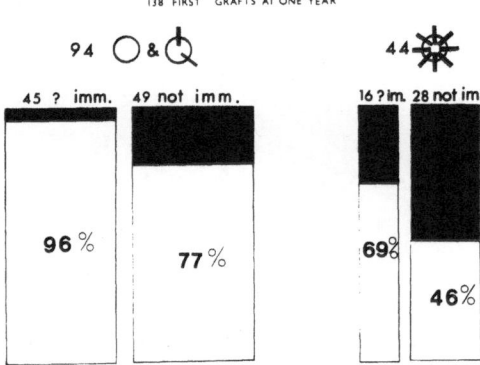

Fig. 14. Division according to degree of vascularisation.

146

cases shared 3 antigens to allow conclusions to be drawn, but the incidence of rejection was 33% and response to treatment 100%. These groups have been further subdivided according to the level of risk, and at each level the results show a similar trend (data not shown).

Mismatching of antigens from the B series was, if anything slightly more important than mismatching from the A series. Otherwise no particular antigen provoked rejection any more frequently than any other.

As we have found before (Gibbs et al., 1974), rejection was commonest during the first year and especially during the first three months. Episodes were classified as diffuse or linear, being placed in the latter category if there was the slightest hint of a line at any stage. There were 228 episodes in 151 cases, 98 cases rejected once, 38 twice and 15 trice or more often. 127 of the episodes were diffuse of which 46 failed to clear on treatment, and 101 were linear of which 27 failed to respond. When no antigens were shared the ratio of diffuse to linear episodes was 45. 46; when 1 was shared 42 : 37; when 2 were shared 33: 19 and when 3 were shared 3 : 3. Otherwise no differences in the character of rejection episodes, acording to the number of antigens shared, were noted.

The 'transfusion effect' in kidney grafting is hotly disputed. It now seems that cases previously 'immunised' by pregnancy and blood transfusion, provided they do not develop cytotoxic antibodies, fare better than cases not so immunised. In earlier analyses we included previous keratoplasty on the same eye as one of the causes of potential immunisation, and since repeat grafts carry a worsening prognosis at any rate partly due to their mechanical effects, this rather confused the issue. This time we have restricted our enquiries to first time grafts on the eye in question. There were 138 first grafts which had been followed up for one year, and were in patients whose history regarding contralateral grafts, pregnancies and blood transfusions was certainly known. By one year a quarter of them had failed (Fig. 12). If these arc divided into the immune and the non-immune (Fig. 13), only 11% of the former failed compared with 34% of the latter. This difference is very significant $P < 0.01$; and it is not due to there being a higher proportion of high risk cases in the non-immune group, because if we divide them according to the degree of vascularisation (Fig. 14) the trend in each division is the same. If contralateral grafts are excluded and only possible immunisation by pregnancies and blood transfusions incriminated, the pattern is still similar and the difference significant − although less so, $P < 0.05$. These figures take into account failures for any reason. If only failures from irreversible rejection are considered, a similar pattern emerges, but the numbers are smaller and the differences are not quite statistically significant.

DISCUSSION

It is always dangerous to draw firm conclusions from a series of kerato-plasties because of the large number of variables. Ideally, HLA matching should be compared in cases that are in all other respects similar, and this we have not found possible to arrange. However, by assessing prognosis on the number of times a graft has been repeated on the same eye, as well as on the degree of host vascularisation, we hope to have 'trapped', so to speak, most of the features which greatly worsen it, even perhaps some that at present go unrecognised.

Our experience that HLA matching is unimportant in cases at low risk is similar to that of Allansmith and his co-workers in America (Allansmith *et al.*, 1974). Our findings that it is of importance in cases at greater risk is similar to that of Dr. Kok van Alphen et al. in Holland (Kok van Alphen *et al.*,, 1977); indeed by grafting on an emergency basis they achieved excellent matching in severely vascularised cases and their results are most encouraging.

We realise that there are two particular defects in this series. The first is that we have meagre information regarding antibodies. We are now pursuing them more eagerly, and it is of interest that we recently found I.A. antibody in a case that could have been immunised only by a previous keratoplasty – since he was a man and had had no blood transfusions nor any other allografts. The second defect is that only seven of the 300 cases share 3 antigens and none share 4. We now believe that 3 and 4 antigen matches should be provided for medium risk as well as for high risk cases. They might substantially improve the outcome in the medium risk group however little they affect it in the high risk group. It must not be forgotten that even a 4 antigen match is still incompatible, it is not an autograft, so if very good HLA matches are reserved just for cases at very high risk a fair proportion of them will probably still fail, and this could lead to unwarranted pessimism about the value of HLA matching overall.

More exact information awaits the building up and analysis of a large series containing many well matched cases as well as many poorly matched ones, and it is difficult to know how this can be achieved. In our limited experience cryo-preservation gives rather variable results, for we have had a few primary failures as well as successes. High risk cases need donor corneas not only with a good HLA match, but also with a high density of viable endothelial cells, and after the freeze-thaw cycle we cannot be perfectly confident of the latter. M.K. medium allows a few days grace, but grafts still have to be performed on a semi-emergency basis, so administrative problems are not entirely solved.

CONCLUSIONS

This is the fourth time we have analysed our series, the previous numbers being 155 (Gibbs *et al.*, 1974), 200 (Batchelor *et al.*, 1976) and 250 (Gibbs and Casey, 1976). Each time the results have shown the same trend, that the sharing of 2 HLA antigens by donor and recipient is of benefit compared with the sharing of 1 or none. However, it now seems that this is the case only up to a certain level of risk. While it is likely that the sharing of 3 and 4 antigens will raise that threshold, more work needs to be done to evaluate this. The possible role of IA antigen in corneal graft rejection, and the possibility that a 'transfusion effect' might be induced in a patient preoperatively to protect his graft from rejection, are fascinating prospects for future study.

REFERENCES

Allansmith M.R., M. Fine & R. Payne. *Trans. Am. Acad. Ophthalm, Otol.* 78: *445*, (1974)
Barnes, B.A. *Transplantation* 3: *812*, (1965).
Batchelor, J.R. *et al. The Lancet*, (March 13th 1976).
Gibbs D.C., J.R. Batchelor, A. Werb, W. Schlesinger & T.A. Casey. *Trans. Ophthal. Soc. U.K.* 94: *101*, (1974).
Gibbs D.C. & T.A. Casey. Second World Congress on the Cornea, Washington D.C., U.S.A., 1976.
Dr. Kok van Alphen *et al. Dutch Ophthalm. Soc.*, (1977).

Author's address:
Corneo-plastic Unit,
Queen Victoria Hospital,
East Grinstead,
Sussex,
England

DEVELOPMENT IN USE OF CULTURED ENDOTHELIUM IN CORNEAL TRANSPLANTATION

D.M. MAURICE, J.P. McCULLEY AND M.M. PERLMAN

(Stanford, California, U.S.A.)

In cases of endothelial dystrophy it is at present necessary to perform a full thickness keratoplasty. There would be evident advantages in replacing only the affected layer with endothelial cells grown in tissue culture. These are as follows:

1. Cells of known origin and from younger donors could be available.

2. Fewer donor cells and of mixed genetic origin would be used, thus reducing the immunological challenge.

3. Donor material could be available at all times.

4. It may be possible to use the patient's own stromal button for the graft, which would lessen the danger of poor apposition of graft and host.

It has not been established whether cultured cells will recover their morphological and functional characteristics when returned to the eye, and these experiments were designed to test this point in the rabbit. Cells were grown in mass in a manner similar to that described (Perlman and Baum, 1974). Three approaches have been explored.

1. The injection of suspensions of cultured cells into the anterior chamber in the hope that they would attach to the bare Descemet's membrane. This was the approach originally suggested by one of us at the NEI corneal task force (1973). A chemical method of destroying only the endothelial layer of the cornea was devised with this in mind (Maurice and Perlman, 1977). About $5x10^5$ cells suspended in 1 ml of medium were injected into the anterior chamber of a rabbit's eye, which was then held dependent for up to 4 hr. Examination of these animals in the slit lamp on following days showed no evidence of endothelial cell replacement on the posterior surface of the swollen cornea, and histological sections showed only isolated clumps of cells not only on the cornea but also on the lens and iris surface. The failure of cells to grow in these edematous eyes was possibly due to chemical alterations of Descemet's membrane.

2. A rabbit's cornea was isolated and mounted on a ring (Dikstein and Maurice, 1972), its endothelium was rubbed away and cultured cells were allowed to settle on the bared Descemet's membrane by gravity. The tissue was then incubated for 4 days by which time a monolayer of cells was found attached to the surface. It was then used for the preparation of a donor graft by standard methods of keratoplasty. Because the tissue became very edematous during incubation, it was thinned osmotically 24 hrs before

use by replacement of the tissue culture medium with one containing 5% dextran. Of necessity, heparin was given both systemically and locally during the operation in order to prevent the clotting of the aqueous humor. Steroid treatment was continued for several weeks after the operation. With this procedure some grafts into endothelium-free eyes became thin and transparent (Maurice, McCulley, Perlman, 1977). Light and scanning electron microscopy demonstrated an intact, though slightly irregular, endothelial cell layer with complex junctional interdigitation. Grafts from cultured cells labelled with H^3 thymidine made into normal corneas also remained clear and retained their radioactivity. A number of transplants lost their clarity after 7—10 days, however, apparently as a result of fibroblast invasion which occurred in spite of the steroid treatment.

3. Cells were grown as a monolayer on a transparent substrate which was then used to replace the endothelial cell layer of a corneal disc trephined from a rabbit. The most promising substrate tested has been a thin film of cross-linked gelatin. This is prepared by dipping a loop of platinum wire in 3% gelatin solution, drying the film so formed at 4°C and fixing it first in glutaraldehyde vapor and then in 12% glutaraldehyde solution, followed by copious washing. These membranes are physically strong and transparent, although only a few microns thick, have a high hydraulic conductivity and provide an excellent substrate for cell growth.

The major technical problem in introducing these membranes into the eye is to maintain their contact with the posterior surface of the graft. They tend to bridge the gap between the wound edges, as in a detached retina, and on occasion to form wrinkles where they are in contact with the tissue. These spaces between membrane and tissue rapidly fill with fibroblasts, leading to a poor functional result. A technique has been developed which promises some success. The graft is placed on a holder so that its natural curvature is reversed and its Descemet's membrane is coated with a very thin film of warm 10% gelatin. The cell-covered membrane, still on its platinum loop, is quickly pulled down on the tacky surface and is trephined around the edge as soon as the glue is set (about 1 minute). This gives a temporary attachment which, however, is sufficient to maintain contact between the layers during and after the operation. Nevertheless, at the time of this symposium the two operations that have been technically successful have failed to give a good functional result, the grafted button never approaching its normal hydration. Examination by TEM in these cases has shown that the cultured endothelial cells show an apparently normal morphology and are commencing to lay down a fresh Descemet's membrane. However, in each case a continuous monolayer of fibroblastic cells was found to exist on the opposite side of the gelatin layer which would account for the poor functional result.

CONCLUSIONS

Although we have not yet been able to consistently produce successful endothelial cell grafts in the rabbit using cultured material, the experiments are promising in showing that such cells will take up their normal morphology and show evidence of active function in their new environment. The principal difficulty is the control of interference from fibroblasts which either replace the cells or intervene between them and the stroma. If these problems can be solved, we hope to advance to testing human endothelial cultures and eventually to using a culture-keratoplasty technique in patients.

REFERENCES

Dikstein, S. & D. Maurice. The metabolic base to the fluid pump in the cornea. *J. Physiol.* 221: *29*, (1972).

Maurice, D.M., J.P. McCulley & M.M. Perlman. Donor endothelium from tissue culture. *Invest. Ophthalmol. and Vis. Sci.* 15: *103abs*, (1977).

Maurice, D. & M. Perlman. Permanent destruction of rabbit corneal endothelium. *Invest. Ophthalmol. and Vis. Sci.* 16: *647*, (1977).

National Eye Institute: Summary report of the cornea task force. *Invest. Ophthalmol.* 12: *391*, (1973).

Perlman, M. & J. Baum. The mass culture of rabbit corneal endothelium. *Arch. Ophthalmol.* 92: *235*, (1974).

Authors' address:
Division of Ophthalmology
Stanford University Medical Centre
Stanford, California 94305
U.S.A.

POST-OPERATIVE CONTROL OF THE DONOR ENDOTHELIUM IN CORNEAL GRAFTING BY MEANS OF HISTOCHEMICAL STAINING

J. FRANCOIS, V. VICTORIA-TRONCOSO AND H. VERBRAEKEN

(Ghent, Belgium)

INTRODUCTION

The maintenance of the transparency of the corneal stroma depends, on the one hand, on the equidistance of the collagen fibrils, which form a very regular hexagonal mesh (Maurice, 1962) and, on the other hand, on the degree of dehydration of the acid mucopolysaccharides, which constitute the interfibrillar ground substance (Hedbys and Mishima, 1963). The neutralisation of those mucopolysaccharides by cetylpyridinium chloride, as well as their enzymatic digestion prevents corneal oedema. The hydration capacity of the corneal mucopolysaccharides depends above all on the size of the polyanionic surface formed by the free negative charges of the mucopolysaccharide chains. The collagen fibres themselves are incapable of self-hydration or of modifying their volume.

It is accepted today that it is the *endothelium*, which extracts toward the anterior chamber the water, that tends to produce a swelling of the stroma, the swelling pressure being 40 mmHg (Hedbys et al., 1963). The endothelial cells possess, indeed, a sodium ion pump. That pump is thermo-sensitive, as it is inhibited by cold (Davson, 1955; Harris, 1967) and by ouabain (Dickstein and Maurice, 1972). This thermo-sensitivity shows that the dehydration is an active process, the energy for which is supplied by a high-energy nucleotide, namely ATP, the necessary enzyme being adenosintriphosphatase, which can be inhibited by ouabain (Bonting, 1961).

It results from the foregoing that, in perforating corneal graftings, the donor's cornea must have a viable endothelium, the enzymatic systems of which must be intact.

The *corneal epithelium* possesses also a pump of the same type (Green, 1965), but it extracts the water from the pre-corneal film in order to hydrate the stroma. Maurice and Riley (1970) showed experimentally that the cornea can maintain its state of dehydration in the absence of epithelium. Furthermore, the corneal epithelium constitutes the most antigenic layer of the cornea. It is for that reason that we recommend removing the donor's epithelium by peeling it off at the time of the corneal transplantation.

The *corneal stroma* itself plays a rather passive role, because it possesses no mechanism for controlling its hydration and, as a consequence, its transparency. The keratocytes have, moreover, an extremely slow metabolism. A biomicroscopic examination is sufficient to observe the absence of leucomata or other alterations. A graft cloudy because of hydration, but whose endothelium is certainly viable, poses no problem, because such endothelium can eliminate all the water in less than twenty-four hours (Leuenberger, 1978).

In conclusion, it may be said that the corneal endothelium, which contains about 500.000 cells of 5μ in thickness and 20μ in diameter, is very fragile, not only to handling, but also, after death, to the action of the aqueous humour, which has a lytic effect on the cells.

When a lamellar grafting is made, the quality of the endothelium of the graft no longer plays any role. It is for that reason that preference should be given to that operation whenever it is possible.

PERSONAL METHOD

The ocular globes are removed within six hours after the death and placed at the bottom of a sterile flask on a cotton pad, steeped in an isotonic and antibiotic solution (1.000.000 U penicillin and 0.5 g streptomycin per 100 ml of physiological solution). They are conserved at $4°C$ for not more than twenty-four hours, before being utilised.

The two eyes of the donor are examined immediately before the operation, first at the biomicroscope. The better eye, if there is a difference, is chosen for the transplantation. We verify the endothelial viability of the other eye. We have, indeed, been able to establish that, in the case of a pair of eyes from the same donor, of which the corneal endothelium presents no difference at the biomicroscope between the two eyes, the difference in endothelial viability never exceeds 10%, that is to say that, from that point of view, the two eyes of one and the same pair are similar.

Any eyes which, at the biomicroscope, show a cornea guttata, an endothelial dystrophy, too many folds in the Descemet's membrane or inflammatory signs of the anterior segment, are discarded.

The cornea, the endothelial viability of which we wish to study, is sectioned at the level of the limbus and washed for several seconds with physiological saline. It is then immersed in a 1% aqueous solution of Tripan blue for one minute and then washed again with physiological saline. Normally, the endothelium will not be stained. If more than 30% of the endothelial cells are stained, the cornea is discarded.

A positive staining by Tripan blue demonstrates an alteration of the membranes, which become permeable to the dye (Figs. 1 and 2). Therefore, a positively stained cell must be considered as non-viable. In the contrary case, the cornea is immersed for one minute in a 0.1% solution of toluidine blue buffered with 0.06 M phosphate and then in a bath of physiological saline.

Finally, it is examined under the microscope (Wild microscope, x 10 ocular, x 10 objective lens). Ten fields of the endothelium are studied, as indicated in Fig. 3. Each field is rated at 10%. If five fields (50%) are stained, the cornea is discarded. If that is not the case, it is accepted,

156

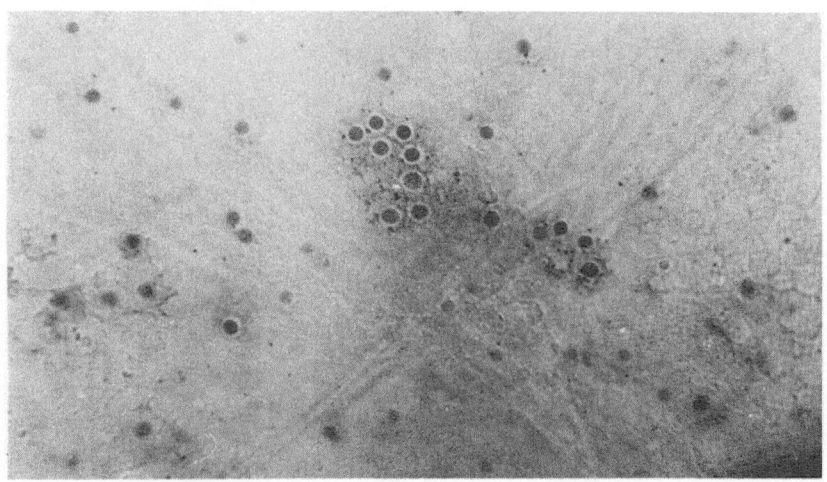

Fig. 1. Group of corneal endothelial cells stained by tripan blue. Folds of Descemet's membrane are seen.

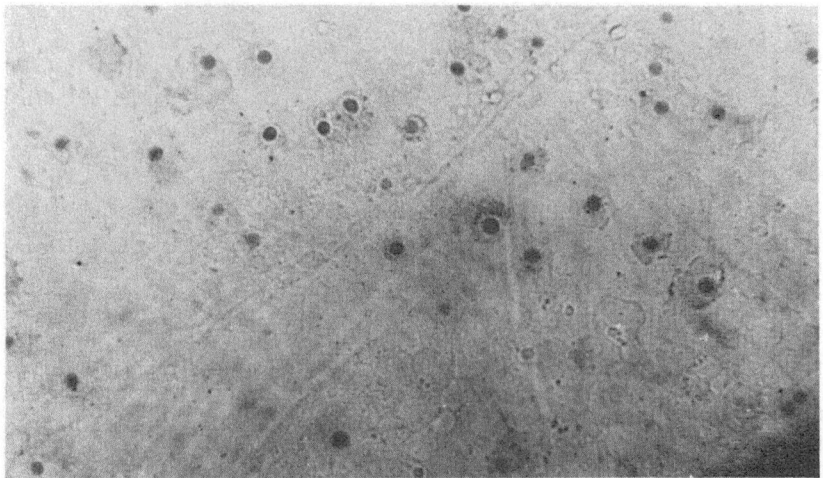

Fig. 2. Corneal endothelial cells. Some isolated cells are stained by tripan blue. Folds of Descemet's membrane.

depending upon the case. For example, for a keratoconus, 50% of viability is sufficient, but for a case already affected by an endothelium disorder such as, for example, Fuch's dystrophy, 80–100% of viability are absolutely necessary.

Toluidine blue permits not only the morphological study of the endothelial cells (Fig. 4), but also the appraisal of the ADN, which is α-metachromatic, and of the ARN, which is β-metachromatic. Sometimes the cells are

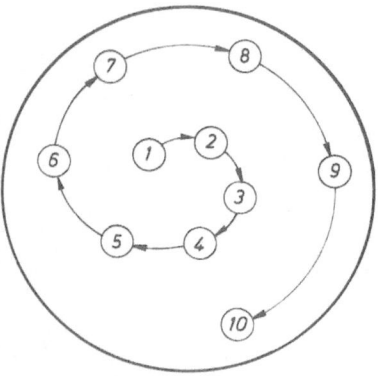

Fig. 3. Areas of the corneal endothelium which are examined.

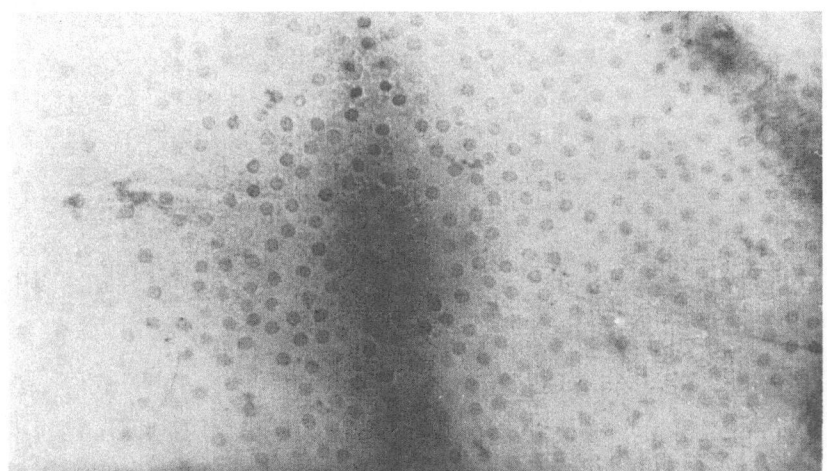

Fig. 4. Normal corneal endothelial mosaic, which is not stained by toluidine blue.

not stained, because of only slight penetration of the dye. In such a case, the cornea can be fixed for ten minutes in 10% formaldehyde, buffered with 0.06 M phosphate and stained again with toluidine blue.

Morphologically, one can find: (1) intercellular vacuolisation (Fig. 5), (2) intracytoplasmic microvacuolisation (Fig. 5), (3) intracytoplasmic macrovacuolisation, (4) increase of the cell volume (Fig. 6), (5) picnosis or karyorrexis (Figs. 6 and 7) or (6) complete cell destruction (Fig. 8).

The lesions are generally not isolated, but affect in most cases several cells of the same field, which must therefore be considered as non-viable (0%).

As soon as it is certain that the endothelium of the graft is viable and in good condition, we begin the operation. The graft is irrigated with 2% mercurochrome and its epithelium is removed. While awaiting the insertion of the graft in the receiving cornea, care is taken that its endothelium is

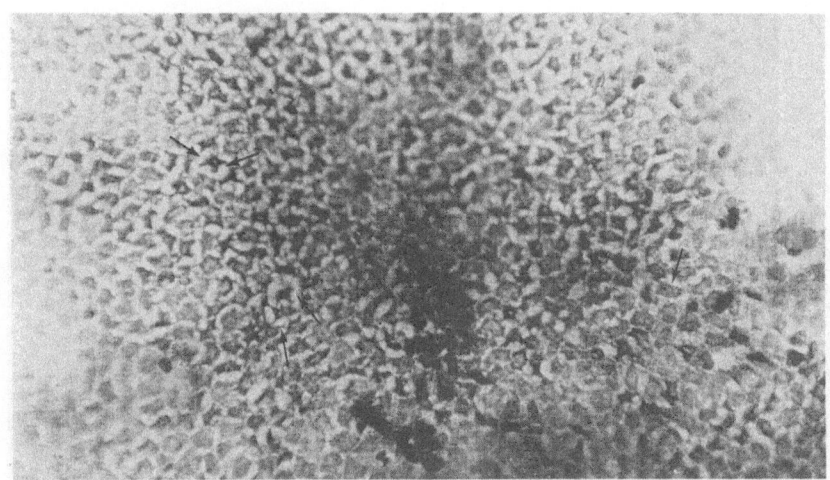

Fig. 5. Corneal endothelium. Oedematous intercellular spaces (arrows). Toluidine blue staining.

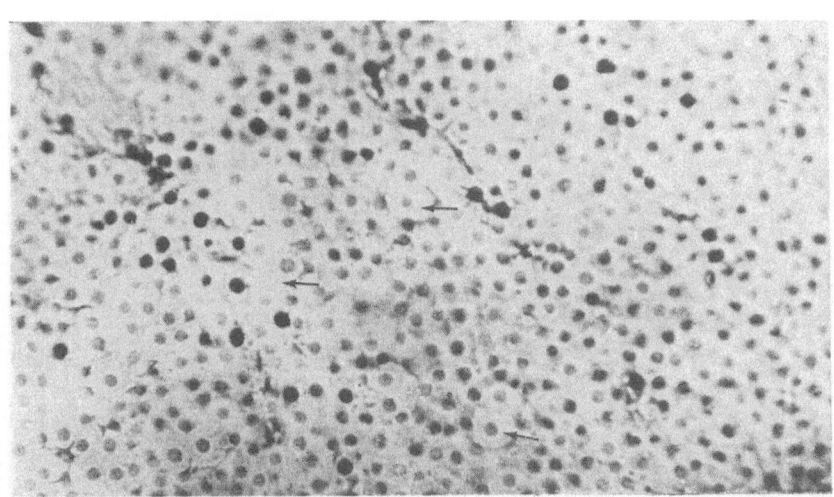

Fig. 6. Endothelial cells with increased volume (arrows). Some nuclei are picnotic. Toluidine blue staining.

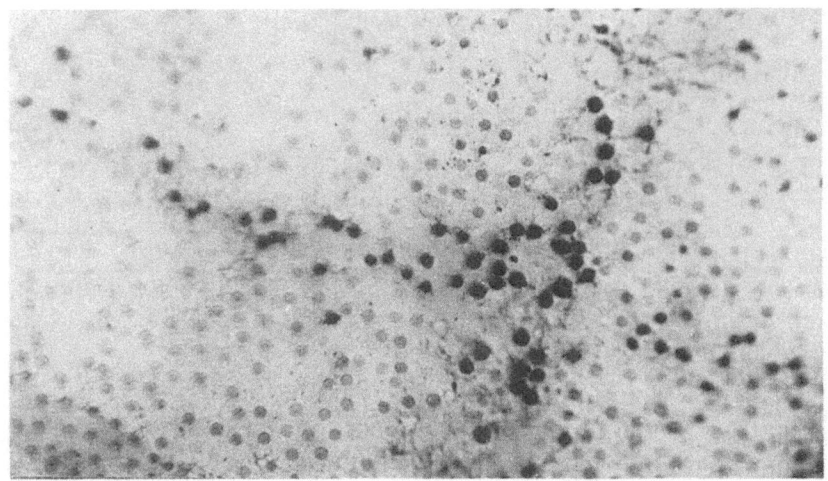

Fig. 7. Area with normal endothelial cells and a sequence of picnotic cells. Toluidine blue staining.

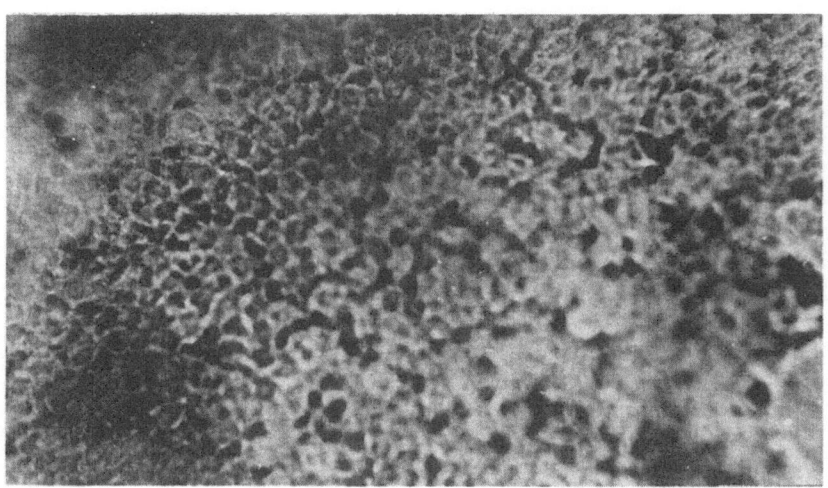

Fig. 8. Destruction of endothelial cells and karyorexis of the nuclei. Toluidine blue staining.

160

constantly directed upward. The trephination of the receiving cornea and the suture of the graft are carried out under the microscope. After having first placed four sutures of 8–0 virgin silk in order to keep the graft in position, we make a continuous suture with 10–0 Perlon. As soon as the anterior chamber has been reformed by an injection of air or physiological saline, the virgin-silk threads are removed. At the end of the operation, a peripheral iridectomy, using the Charleux-Etienne technique, is performed.

Two days before the operation, an immuno-suppression treatment is instituted (3 x 50 mg of imuran per day) and continued in general for two months. The purpose of this treatment is to prevent the rejection of the graft.

On the two days immediately following the operation, we apply atropine and aureomycin locally. Beginning on the third day, we instil maxitrol four times daily. Also from the third day, we inspect the graft every day at the biomicroscope (Figs. 9 and 10). After a month, the endothelial mosaic is controlled by means of the specular microscope equipped with a x 5 or a x 10 ocular (Syber, Gainesville, Florida).

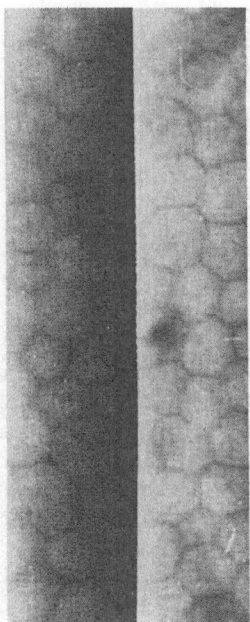 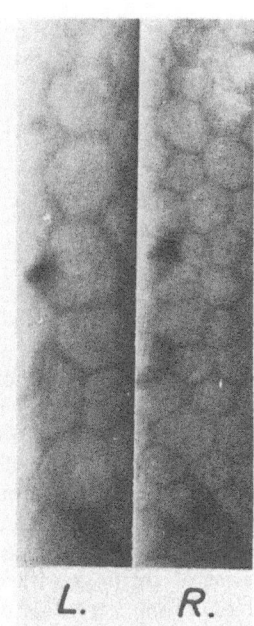

Fig. 9. Corneal endothelial mosaic after perforating grafting in a case of keratoconus (70% of the endothelial cells of the donor were viable).

Fig. 10. Fuchs' endothelial dystrophy. L = left eye, R = right eye.

RESULTS

It is necessary to consider, on the one hand, the post-operative oedema which occurs during the first days and which depends upon the condition of the donor endothelium and, on the other hand, the long-term condition of the endothelial mosaic. When a corneal oedema appears two or three weeks after the operation, it is no longer due to a deficient endothelium, but to a rejection phenomenon.

We have compared forty consecutive perforating graftings for which we had used the endothelial control technique, with forty consecutive perforating graftings without that control (Table I).

Table 1. Perforating corneal graftings. Results during the three first postoperative weeks.

Disease	Perforating graftings without endothelial control			Perforating graftings with endothelial control		
	No.	Good result	Bad result	No.	Good result	Bad result
Keratoconus	14	12	2	15	15	0
Endothelial dystrophy of Fuchs	3	1	2	3	3	0
Postherpetic leucoma	9	7	2	10	10	0
Traumatic corneal perforations	1	1	0	5	5	0
Interstitial keratitis	4	4	0	2	2	0
Corneal burnings	2	2	0	–	–	–
Macular dystrophy of the cornea	3	3	0	1	1	0
Trachomatous leucoma	1	0	1	–	–	–
Leucoma after corneal ulcer	3	3	0	3	3	0
Megalocornea	–	–	–	1	1	–
Total	40	33	7	40	40	0

In the series of graftings without control, we had seven cases in which an early corneal oedema occurred within the two weeks following the operation and gave rise to an opacification of the graft (17.5% of the cases). The earliness of the onset of the oedema proves that it was due to the deficient endothelium of the graft. It should be observed that this complication was seen, among others, in two cases of keratoconus out of fourteen (14% of the cases), although this affection has the best operative prognosis.

In our series of graftings with controlled viability of the endothelium, we did *not have one single case* of corneal oedema during the first two weeks. The difference between the results is above all evident when one considers the cases of Fuch's endothelial dystrophy and of vascularised postherpetic leucoma, of which the operative prognosis is bad. Even in those cases we had no failure, whereas in the other series, without control, the unsuccessful cases amounted to 66% for Fuch's dystrophy and to 22% for herpetic leucoma.

As regards the endothelial mosaic, this remained normal in those cases wherein the endothelium of the receiver was normal, and expanded in those cases wherein it was pathological (Fuchs' dystrophy for example).

By way of example, we have for two years observed a patient suffering from Fuchs' endo-epithelial dystrophy (Figs. 11 and 12). His right eye was operated on for cataract, while a perforating grafting was made in the same session. At the left eye we performed a grafting first and extracted the cataract afterwards. For both eyes, the graft displayed an endothelium which was 100% viable. The visual acuity is now 7/10 at the right eye and 8/10 at the left. The dystrophy has not recurred. The endothelial mosaic is normal at the specular microscope, although it is more expanded in the left than in the right eye. The corneal thickness also is normal.

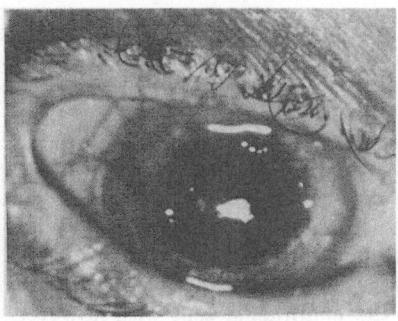 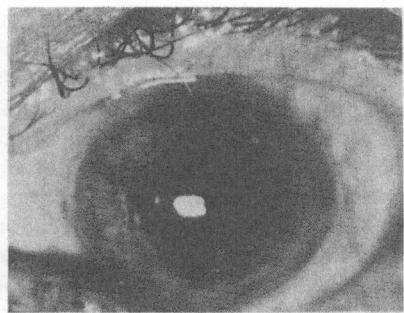

Fig. 11. Fuchs' endothelial dystrophy. Right eye. Postoperative result after 2 years.

Fig. 12. Fuchs' endothelial dystrophy. Left eye. Postoperative result after 26 months.

DISCUSSION

The failure of a corneal transplantation may be due to four main causes:

1. An infection.

2. A primary endothelial failure, which manifests itself as an oedema of the graft, appearing during the first few postoperative days. That failure is due to the fact that the endothelium was in a bad condition before the transplantation, that is to say, that it was not viable. The only exception to this rule is a vascularised receiving cornea.

3. An immunological rejection is distinctly longer delayed in the case of a first grafting. It does not occur before two or three weeks. It can be immediate, when it concerns a second or a third grafting. In such a case, the endothelial failure is secondary to the immunological processs, which affects the whole of the cornea. It is for this reason that we give an immuno-suppressor treatment, which is above all indicated in the cases of vascularis-ed corneas and repeated surgery. A perfectly viable endothelium, however, will reduce the risk of failure.

Let us recall that the rejection of a graft is an immunological phenomenon of the cellular type, depending upon clones of immunocompetent lympho-cytes, which explains why the reaction is late.

4. The reappearance in the graft of a pre-existing disorder of the receiving

163

cornea, such as Fuchs' endothelial dystrophy or macular dystrophy of the cornea. In such cases, one can:

a) Perform a trephination of such a diameter that nearly all the lesions visible at the biomicroscope are eliminated.

b) Use a graft of which the endothelium is 100% viable.

With regard to the condition of the endothelial mosaic, the result at the specular microscope is different, depending upon the previous condition of the endothelium. Thus, in a case of bilateral Fuchs' dystrophy, in which we have grafted corneas of which the endothelium was 100% viable, we observed after two years that the mosaic of the left eye, the more affected, was expanded, whereas that of the right eye was less so, although more than normally (Fig. 10). We attribute that phenomenon to the fact that the viable cells of the donor stretch out peripherically in order to cover the ring of the receiving cornea, the endothelial cells of which are degenerating. The larger the number of pathological cells, the larger the area to be covered and the greater will be the expanding of the donor's endothelial cells.

In the case of keratoconus or of any other corneal disorder without any endothelial alteration, corneal graftings are generally successful. That is why we have not closely studied the endothelial mosaic in those cases. We may nevertheless say that, in cases of keratoconus operated on after control of the endothelial viability of the donor, the endothelial mosaic was normal after the operation. The expanding of the endothelial cells was, however, more marked when the endothelium of the graft had a lesser viability. It may be that if the donor's endothelium were not completely viable, the endothelium of the receiver would have to expand in order to cover the donor's non-viable areas, with the result that the endothelial mosaic would appear expanded at the specular microscope. Thus the control of the endothelium is useful also in the favourable cases, because a good viability of the latter gives a mosaic with less expanded and smaller cells. It must not be forgotten, indeed, that the replacement of the endothelial cells occurs by creeping and expanding of the cells that are still viable, and not by mitosis, except in childhood. That is why the rabbit is a bad animal for experiments, if we want to study the corneal endothelium, because in that animal the endothelial cells divide by mitosis.

In any case, our results show indisputably that it is indispensable to verify the endothelial viability of the corneal graft.

SUMMARY

It is indispensable to verify the endothelial viability of the corneal graft that is to be transplanted. In a series of forty graftings without such control, we had a quasi-immediate oedema with subsequent opacification of the graft in 17.5% of the cases, whereas in a series of forty graftings with control, we had no one single case of corneal oedema during the two first postoperative weeks.

REFERENCES

Bonting, J. Studies on sodium-potassium-activated adenosintriphosphatase. I. Quantitative distribution in several tissues of the cat. *Arch. Biochem. Biophy.* 95: *416–420*, (1961).

Davson, H. The hydration of the cornea. *Biochem. J.* 59: *24–28*, (1955).

Dickstein, S. & D.M. Maurice. The metabolic basis of the fluid pump in the cornea. *J. Physiol.* (London) 221: *99*, (1972).

Green, K. Ion transport in isolated cornea of the rabbit. *Amer. J. Physiol.* 209: *1311–1316*, (1965).

Harris, J.E. Current thoughts on the maintenance of corneal hydratation 'in vivo'. *Arch. Ophthal.* (Chicago) 78: *126–132*, (1967).

Hedbys, B.O., S. Mishima & D.M. Maurice. The inhibition pressure of the corneal stroma. *Exp. Eye Res.* 2: *99–111*, (1963).

Hedbys, B.O. & S. Mishima. The thickness-hydration relationship of the cornea. *Exp. Eye Res.* 5: *221–230*, (1966).

Leuenberger, P.M. Morphologie fonctionnelle de la cornée. *Adv. Ophthal.* 35: *94–166*, (1978).

Malbran, E., R. Fernandez-Meijide & V. Victoria-Troncoso. Estudios sobre la viabilidad del endotelio corneal. *Arch. Oftal.* (Buenos Aires) 4: *143–152*, (1970).

Maurice, D.M. The cornea and sclera. In Davson's: The eye, vol. 1, pp. 289–368, Academic Press, N.Y./London, 1962.

Maurice, D.M. & M.V. Riley. The cornea. In Graymore's: Biochemistry of the eye, Academic Press, New York, 1970.

Author's address:
Ophthalmological Clinic
University of Ghent
De Pintelaan, 135,
B-9000 Gent
Belgium.

ENDOTHELIAL CELL LOSS DURING PENETRATING KERATOPLASTY

WILLIAM M. BOURNE

(Rochester, Minnesota, U.S.A.)

The specular microscope was first described by Maurice (Maurice, 1968) in 1968 for viewing the endothelium of the intact cornea in vitro. The instrument has been subsequently changed (Laing *et al.*, 1975; Bourne and Kaufman 1976) in order to develop a microscope that can be used in the routine examination of the corneal endothelium. In 1976, the objective lens of the specular microscope was modified to obtain a long working distance of 9 mm. A specialized corneal storage container was used that allows a view of the endothelium of donor corneas before their transplantation (Bourne, 1976). This technique of donor examination has enabled efficient screening of donor corneal tissue for subtle endothelial abnormalities. In addition, a comparison may be made with the appearance of the donor endothelium after its transplantation, thus allowing an estimate of the endothelial damage that occurred at keratoplasty. Because most damaged endothelial cells in humans are not replaced by cell division, but rather the endothelium heals by enlargement of the remaining cells (Bourne *et al.*, 1976), an estimate of the cell loss from keratoplasty can be made by comparing the average number of central endothelial cells per square millimeter in the donor cornea before and after its transplantation.

I studied the endothelium of 27 consecutive clear penetrating corneal transplants before and after transplantation. Examination of all donor corneas was performed before keratoplasty by use of the special corneal storage container in which the cornea was kept in McCarey-Kaufman medium (McCarey and Kaufman, 1974) at 4° C. The endothelium of these donor coreas was observed with the modified specular microscope without opening the storage container. The donor corneas were stored in the McCarey-Kaufman medium for periods ranging from 6 to 63 hours (Mean 37 hours). Several corneas were refused as donors on the basis of their specular microscopic pattern alone.

The transplanted corneas were examined with the clinical specular microscope within one week after keratoplasty. The central endothelial cell density was computed by counting the endothelial cells in three different photographic fields of known area from one cornea and averaging the results. The endothelial cell loss in percent was computed for each transplant by comparing the endothelial cell counts before and after keratoplasty. The reproducibility of the counting method was tested and found to be acceptable. Different variables were compared by either Spearman's rank correlation corrected for ties or the rank-sum test; $P < 0.05$ was considered to be statistically significant.

The mean endothelial cell loss that occurred during the 27 transplants was 23%. This was surprisingly low and less than the endothelial cells loss occurring during intraocular lens implantation reported recently (Forstot et al., 1977). The mean endothelial cell density for the 27 corneal transplants postoperatively was 2,152 cells/mm^2. This is also nearly double that of several previously reported series of endothelial cell counts in corneal transplants (Bron and Brown, 1974; Laing et al., 1976; Bourne and Kaufman, 1976). The low endothelial cell loss shown in this study may be due to improved surgical technique or better methods of donor tissue preservation (or both). The fact that fairly young donor tissue was used (mean age 34 years) also may have been a factor.

RESULTS

The results of the endothelial studies in all 27 patients showed a significant association between the presence of a lens postoperatively and the cell loss occurring at keratoplasty ($P < 0.01$). Thus, aphakic transplants (all eyes that were aphakic after transplantation) had significantly less endothelial cell loss from thekeratoplasty procedure than did phakic grafts. The cell loss in eyes that were aphakic before the procedure did not differ significantly from that in eyes undergoing combined penetrating keratoplasty and intracapsular cataract extraction.

The finding of less endothelial cell loss in aphakic corneal transplants is reasonable from a mechanical point of view and is possibly due to the deeper anterior chamber present during the operation, which causes less damage to the donor endothelial cells from rubbing against the recipient iris and lens. Supporting this explanation is the fact that the phakic transplant with the least cell loss (case 8) had an enlarged 15-mm cornea from congenital glaucoma. A 9-mm transplant was performed, and the postoperative depth of the anterior chamber was 4.0 mm, which is much deeper than the normal phakic anterior chamber depth of 3.2 mm (Tomlinson and Leighton, 1973). This finding of less endothelial cell loss in aphakic corneal transplants confirms the results of a comparison in two patients with mated donor corneas which were reported earlier (Bourne et al., 1976).

Because of the large difference in phakic and aphakic grafts, the two groups were analyzed separately. In the phakic transplants, less cell loss was associated with shorter death to enucleation times ($P = 0.05$). More endothelial cell damage occurs with longer exposure to postmortem aqueous humor, (Friedland and Forster, 1976; Breslin and Ng, 1976) and such corneas may be more susceptible to cell loss.

When the phakic and aphakic groups were separated, no significant association was demonstrated between endothelial cell loss and preoperative cell count, donor age, storage times, vitrectromy, or corneal thickness at the first postoperative week.

The preoperative cell count was related to donor age (younger donors more cells, $P < 0.01$). A similar correlation between age and endothelial cell density has been reported previously (Bourne and Kaufman, 1976; Laing *et al.*, 1976). Multiple regression analysis showed that the single most important variable affecting cell loss was the presence of a lens postoperatively (phakic versus aphakic). A second significant, but less important, factor was the graft size.

SUMMARY

I studies the central donor endothelium of 27 clear, penetrating corneal transplants with the specular microscope before and after keratoplasty (Bourne and O'Fallon, 1978). The donor corneas were examined first in vitro while they were immersed in McCarey-Kaufman preservation medium before transplantation. This preoperative examination proved to be valuable for screening donor corneas, several of which were not used on the basis of the specular microscopic appearance alone. I examined the donor endothelium, again within one week after keratoplasty and calculated the number of endothelial cells per square millimeter from photographs. The reproducibility of the counting method was acceptable. Comparison of the examinations before and after transplantation on each patient showed that, on the average, 23% of the donor endothelial cells were lost during keratoplasty. The 12 phakic transplants lost significantly more endothelial cells than did the 15 aphakic grafts (37% versus 12%). A possible explanation for the increased cell loss in phakic keratoplasties is the shallow anterior chamber present during the initial placement of the graft. Phakic grafts that were larger or had shorter time intervals between donor death and enucleation lost fewer cells.

REFERENCES

Bourne, W.M. Examination and photography of donor corneal endothelium. *Arch. Ophthalmol.* 94: *1799*, (1976).

Bourne, W.M. & H.E. Kaufman. Specular microscopy of human corneal endothelium in vivo. *Am. J. Ophthalmol.* 81: *319*, (1976).

Bourne, W.M. & H.E. Kaufman. The endothelium of clear corneal transplants. *Arch. Ophthalmol.* 94: *1730*, (1976).

Bourne, W.M., B.E. McCarey & H.E. Kaufman. Clinical specular microscopy. *Trans. Am. Acad. Ophthalmol. Otolaryngol.* 81: *743*, (1976).

Bourne, W.M. & W.M. O'Fallon. Endothelial cell loss during penetrating keratoplasty. *Amer. J. Ophthalmol.* 85: *760*, (1978).

Breslin, C.W. & W. Ng. The endothelial function of donor corneas: effects of delayed enucleation and refrigeration. *Invest. Ophthalmol.* 15: *732*, (1976).

Bron, A.J. & N.A.P. Brown. Endothelium of the corneal graft. *Trans. Ophthalmol. Soc. U.K.* 94: *863*, (1974).

Forstot, SL., W.L. Blackwell, N.S. Jaffe & H.E. Kaufman. The effect of intraocular lens implantation on the corneal endothelium. *Trans. Am. Acad. Ophthalmol. Otolaryngol.* 83: *195*, (1977).

Friedland, B.R. & R.K. Forster. Comparison of corneal storage in McCarey-Kaufman medium, moist chamber, or standard eye-bank conditions. *Invest. Ophthalmol.* 15: *143*, (1976).

Laing, R.A., M.M. Sandstrom, A.R. Berrospi & H.M. Leibowitz. Morphological changes in corneal endothelial cells after penetrating keratoplasty. *Am. J. Ophthalmol.* 82:

459, (1976).

Laing, R.A., M.M. Sandstrom, A.R. Berrospi & H.M. Leibowitz. Changes in the corneal endothelium as a function of ages,*Exp. Eye Res.* 22: *587*, (1976).

Laing, R.A., M.M. Sandstrom & H.M. Leibowitz. In vivo photomicrography of the corneal endothelium. *Arch. Ophthalmol.* 93: *103*, (1975).

Maurice, D.M.: Cellular membrane activity in the corneal endothelium of the intact eye. *Experientia* 24: *1094*, (1968).

McCarey, B.E. & H.E. Kaufman. Improved corneal storage. *Invest. Ophthalmol.* 13: *165*, (1974).

Author's address:
Department of Ophthalmology
Mayo Clinic
Rochester, Minnesota
U.S.A.

CHEMICAL BURN OF THE RABBIT CORNEA
MORPHOMETRIC STUDIES OF THE CORNEAL STROMA

Y. POULIQUEN, J.P. GIRAUD, M. HIRSCH,
G. RENARD, M. CORDOVA, M. SAVOLDELLI, AND O. MARQUET

(Paris, France)

ABSTRACT

In the rabbit, the corneal burn with a Na OH, 0,5 N solution lead to a diffuse but crowded and durable opacity of this cornea. The ultrastructural observation of this corneal stroma with time shows apparent changes in the fibrillar diameters, alterations of the centered hexagonal fibrillar stacking, with an increase of the interfibrillar distances or sometimes, an agglutination of neighbour fibrils.

But the quantitative study only allows a significant gathering of these facts and reveals that during the first 30 days, the homogeneity is preserved as for the mean fibrillar diameter : 300 ± 85 A (normal 300 ± b 50 A).

After the 30th day, the mean value remains approximately the same but with a standard deviation more than 2 times higher, showing an actual heterogeneity : 300 ± 200 A particularly in the anterior part of the cornea.

The interfibrillar distances inclusively, are generally greater than normally : 625 ± 200 A, specially during the three first weeks after the burn. However, there exist some zones where the normal fibrillar arrangement is maintained : 540 ± 100 A, even in the earliest stages. Some lakefree zones are observed.

At last, a small difference between the anterior and posterior parts of the injury is pointed out.

INTRODUCTION

The experimental burn of the rabbit cornea with a Na OH solution, forms a lasting corneal lesion, of variable intensity according to the caustic concentration. With a 0,15 N solution a lesion originally ulcerated was obtained which does not advance towards the perforation but towards a whitish durable scar, of the corneal stroma.

Somewhere else Renard *et al.* (1976) observed the epithelial and endothelial lesions with a scanning microscope. Our purpose here is to study the ultrastructural aspect of the corneal stroma and quantify the abnormalities during the first two months.

MATERIAL AND METHODS

We used albinos rabbits, New Zealanders, weighing approximately 2.5 Kgs.

The two eyes were burned and sampled at days 1, 3, 5, 12, 21, 30 and 60.

A choice was made between three Na OH concentrations: 0,25 N, 0,50 N and 0,75 N.

The 0,75 N — concentration was too aggressive (perforation), the 0,25 N concentration was too weak. The 0,50 N concentration was the most constantly, producing an opaque corneal lesion, lasting, evolving towards cicatrisation, without perforation, sometimes with an associated ocular hypertony.

The application of the Na OH, 0,50 N solution was performed by instillation with a one minute contact followed by an abundant rinsing with distilled water.

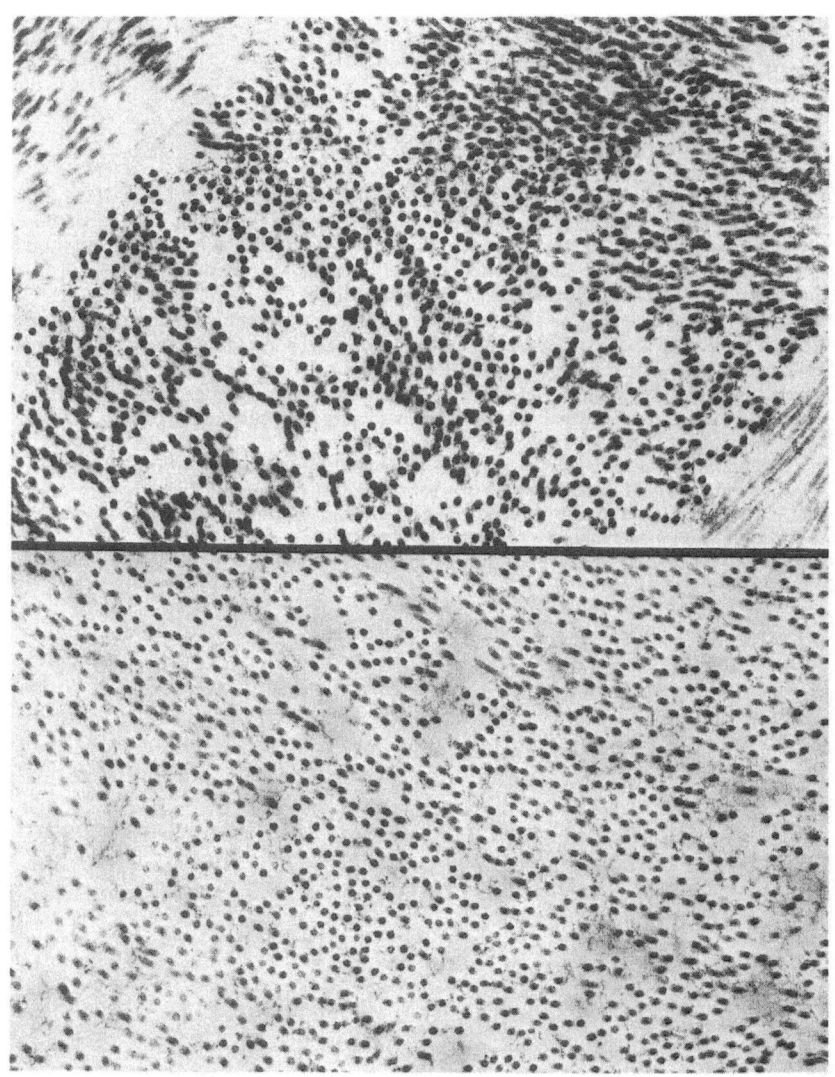

Fig. 1. (TEM x 34800) two aspects of the corneal stroma, first day after the burn. Interfibrillar spaces are increased. Fibrillar diameters are homogeneous.

The corneas quickly become opaques and remain so. They have been sampled at forecast days, fixed in 1,5% glutaraldehyde. Then, the central zone has been excised and maintained 1h 30 in glutaraldehyde and rinsed in PO_4 Buffer 0,1 M, pH 7,4.

A second fixation with Osmium tetraoxyde at 1% in PO_4 Buffer is still performed and finally embedded in Araldite-epon.

The blocks of the central zone of each cornea (4 mm) were cut with a Reichert ultramicrotome OMU2.

For each time delay, approximately 40 pictures were taken with the Electron-microscope, from epithelium to endothelium (x 20,520 Magnification) after calibration of the microscope Philips EM 300.

In average, 30 pictures out of 40 could be analyzed and measured for each delay.

The measured zones were determined by the fibrillar orientation in the slices: perpendicularly to their main axis even for grouped or dispersed fibrils. Their mean diameter and distances were measured (700–1000 for each picture) and the statistical studies performed as usual (Giraud et al., 1975).

RESULTS

1. Iconographic sights of the Burn following time (Figs. 1, 2 and 3).

The careful observation of the picture at different delays of the burn points out the following abnormalities. A dispersion of the fibrils in a fundamental substance clear and loose with an apparence of increased inter-

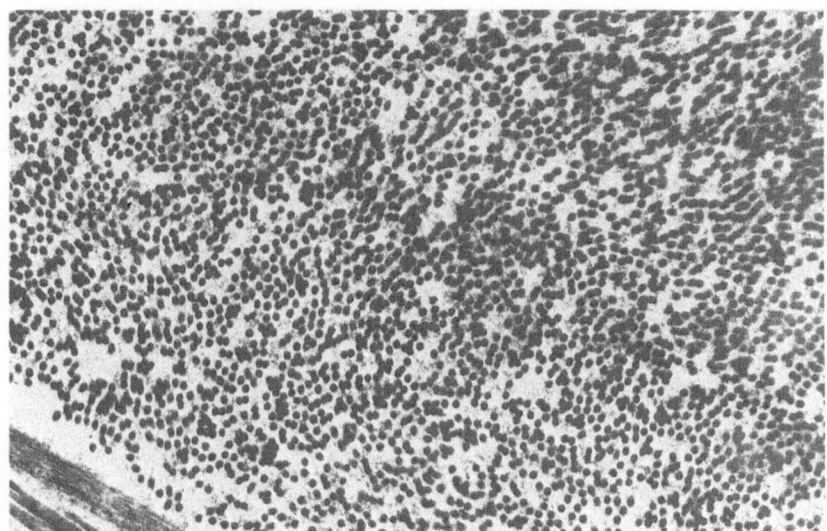

Fig. 2. (TEM x 34800) three days after the burn. Note the heterogeneous interfibrillar spaces and connected fibrils.

173

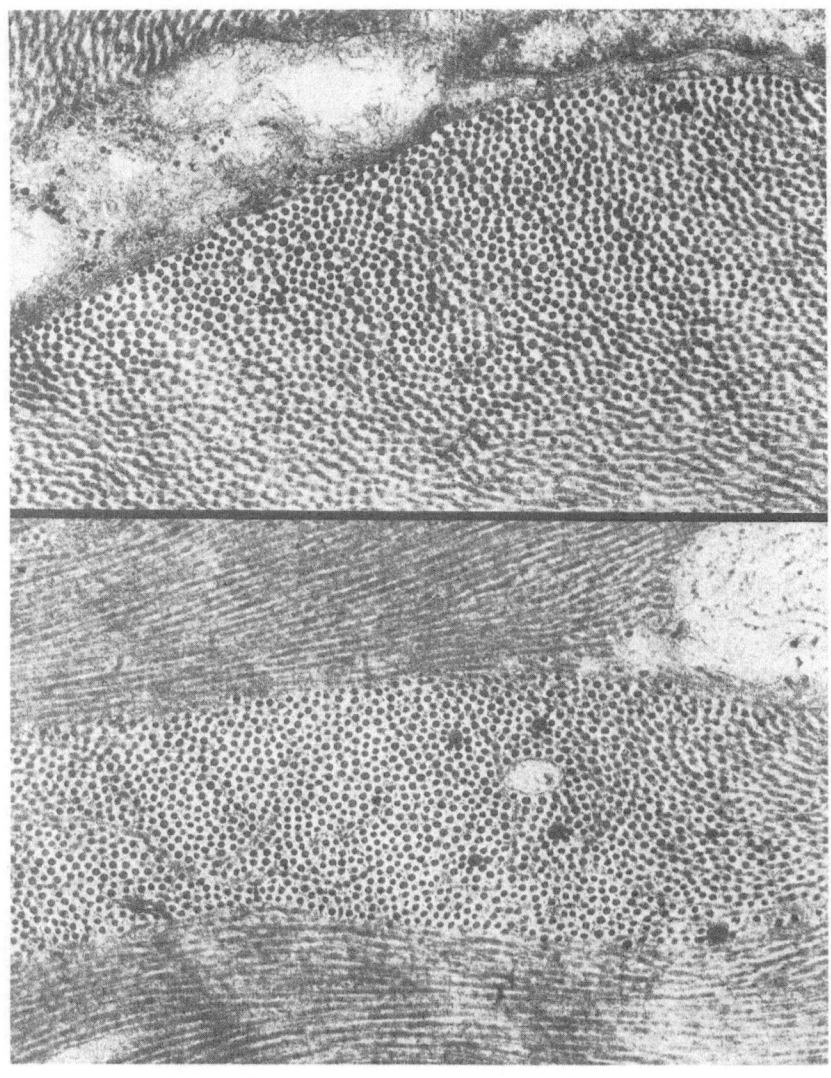

Fig. 3. (TEM x 34800) two aspects of the corneal stroma, one month after the burn. Interfibrillar spaces are more regular, diameters are heterogeneous. Note sometimes 'Rosette' disposition of the fibrils.

fibrillar distances, especially in the early times and sometimes real inter-fibrillar lakes. However, some zones have a normal appearance.

The mean fibrillar diameter is homogeneous in the early times. After the 30th day some heterogeneous fibrillar zones are stated and sometimes one can observe some fibrillar clustering (early and late times).

The differences between the anterior and posterior stroma zones do not appear to be evident.

2. Quantitative studies
A. Fibrillar diameters:
The linear regressions study does not show any variation of the mean fibrillar diameter with time and no difference is seen between anterior and posterior stroma, but the regression process is surely a deep smoothing one (Fig. 4).

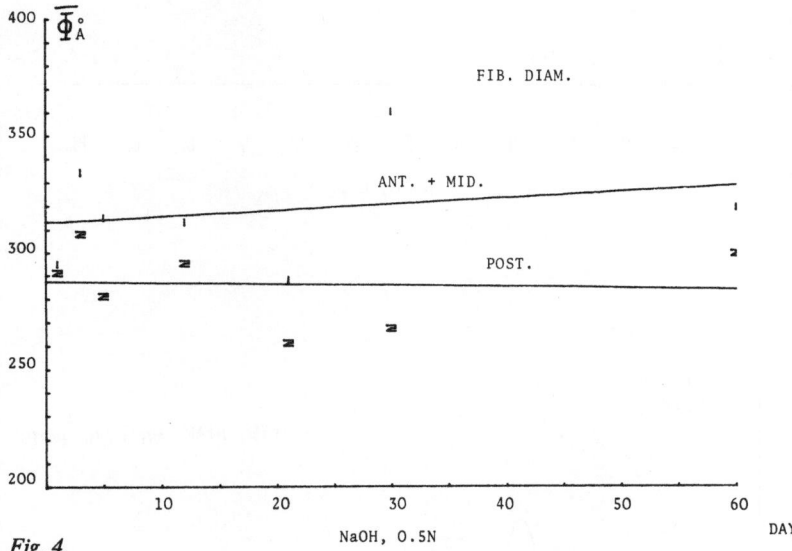

Fig. 4.

Therefore we have proceeded to a test against zero for each difference of the fibrillar diameter means of the anterior and posterior parts of the stroma for each delay (Fig. 5).

Except for D 1 and D 60, the stated difference is significantly different from zero at the 0.05 level for each time delay.

The fibrils in spite of some apparent desorder in diameter are always of approximately 300 Å. Only the standard deviation varies. Before D 21, it is 85 Å, 200 Å at D 30 for anterior and posterior zones, and 200 Å at D 60 for anterior stroma only (Figs. 6 and 7).

B. Interfibrillar distances
The linear regressions do not show again any difference for the interfibrillar distances (Fig. 8). Therefore whe have plotted their standard deviation for each time delay.

175

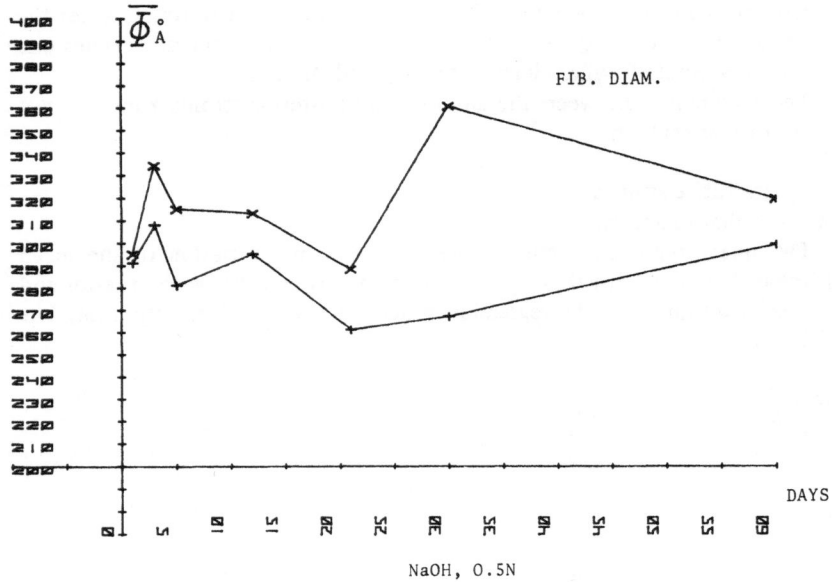

Fig. 5

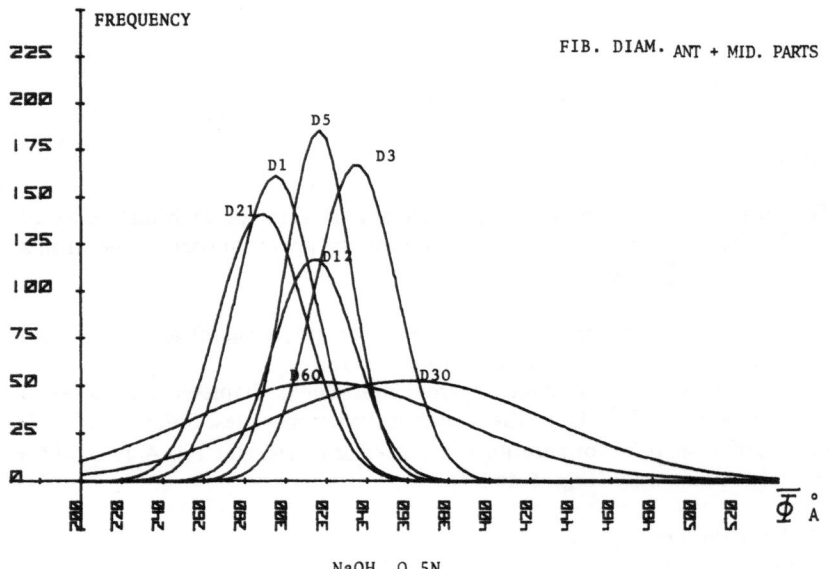

Fig. 6.

176

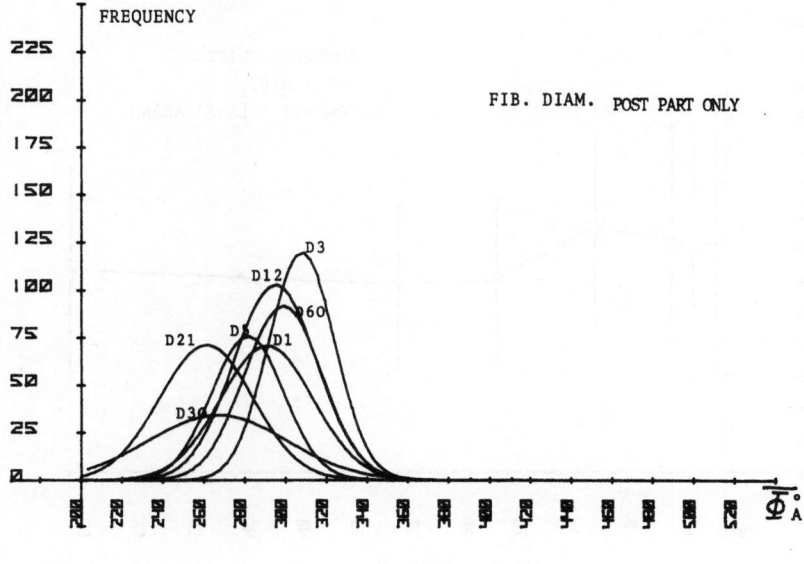

Fig. 7

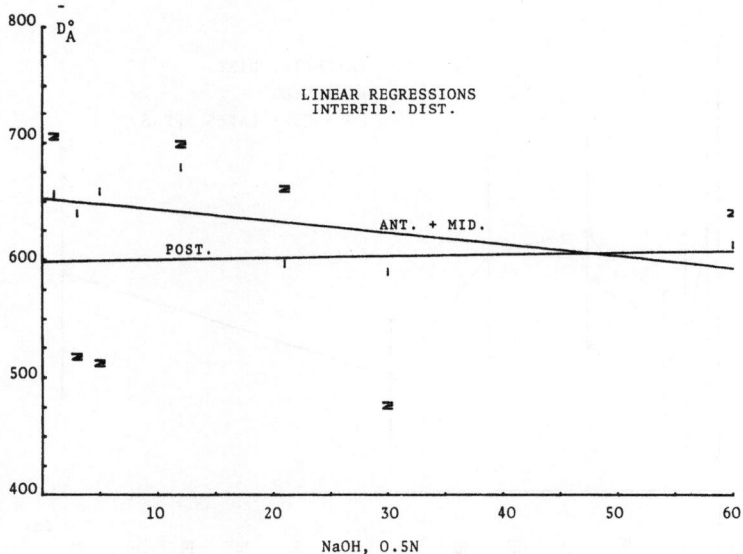

Fig. 8.

177

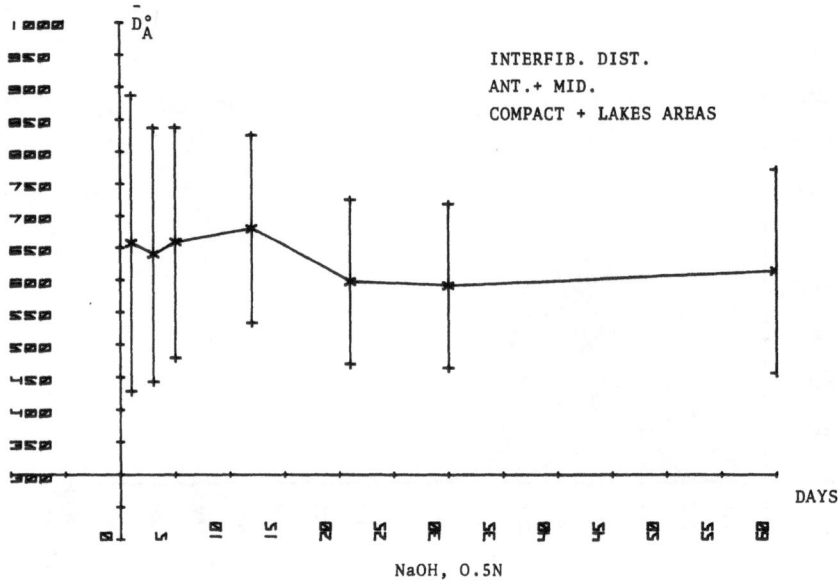

Fig. 9.

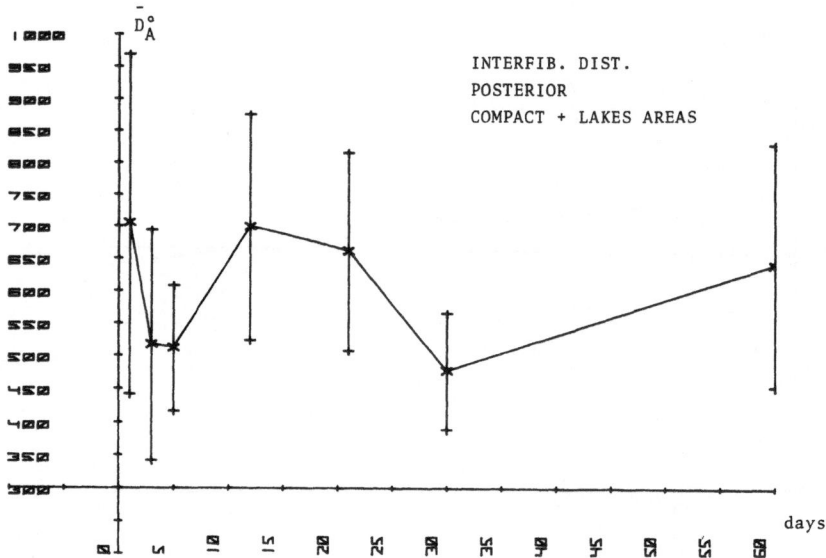

Fig. 10.

178

One observes tor the anterior stroma an average mean value approximately 625 Å with a standard deviation of 200 Å (Fig. 9). For the posterior stroma the mean-values are quasi similar but with a greater variability (Fig. 10). If one suppresses the lakes zones, one finds again the mean values and the standard deviation of the normal cornea (Fig. 11).

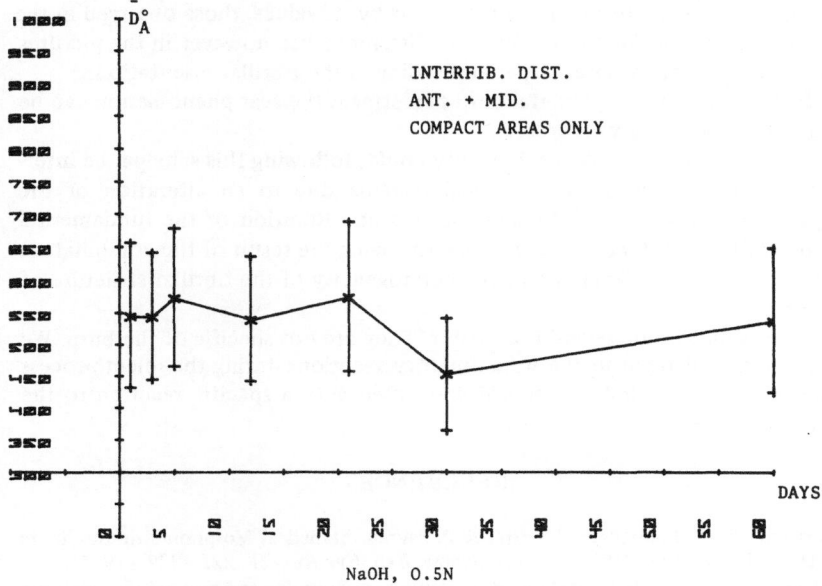

INTERFIB. DIST.
ANT. + MID.
COMPACT AREAS ONLY

DAYS

NaOH, 0.5N

Fig. 11.

DISCUSSION

In a diffuse corneal lesion, where one attempts to follow the evolution with time, it is impossible to restrict oneself to the subjective observation of the electron microscope pictures. The quantimetric analysis, at the contrary, produces a smoothing of the biological phenomenous. It states here only the trends of the fibrillar evolution and their distribution.

They are approximately homogeneously distributed in the anterior and posterior stroma.

They keep until D 21 a remarkable homogenicity in diameter. The mean diameter is normal with a standard deviation almost normal. On the other hand, the interfibrillar distance at this time is greater than during the following time delays.

However, the zones where the interfibrillar distances are greater than normal are mixed with the normal ones suggesting the existence of a phenomenon which, during the first three weeks fibrillar diameter, the standard deviation and determine a certain spacing between the fibrils whereas elsewhere he does not determine it.

It is probable that an interstitial oedema alone can be compatible with these observations.

A lytic action should lead certainly to a more complete modification of the fibrillar diameters.

Later on, the standard deviation of the mean fibrillar diameter is much greater. After D 30, it is 200 Å, pointing out the heterogeneity as being parallel with an increase of the interfibrillar distances.

This heterogeneity of the fibrils recalls by its values, those observed in the experimental scar of the rabbit. The difference lies however in the pictures which shows for the later a spatial puzzling in the fibrillar orientation.

In the type of experimental burn performed, the scar phenomenon can be considered as being well-ordered.

Then, the primitive corneal opacity could, following this schema, be interpreted as the result of a corneal oedema due to an alteration of the epithelium and the endothelium or also an alteration of the fundamental interfibrillar substance, the late opacity being the result of the combination of this residual oedema and of the heterogeneity of the fibrillar structure of the stroma.

It remains to understand the cluster. They are not specific of the burn. We have observed them in the inflammatory reactions during the reject process this let us think that we are not concerned with a specific reaction to the caustic applied.

REFERENCES

Giraud, J.P., Y. Pouliquen, G. Offret & P. Payrau. Statistical Morphometric Studies in Normal Human an Rabbit Corneal Stroma. *Exp. Eye Res.* 21: *221–229*, (1975).
Renard, G., M. Hirsch, O. Marquet & Y. Pouliquen. Scanning and transmission electron microscopic study of alkaliburned cornea. Association for Eye Research, 17th meeting Guilford 8–12 Sept., 1976.

Author's address:
Laboratoire de la Clinique Ophtalmologique de l'Hotel Dieu,
Place du Parvis Notre Dame,
75004 Paris,
France

Docum. Ophthal. Proc. Series, Vol. 20

ATYPICAL LATTICE DYSTROPHY OF THE CORNEA
A CLINICAL AND HISTOLOGICAL STUDY

ATSUSHI KANAI, MINORU TANAKA, TATSUO YAMAGUCHI
AND AKIRA NAKAJIMA

(Tokyo, Japan)

INTRODUCTION

Primary amyloid dystrophy of the cornea can be classified as both lattice dystrophy and gelatinous drop-like dystrophy. Many papers have been reported since Biber first described the lattice dystrophy of the cornea, which he called gitterige keratitits in three unrelated females in 1890. The lattice dystrophy is transmitted as autosomal dominant. On the other hand, the gelatinous drop-like dystrophy is being inherited recessively.

The clinical and histopathological study that we conducted in recent years revealed affected cases of the atypical lattice dystrophy in two unrelated pedigrees covering four generations.

CLINICAL STUDY

a. Family 'S'

The pedigree of family 'S' covering four generations is shown in Fig. 1. No consangunious marriage was found from this pedigree. Seventeen members were found to be affected and a further two reported to be affected. The youngest case who was available for examination was a four-year-old boy.

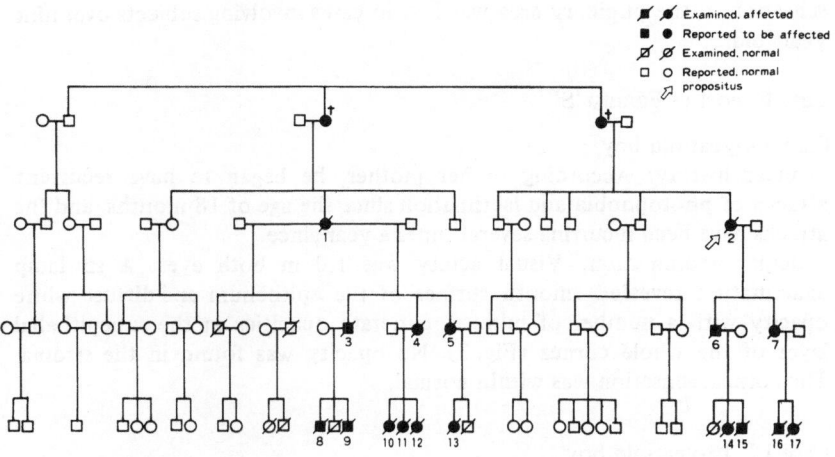

Fig. 1. Pedigree of family 'S'.

The eldest case was 75-year-old female in this family. Fig. 2 shows the summary of corneal alterations in seventeen affected members who were available for examination.

,Onset of corneal attack was between the age of 10 to 20 in elder group cases. However, for the third or fourth generation group, onset of these attacks were generally at a younger age. Seven affected cases involving four to 13-year-old showed that they were not suffering from lattice dystrophy, but from recurrent erosions of the cornea.

Case	Age	Sex	Onset of attack	V.A	Epithelial irregularity	Subepithelial opacity Diffuse	Subepithelial opacity ring form	Stromal linear opacity	Reduced corneal sensation
1	72	F	15	R 0.01 L 0.01	+	+	+	+	+
2	75	F	20	R 0.01 L 0.01	+	+	+	+	+
3	38	F	16	R 0.3 L 0.1	+	+	+	+	+
4	33	F	6	R 0.3 L 0.3	+	+	+	+	+
5	28	F	5	R 0.6 L 0.6	−	+	+	+	+
6	52	M	20	R 0.1 L 0.1	+	+	+	+	+
7	40	F	3	R 0.4 L 0.4	+	+	+	+	+
8	12	M	3	R 1.0 L 1.0	−	+	−	−	+
9	4	M	1.6	R 1.0 L 1.0	−	+	−	−	−
10	9	F	3	R 0.8 L 0.7	−	+	−	−	−
11	7	F	3	R 1.0 L 1.0	−	+	−	−	+
12	6	F	3	R 1.0 L 1.0	−	+	−	−	+
13	5	F	3	R 1.0 L 1.0	−	+	−	−	−
14	25	F	11	R 0.6 L 0.6	−	+	+	+	+
15	21	H	4	R 0.7 L 0.8	−	+	+	+	+
16	16	F	3	R 1.2 L 0.8	−	+	+	+	+
17	13	M	3	R 1.0 L 1.0	−	+	+	−	+

Fig. 2. Summary of corneal alterations in family 'S'.

Stromal linear opacities were found in cases involving subjects over 16 years old. Visual disturbance was noted at the end of the first decade, and visual acuity was found to be under 0.1 in cases of over fifth decade. Corneal sensation in the pupillary area was lost in cases involving subjects over nine years old.

Case Report in Family 'S'

Case 9 4-year-old boy.

Ocular history: According to her mother, he began to have recurrent attacks of photophobia and lacrimation since the age of 18 months, and the attacks have been recurring several times a year since.

Ocular examination: Visual acuity was 1.0 in both eyes. A slit-lamp examination revealed smooth surface of the epithelium and diffuse white opacity with a number of minute, punctate opacities in the subepithelial layer of the whole cornea (Fig. 3). No opacity was found in the stroma. The corneal sensation was within normal.

Case 17. 13-year-old boy.

Ocular history: According to her mother, he began to have attacks of red,

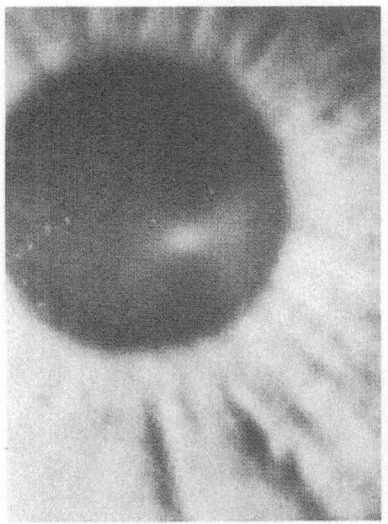

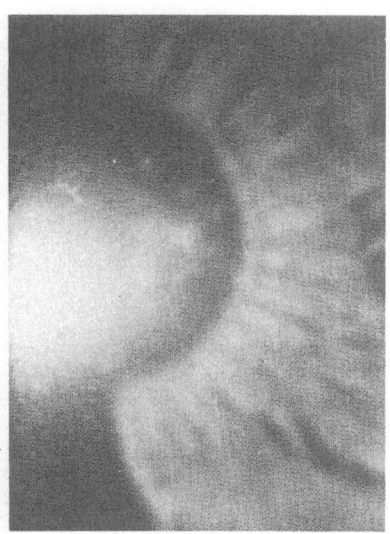

Fig. 3.   A slit-lamp photograph of
          Case 9 in family 'S'.

Fig. 4.   A slit-lamp photograph of
          Case 17 in family 'S'.

sore eyes at the age of three. These attacks recurred regularly at yearly
interval for five years.

Ocular examination: Visual acuity was 1.0 in both eyes. A slit-lamp
examination revealed smooth surface of the epithelium and diffuse white
opacity with minute, punctate opacities in the subepithelial layer of the
whole cornea. Several small ring opacities in the Bowman's membrane and
adjacent stroma were seen in pupillary area. Corneal sensation was reduced
in pupillary area (Fig. 4).

Case 14. 25-year-old female.
Ocular history: Her ocular attacks begat at the age of 10 and recurred
every two months until the age of 20. During the past few years before she
came to our clinic, her attacks of sore eyes had occurred only once or twice
a year.

Ocular examination: Visual acuity was 0.6 in the right eye and 0.5 in the
left eye. A slit-lamp examination revealed the smooth surface of corneal
epithelium and diffuse opacity in the subepithelial layer of the whole
cornea. Several dense small ring opacities appeared to involve both Bowman's membrane and adjacent stroma in the pupillary area. Fine translucent
dotted lines were found in the anterior third of the corneal stroma, except
in the peripheral limbus, by the retro-illumination of slit-lamp. The corneal
sensation was reduced in the pupillary area (Fig. 5).

Case 4. 33-year-old female.
Ocular history: She reported that her eyes began to have trouble when she
was about 17 years old, and that she had experienced short attacks of ocular

183

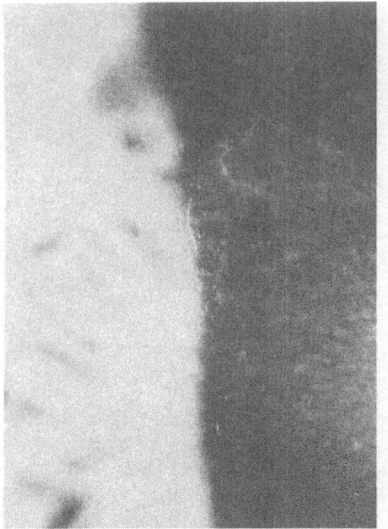
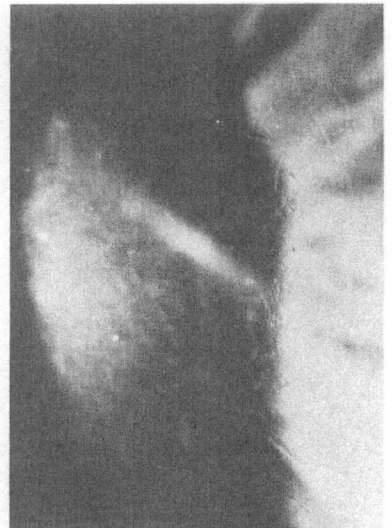

Fig. 5. A slit-lamp photograph of Case 14 in family 'S'.

Fig. 6. A slit-lamp photograph of Case 4 in family 'S'.

pain and lacrimation two or three times a year. These attacks stopped about five years ago.

Ocular examination: Visual acuity was 0.4 in both eyes. A slit-lamp examination revealed the irregular surface of corneal epithelium in the pupillary area, and diffuse opacity in the subepithelial layer of the whole cornea. Several dense ring opacities were present in both Bowman's membrane and adjacent stroma in the pupillary area. Network of fine translucent dotted lines with diffuse opacity were present in the all layers of the stroma (Fig. 6).

Case 2. 75-year-old female.

Ocular history: She began to have recurrent attacks of photophobia and lacrimation when she was 20 and noted blurred vision since she was 40.

Ocular examination: Visual acuity was 0.01 in the both eyes. A slit-lamp examination revealed rough surface of corneal epithelium with irregular thickness in the pupillary area. Fluorescein application produced no stain in both corneal surface. Diffuse opacity in the subepithelial layer of the whole cornea was present with several small dense macular opacities in pupillary area. Network of fine translucent dotted lines with ground-glass appearance was present in all layers of the stroma including peripheral limbus. Corneal sensation was lost in the peripheral limbus as well as in the central opacity area (Fig. 7).

b. Family 'O'

The pedigree of family 'O' covering four generations is shown in Fig. 8. Twenty-five were found to be affected and a further eight were reported to

184

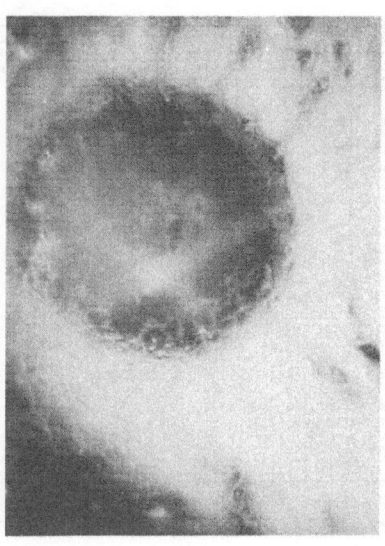

Fig. 7. A slit-lamp photograph of
Case 2 in family 'S'.

be affected. No consanguineous marriage was found from this pedigree. The
youngest case was a four-year-old and the eldest case was a 69-year-old.
Fig. 9 shows the summary of corneal alterations in 25 affected members.
Onset of corneal attack began at the age of 18 months in three cases. Ten
affected cases ranging from four to 12 years old were shown to be suffering
from corneal recurrent erosions. Stromal linear opacities were found in
subjects over 15 years old. Visual acuity was under 0.1 in cases of over
fourth decade. Corneal sensation in the pupillary area was lost in cases over
five years old.

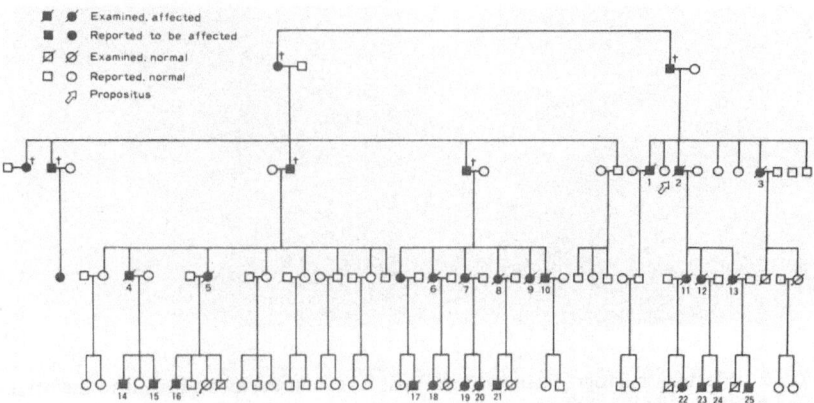

Fig. 8. Pedigree of family 'O'.

Case	Age	Sex	Onset of attack	V.A	Corneal alterations				Reduced corneal sensation
					Epithelial irregularity	Subepithelial opacity		Stromal linear opacity	
						Diffuse	ring form		
1	69	M	18	R 0.04, L 0.04	+	+	+	+	+
2	65	M	15	R 0.1, L 0.06	+	+	+	+	+
3	59	F	27	R 0.02, L 0.02	+	+	+	+	+
4	44	M	6	R 0.1, L 0.5	+	+	+	+	+
5	40	F	17	R 0.02, L 0.02	+	+	+	+	+
6	39	F	11	R 0.2, L 0.04	+	+	+	+	+
7	37	F	3	R 0.2, L 0.1	+	+	+	+	+
8	35	F	15	R 0.2, L 0.5	+	+	+	+	+
9	32	F	17	R 0.7, L 0.9	+	+	+	+	+
10	28	M	9	R 0.5, L 0.2	+	+	+	+	+
11	36	F	3	R 0.3, L 0.6	+	+	+	+	+
12	33	F	3	R 0.2, L 0.4	+	+	+	+	+
13	31	F	26	R 0.7, L 0.8	+	+	+	+	+
14	15	M	2.6	R 0.8, L 1.2	−	+	+	+	+
15	9	M	2	R 1.2, L 0.9	−	+	−	−	+
16	12	M	3	R 1.0, L 1.0	−	+	−	−	+
17	19	M	3	R 0.9, L 0.4	+	+	−	+	−
18	10	F	3	R 1.0, L 1.0	−	+	−	−	+
19	11	F	2	R 1.2, L 1.2	−	+	−	−	+
20	7	F	2	R 0.9, L 1.0	−	+	−	−	−
21	8	M	1.6	R 1.2, L 0.9	−	+	−	−	−
22	5	F	1.6	R 1.0, L 1.0	−	+	−	−	+
23	6	M	1.6	R 0.9, L 0.9	−	+	−	−	+
24	4	M	2		−	+	−	−	−
25	4	M	2		−	+	−	−	−

Fig. 9. Summary of corneal alterations in family 'O'.

HISTOPATHOLOGICAL STUDY

Six full thickness disc (Cases 1 and 2 in family 'S'; Case 2 and Case 5, both eyes of Case 3 in family 'O' and three lamellar discs (Case 10 and both eyes of Case 2 in family 'O') of corneal tissue were studied histochemically and electron microscopically. The sections stained with congo-red showed

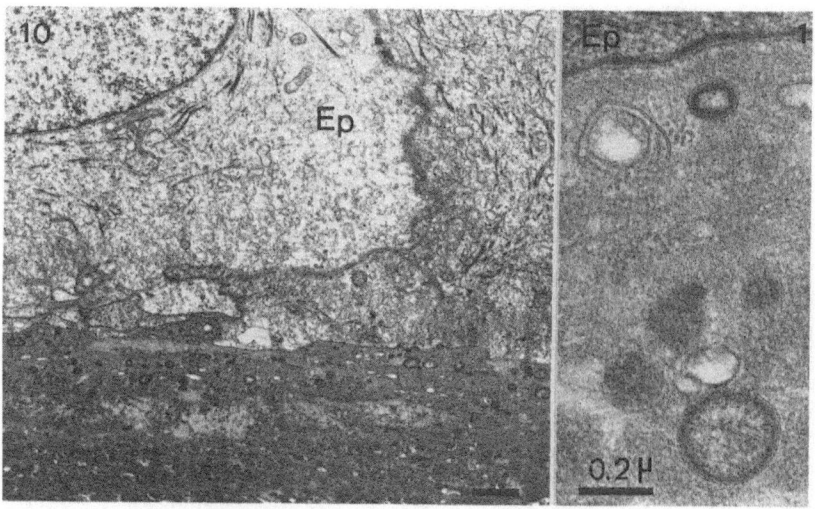

Fig. 10. Electron micrograph shows basal cells layer and the area adjacent to the basal cell. Ep: Basal cell (X 8,000).
Fig. 11. The area adjacent to the basal cell (Ep) shows dense substance with many cellular process-like materials (X 75,000).

186

positive staining in stromal lesions in all discs. Luxol fast blue stain was positive in subepithelial layer. No paticular alterations were observed in the epithelial cells. Different densities were found in the basal cell cytoplasm. These basal cells contained many small bundles of keratofibrils. The basement membrane was absent in some area (Fig. 10). The area adjacent to the basal epithelial cell contained dense substance about 4 μ in thickness with many cellular process-like material (Fig. 11). Altered Bowman's membrane was seen between dense substances. Fine dense fibrils were present in Bowman's membrane (Figs. 12, 13). The most characteristic figures in stromal lesion were small vacuoles and the irregular shaped, electron dense deposits which measure up to about 5 μ in diameter (Fig. 14). Electron dense deposits consisted of the accumulation of about 80–100Å and these fibrils revealed tubular structure. Multiple small vacuoles were present in the anterior stroma and scattered in the middle and posterior stroma (Figs. 15, 16). Some vacuoles contained dense substances. Dense fibrils were present around small vacuoles in some area. Vacuoles were also present adjacent to Descemet's membrane. Some vacuoles contained dense material. The Descemet's membrane and endothelial cell appeared normal (Fig. 17).

DISCUSSION

Many pedigrees of lattice dystrophy of the cornea have been published to demonstrate the dominant non-sex-linked transmission of this diseases (Freund, 1903; Hermann, 1946; Stansbury, 1948; Dark and Thomson,

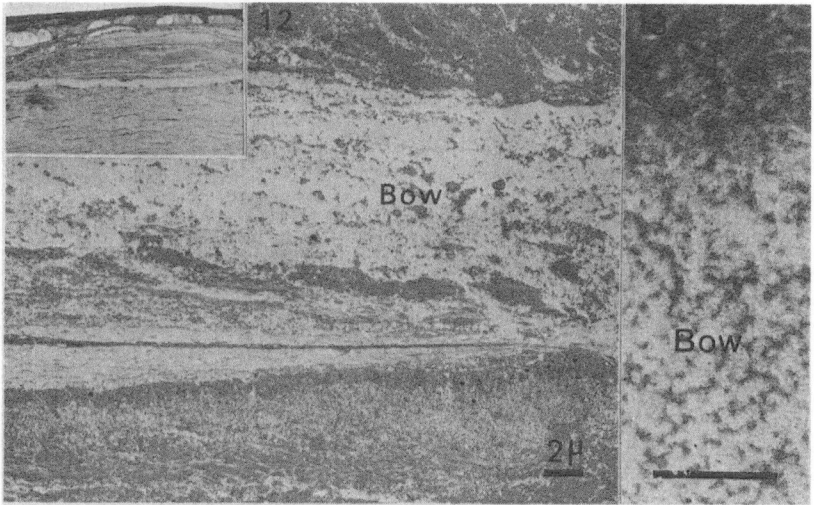

Fig. 12. Altered Bowman's membrane (Bow) is seen between dense substances (X 3,500). insert: Light microscopical section. Toluidin blue stain (X 25).
Fig. 13. Higher maginification of altered Bowman's membrane (Bow) shows the presence of dense fibrils (X 23,000).

1960). Nineteen members in family 'S' and 33 members in family 'O' were affected in four generations. The sex incidence was equal.

The clinical picture in these two families confirms that observed cases followed a uniform evolution of the corneal changes. Onset of corneal

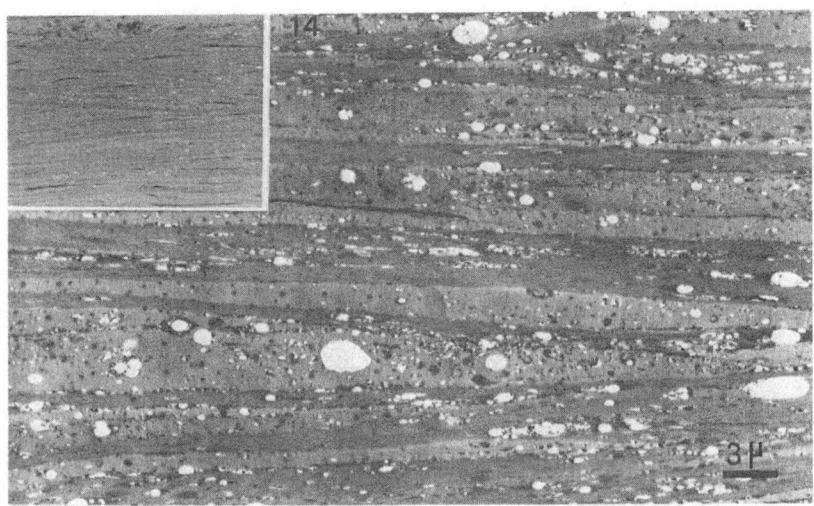

Fig. 14. Electron micrograph of the anterior stroma shows multiple small vacuoles (X 3,300). Insert: light microscopical section. Toluidin blue stain (X 40).

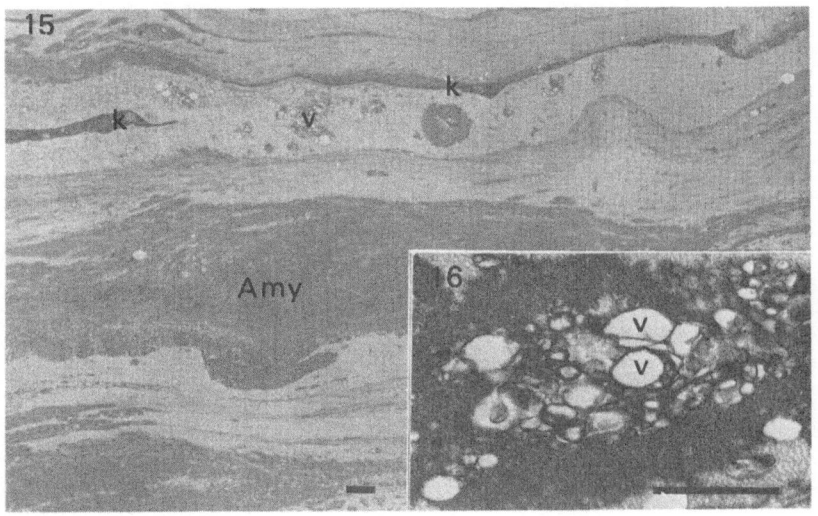

Fig. 15. The irregular shaped electron dense deposits (amy) are seen in the whole stroma. V: Vacuoles, K: keratocyte. (X 5,000).
Fig. 16. Amyloid fibrils are present around small vacuoles (V). (X 23,000).

attack was between the age of 10 to 20 in older cases. However, for the third or fourth generation groups, onset of these attacks first came as early as 18 months in three cases but generally at older but pre-kindergarden ages.

It is characterized that corneal symptoms begin as a type of recurrent erosions associated with photophobia and lacrimation. Diffuse opacity is present beneath the epithelial layer of whole cornea. While the cornea attacks are repeated, many minute punctate-form opacities and several small dense ring opacities are combined at the depth of Bowman's membrane. Corneal sensation in pupillary area is reduced at this stage in most cases. The recurrent attacks tend to become less frequent from this stage, and visual acuity begins to decrease progressively over the course of the disease. As corneal opacity of the pupillary area is increasing in the subepithelial layer, fine transculent dotted lines begin to be formed in the anterior third of the stroma, except in the peripheral limbus. This can be observed by the retro-illumination of a slit-lamp. In the terminal stage, irregular corneal surface is present in the pupillary area. Disciform opacity in the subepithelial layer reaches to the anterior stroma, and it combines with small dense macular opacities. Fine translucent dotted lines increase in number, and they are distributed in a reticular form in all layers of the stroma. At the same time, diffuse opacity also spreads throughout the anterior stroma. Corneal sensation is lost in the peripheral limbus as well as in the central opacity area (Fig. 18). Most cases are required to receive the lamellar or penetrating kera-toplasty.

The characteristic corneal feature of lattice dystrophy is linear opacities in the stroma. Linear opacities were found in cases involving subjects over 16

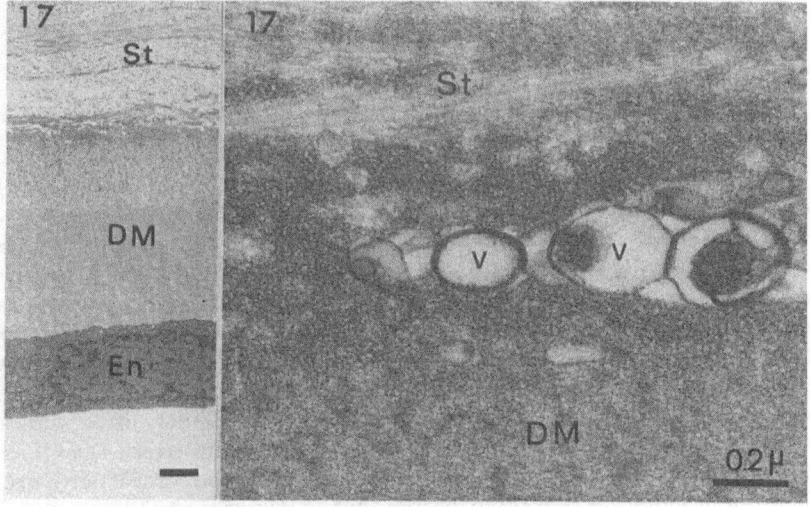

Fig. 17. Vacuoles are present adjacent to Descemet's membrane (DM) Some vacuoles contain dense material. The endothelial cell appears normal. St: stroma. (a: x 6,500, b: x 75,000).

Corneal changes in various stages

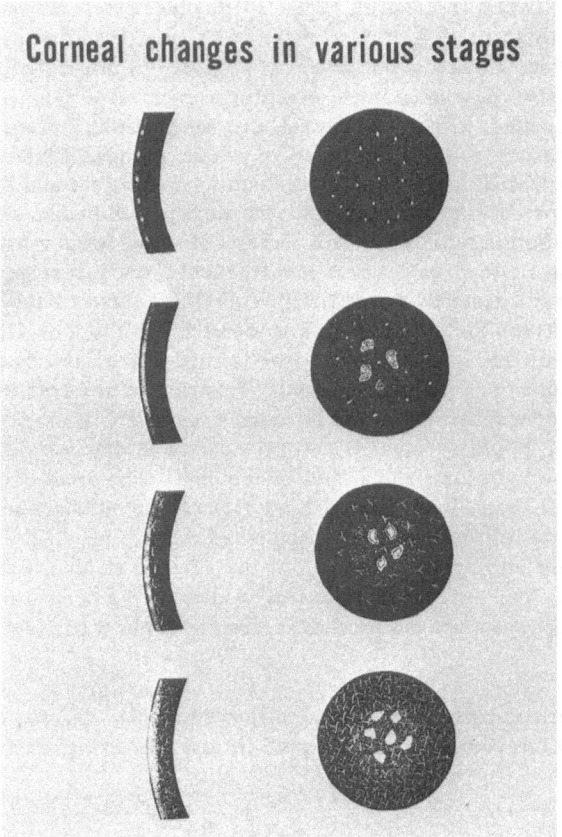

Fig. 18. The illustration shows each stage in corneal alterations of our present cases.

years old in family 'S' and 19 years old in family 'O'. Ramsay (1957) reported linear opacities were present as early as at the age of two years. Bucklers (1937) described the lattice lines, when cut in optical section, as optically empty channels outlined by fine bright edges giving a double-contoured appearance. Ramsay (1957) has noted that large lines contain fine granular material. In contrast to these descriptions, Dark and Thomson (1960) have mentioned that the lattice lines in optical section appeared as solid relucent trunks and have shown them to be fluorescent in ultraviolet light. Double-contoured relucent branching lines are found, often with a radial disposition, interlacing and overlapping at different levels. They form an irregular latticework resembling the arrangment of the corneal nerve net. The lines cannot be traced to be the limbus. On the other hand, linear opacities which we could observe from our cases showed different diameter and distribution compared with that of typical case. Fine small lines of reticular form in present cases show translucent double-contoured material

190

and are thinner than those of the typical ones. These small lines can be observed by the retro-illumination (Fig. 19). They are distributed throughout the stroma, including the limbus area.

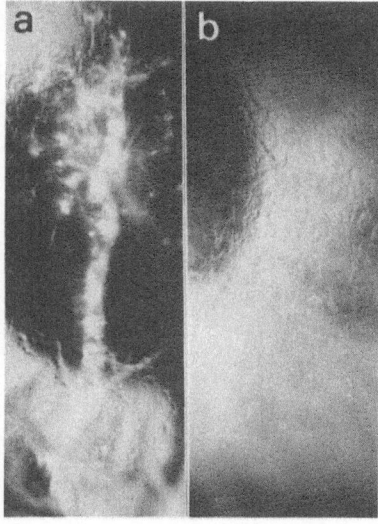

Fig. 19. Slit-lamp photographs of typical linear opacities (a) and atypical linear opacities in our cases (b).

SUMMARY

Pedigrees of two unrelated families suffering from atypical lattice dystrophy have been presented.
1. It is characterized in youth by frequent recurrent erosions of corneal epithelium.
2. Linear opacities in the stroma were found in cases involving subjects over 16 years old in family 'S' and over 15 years old in family 'O'.
3. Linear opacities are characterized as reticular form of fine translucent dotted lines in the whole stroma including the peripheral limbus.

REFERENCES

Biber, H. Uber einige seltense hornhauterkrankungen. Die oberflachliche gitterige keratitis. Inaugural Dissertation, pp. 35–42, Zurich, A. Diggelmann (1980).
Bucklers, M. The three forms of familial corneal degeneration and their hereditary transmission. *Arch. Ophth.* 18: *331*, (1937).
Dark, A.J. & D.S. Thomson. Lattice dystrophy of the cornea. A clinical and microscopic study. *Brit. J. Ophthal.* 44: *257* (1960).
Freund, H. Die gitterige hornhauttrubung. *Arch. of Ophth.* 57: *377* (1903).
Hermann, C. La dystrophie grillagee de la cornee. *Ophthalmologica* 112: *350* (1946).

Ramsay, R.M. Familial corneal dystrophy lattice type. *Trans. Amer. Ophthal. Soc.* 55: *701* (1957).

Stansbury, F.C. Lattice type of hereditary coreal degeneration. Report of five cases, including one of a child of two years. *Arch. Ophthal.* 40: *189* (1948).

Authors' address:
Department of Ophthalmology
Juntendo University
3-1-3 Hongo Bunkyo-Ku
Tokyo
Japan

MANAGEMENT OF KERATOCONUS

MOTOKAZU ITOI

(Kyoto, Japan)

INTRODUCTION

The incidence of keratoconus among Japanese people is roughly estimated at 1 in 10,000; since there are approximately 100 million people in Japan, this means there should be about 10,000 cases of keratoconus in Japan (Itoi *et al.*, 1974). About one tenth of this number have visited our clinic as new patients in the past five years, thus making our place one of the largest keratoconus centers in the world. This paper reports on our experience in the management of keratoconus.

KERATOCONUS AMONG JAPANESE

Japanese keratoconus (Itoi and Futenma, 1975; Itoi, 1976) is somewhat different from Caucasian keratoconus. About two thirds of Japanese keratoconus patients are male, while most Caucasian patients are female (Duke-Elder, 1965). About half of Japanese keratoconus patients have what we call an anterior-type keratoconus, which is similar to the form found in Caucasians; the remaining half, however, have what is called a posterior-type keratoconus, as shown in Figure 1. 97% of the anterior-type keratoconus cases have both eyes affected, while only 39% of the posterior-type are bilateral. Posterior-type keratoconus breaks out later than anterior-type keratoconus; it often appears after the age of 20, sometimes even after the age of 35.

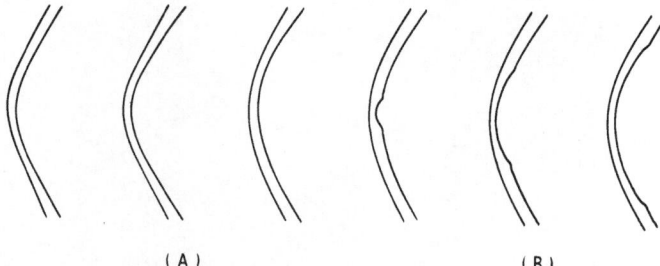

(A)   (B)

Fig. 1. Anterior-type Keratoconus (A) and Posterior-type Keratoconus (B).

The apex of the cone of posterior-type keratoconus is usually far from the pupillary area, as shown in Figure 2. It progresses faster and has a greater chance of Bowman's or Descemet's rupture than does the anterior type.

Besides anterior-type and posterior-type keratoconuses, there are atypical keratoconuses, as shown in Figure 3.

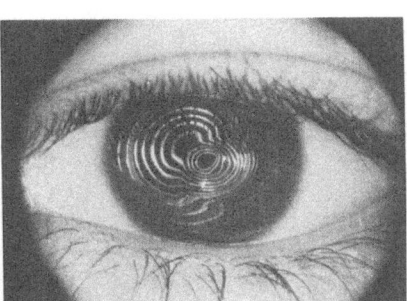

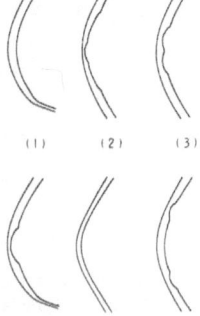

Fig. 2.
Fig. 3.

Fig. 2. Posterior-type keratoconus, the apex of the cone is far from the pupillary area.
Fig. 3. Keratoconus-like diseases: (1) (pellucid) marginal degeneration; (2) concentric double keratoconus; (3) double keratoconus; (4) posterior keratoconus with marginal degeneration; (5) keratoconus with thin cornea; (6) multiple keratoconus.

MANAGEMENT OF KERATOCONUS

When a keratoconus patient comes to our clinic, besides routine examinations, we perform photokeratometry, using the apparatus we have developed (Fig. 4). The photokeratometer can cover the whole cornea, from limbus to limbus, and from the photo taken by it, the corneal shape can be

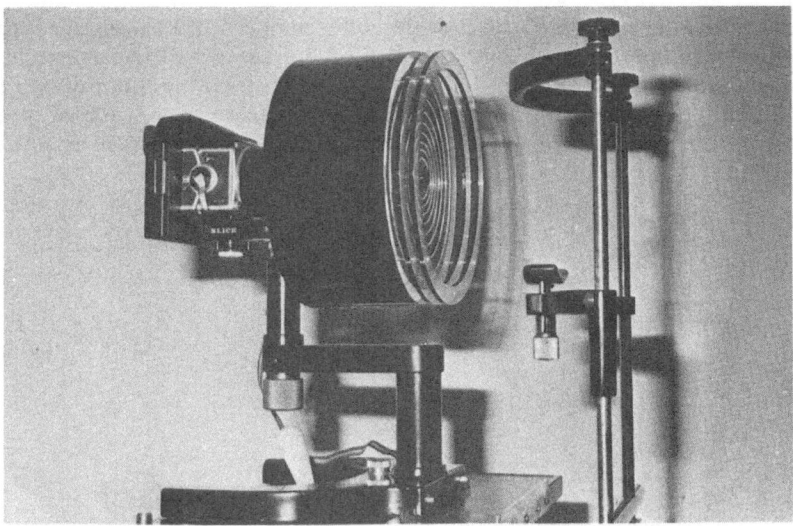

Fig. 4. The new photokeratometer which can cover the whole cornea, from limbus to limbus.

194

determined through the use of an automatic photoreader and a computer (Hewlett-Packard System 45). Figure 5 shows the corneal shape printed out by the computer (Itoi and Maruyama, in press).

Sometimes, in posterior-type keratoconus patients, visual acuity after contact-lens correction is less than expected from knowledge of the corneal condition alone. In these cases, we measure the contrast-sensitivity function (or the modulation-transfer function) with the apparatus we have developed (Fig. 6).

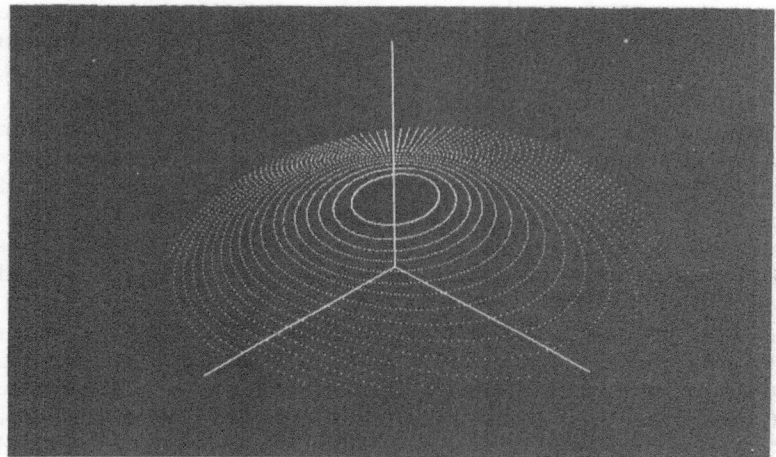

Fig. 5. The shape of the conical cornea printed out by the computer.

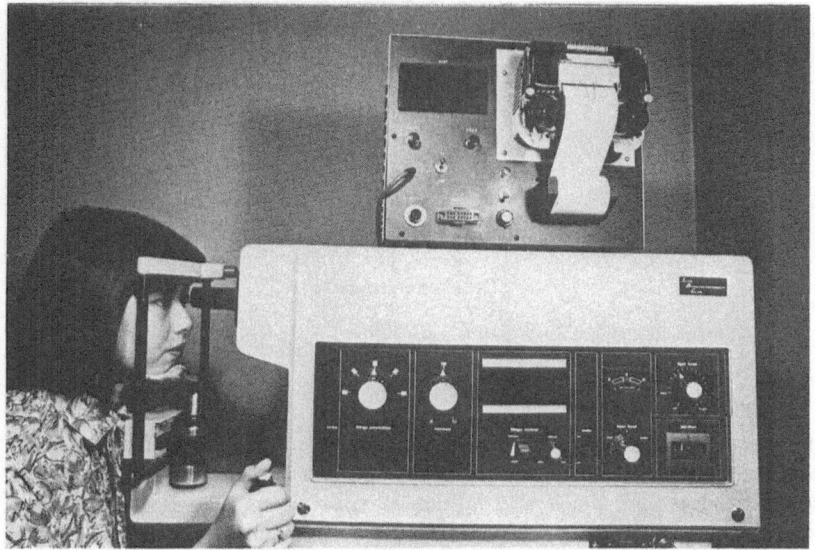

Fig. 6. Measurement of the contrast-sensitivity function using the apparatus we have developed.

Measurement of the contrast-sensitivity function can reveal valuable information about visual functions other than visual acuity (Itoi *et al.*, 1975). When the contrast-sensitivity function has an abnormal attenuation, there is a suppression of the visual function between the retina and the brain. When there is no attenuation of the contrast-sensitivity function, we seriously attempt again to fit contact lenses, and we have so far always succeeded in finally giving the patients good vision.

In general, neither soft contact lenses nor a combination of soft and hard lenses is satisfactory for Japanese keratoconus patients, because the apex of the cone is usually outside the pupillary area and thus, patients cannot see well because of the remaining astigmatism. Aspherical hard lenses are also unsatisfactory, because usually they do not fit over the center of the cornea, and the patient cannot see well through the small optical part of the lens.

One cannot expect good results with conventional hard spherical lenses on keratoconus patients. Therefore, the only way is to fit spherical hard lenses which are beveled specially for each patient. This beveling should be designed so as to fit the corneal shape and to facilitate the exchange of tear fluid. Usually, the lens is designed so as to touch at three points; in advanced cases of keratoconus, however, the lens is fitted by a two-point touching method (Nakayana *et al.*, 1978).

As shown in Table 1, out of the 1,583 keratoconus-affected eyes in our 900 new patients during the past five years, we were able to fit about 860 eyes directly with specially-beveled spherical lenses; another 450 eyes were able to be fitted with contact lenses after thermokeratoplasty. Thus, over 80% of these 1,583 eyes are now functioning well with individually-designed contact lenses.

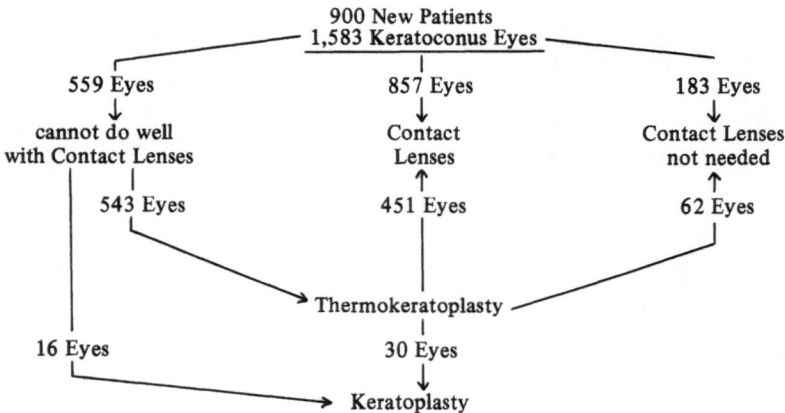

If the contact-lens-corrected visual acuity is over 20/30, and if the patient can wear contact lenses for more than 10 hours a day, we usually prescribe contact lenses and check the patient at intervals of 3 to 6 months afterwards. If the patient cannot do well with contact lenses, we suggest that he have thermokeratoplasty; only if the keratonconus is too advanced for thermokeratoplasty, do we suggest keratoplasty.

RATIONALE OF THERMOKERATOPLASTY

As mentioned above, it is assumed that there are about 10,000 keratoconus cases in Japan. We also assume that at least 6,000 keratoplasties would normally be indicated for these 10,000 cases. However, because of the shortage of eyes in Japanese eye-banks, only a small fraction of this number could actually receive keratoplasties.

This problem motivated our joint development of a thermokeratoplastic procedure with Drs. Gasset, Shaw, Kaufman, Sakimoto, and Ishii (1973). The original procedure was then modified by Futenma and myself (1973), and we have now treated 520 cases of keratoconus using our modified thermokeratoplastic procedure.

THERMOKERATOPLASTY

The cornea is composed of a framework of collagen fibrils, and if a collagen fibril is heated up gradually, it suddenly begins to shrink when a certain temperature, close to 70°C, is reached. Thus, if the corneal surface is heated to about 70°C, the cornea flattens because of the thermal shrinkage of the underlying collagen fibrils, but the cornea usually becomes opaque afterwards because of damage to the corneal cells in the process. However, if the corneal surface is heated up to 90°C for only one second, the corneal cell damage is reversible, and the cornea can be flattened without opacity resulting. As reported elsewhere, a thermokeratoplasty has been developed based on these facts for the treatment of keratoconus (Gasset *et al.*, 1973).

Figure 7 shows the apparatus for thermokeratoplasty, consisting of a heat

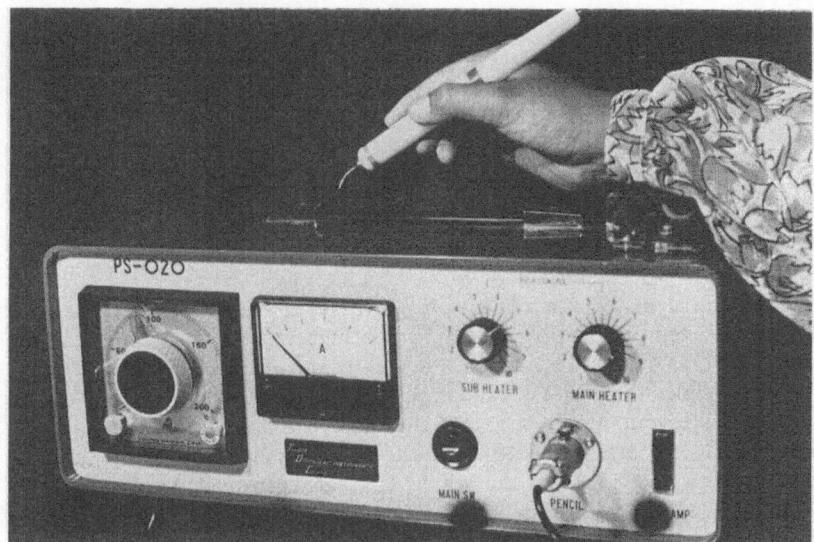

Fig. 7. The apparatus for thermokeratoplasty. The heat applicator's tip temperature is finely regulated by a servomechanism in the control box.

applicator, called a thermopencil, and its control box. The heat applicator's tip temperature is finely regulated by a servomechanism in the control box.

Before thermokeratoplasty is performed, the patient's eye is anaesthetized by a topical administration of 4% oxybuprocaine hydrochloride. Then, the patient's eye is irrigated with chilled saline solution for 10 minutes to lower the corneal temperature, thus minimizing thermal damage to the endothelium.

Usually, thermokeratoplasty is performed using a slitlamp, as shown in Figure 8. First, the localization of the apex of the cone is determined by slitlamp observation. Then, a gentle touch of extremely brief duration is made on the apex by the thermopencil, the tip of which should not be pressed against the cornea. After again bathing the corneal surface with cold saline solution, another gentle touch is made to the area next to that of the first touch. This procedure is repeated several times.

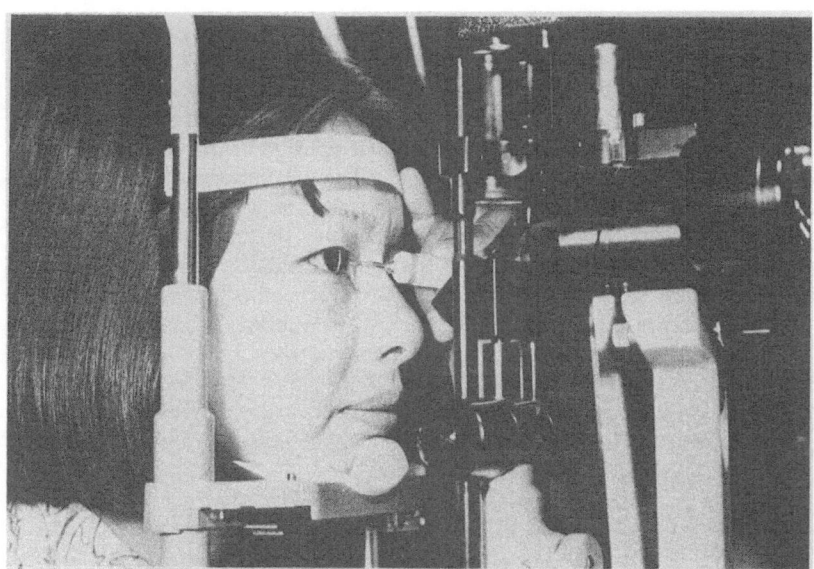

Fig. 8. Thermokeratoplasty is performed using a slitlamp.

When the apex of the cone is inside the pupillary area, the cornea is heated to a temperature of 75–85°C. The higher the temperature, and the larger the area of heat application, the greater the effect of flattening, but at the same time, there is a greater risk of corneal opaqueness. The key to success lies in our modification of the original thermokeratoplastic procedure which had attempted to make the corneal shape normal by applying heat at 100°C or more to the whole cone area. Instead, we aim only to remodel the cornea sufficiently for contact-lens fitting by using a lower temperature of around 80°C and by treating only the area around the conical apex. This is our major modification of the original thermokeratoplastic procedure.

After the operation, an antibiotic ointment is administered, and the patient wears an eye patch for 2 or 3 days until the epithelium of the treated area recovers, after which point the patient can wear contact lenses.

There have been no cases of infection, iritis, or corneal ulceration after thermokeratoplasty. The most serious complication has been corneal opaqueness, which usually does not take place in patients with not-too-advanced keratoconus if heat is applied according to the methods described above. However, in advanced keratoconus with a thin and/or scarred cornea, there is still some chance of corneal opaqueness.

After thermokeratoplasty, average visual acuity with contact-lens correction is about 0.8, or 20/25; in a patient with advanced keratoconus, it is 0.6, or 20/35. The chi square test shows a statistically significant difference in visual acuity between our patients who received thermokeratoplasty and those who were not treated (Itoi, 1978).

Thermokeratoplasty has several advantages over the usual keratoplasty: it is a simple procedure without serious complications and does not require a donor eye; the patient can start using a contact lens a few days afterwards. However, average visual acuity after thermokeratoplasty is a little less than that after keratoplasty, and in a few cases, thermokeratoplasty failed to stop the progress of the cone.

Thermokeratoplasty is a procedure which does not replace keratoplasty, but is to be tried before it. We tell patients who are waiting for keratoplasty that they can try thermokeratoplasty if they so wish, and if the result is satisfactory, they can then cancel their keratoplasty operations. If it is not, they can have keratoplasty as scheduled.

As shown in Table 1, out of 543 eyes receiving thermokeratoplasty, only 30 eyes required keratoplasty afterwards because of poor results.

RESULTS AND CONCLUSION

In the past five years, we have examined 900 new patients with 1,583 keratoconus eyes. Of these, 183 eyes did not require any treatment, 857 eyes could be managed just by contact lenses beveled specially for each patient, and 559 eyes required surgery. Thermokeratoplasty was tried first on 543 of the surgical cases, with keratoplasties given to the others. Of these 543 thermokeratoplasties, only 30 later required keratoplasty because of poor results.

We believe our experience justifies the conclusion that thermokeratoplasty should be the initial surgical treatment for keratoconus, with keratoplasty used only as a last resort.

REFERENCES

S. Duke-Elder, (ed). System of Ophthalmology, Vol VIII, p. 967. Henry Kimpton (1965).

A.R. Gasset, E.L. Shaw, H.E. Kaufman, M. Itoi, T. Sakimoto & Y. Ishii. *Trans. Amer. Acad. Ophthal. Otolaryng.* 77: 441–445 (1973).

M. Itoi. Keratoconus-Experience with 550 Cases. *Acta Soc. Ophthal. Jap.* 80: *952–931*, (1976).

M. Itoi. Thermokeratoplasty for the Treatment of Keratoconus-Experience with 500 Cases. *J. Clin. Ophthal.* (Japan) 32: *371–376* (1978).

M. Itoi and M. Futenma.. Thermokeratoplasty. *Ophthalmology (Japan)* 15: *935–940* (1973).

M. Itoi & M. Futenma. Anterior and Posterior-Type Keratoconus. *Acta Soc. Ophthal. Jap.* 79: *652–659* (1975).

M. Itoi, H. Kuribayashi & T. Yamaguchi. Thermokeratoplasty-Experience with 180 Cases.

M. Itoi and S. Maruyama. A New Photokeratometry System. *Folio Ophthal. Jap.,* to be published (1978).

M. Itoi, Y. Sugimachi, M. Futenma & H. Ohzu. Modulation Transfer Function in Patients with Corneal Disease.

C. Nakayama, H. Kuyama & M. Itoi. Contact Lens Fitting for Keratoconus Patients. Fourth International Medical Contact Lens Symposium, Kyoto, May, 1978.

Author's address:
Department of Ophthalmology
Kyoto Prefectural University of Medicine
Kyoto
Japan

Docum. Ophthal. Proc. Series, Vol. 20

OCULAR SURFACE EVALUATION*

RICHARD A. THOFT AND JUDITH FRIEND

(Boston, Mass., U.S.A.)

INTRODUCTION

Under normal circumstances, the island of corneal epithelium surrounded by the relatively great expanse of conjunctiva is self sufficient. It replicates itself weekly, deriving its nutrition from the aqueous humor. However, in cases where this island of cells is destroyed, as in chemical burns, repopulation of the corneal surface takes place from the surrounding conjunctiva. Previous work has demonstrated that conjunctival epithelium will transform histologically into corneal epithelium in 3 to 5 weeks, but that biochemical and functional transformation are considerably delayed (Friedenwald, 1951; Maumanee and Scholz, 1948; Thoft and Friend, 1977; Friend and Thoft, 1978). The glycogen content, lactate dehydrogenase (LDH) activity, and healing rates are less in conjunctivally derived corneal epithelium, as compared to normal corneal epithelium, for at least 6 weeks following regeneration of the corneal surface. In addition, chemical injury to the conjunctiva which serves as the source of the regenerating epithelium further retards the transformation of the cells, leading to a prolonged period of corneal surface vulnerability following total epithelial loss.

Since many chemical burns involve damage to the conjunctiva as well as to the cornea, it seems possible that this slow and incomplete transformation of conjunctival cells to corneal epithelial cells may be responsible in part for the notoriously bad prognosis associated with chemical burns. Not only do the initial injuries heal slowly, with inevitable scarring and vascularization, but subsequent attempts at keratoplasty are subject to the same healing problems. The use of healthy conjunctiva from eyes (Thoft, 1977) has been found to permit rapid resurfacing of chemically burned eyes, and has provided additional support for the proposal that the surface healing problems may be partially due to primary abnormality of cells derived from the injured conjunctiva. This thesis, which invokes a primary metabolic abnormality of the cells, rather than an unfavorable environmental influence on them, suggests that one should evaluate the ability of conjunctival cells to transform into corneal epithelial cells before they are called on to do so.

* This work was supported in part by Research Grant EY-01830, Program Project EY-00208, Institutional National Research Service Award EY-07018, and Biomedical Research Support Grant #PHS 5S07RR05527 from the National Eye Institute, National Institutes of Health; and in part by the Massachusetts Lion Eye Research Fund, Inc.

An example of deficient resurfacing is shown in the next figures. In Figure 1, one month after injury, modest scarring and epithelial irregularity, with vascularization are seen. Four months later, as seen in Figure 2, the

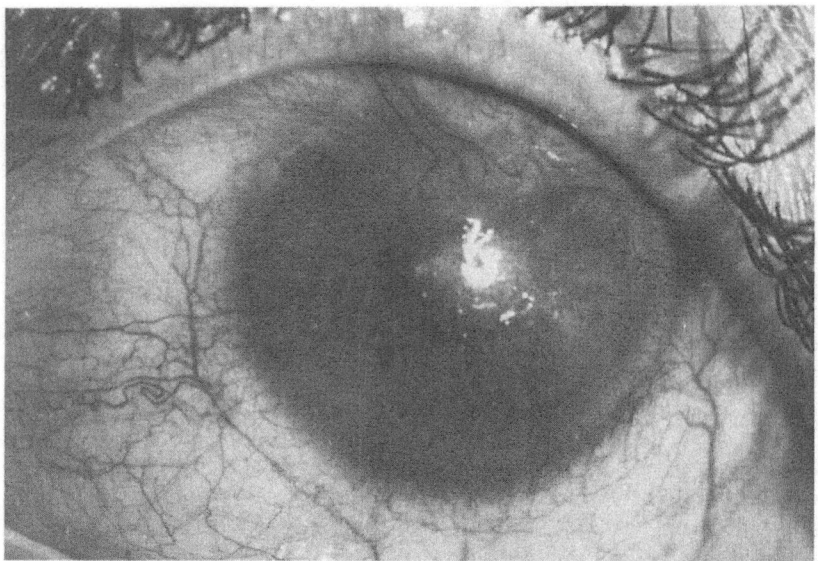

Fig. 1. One month after a chemical burn, surface shows modest scarring, some epithelial irregularity and mild vascularization.

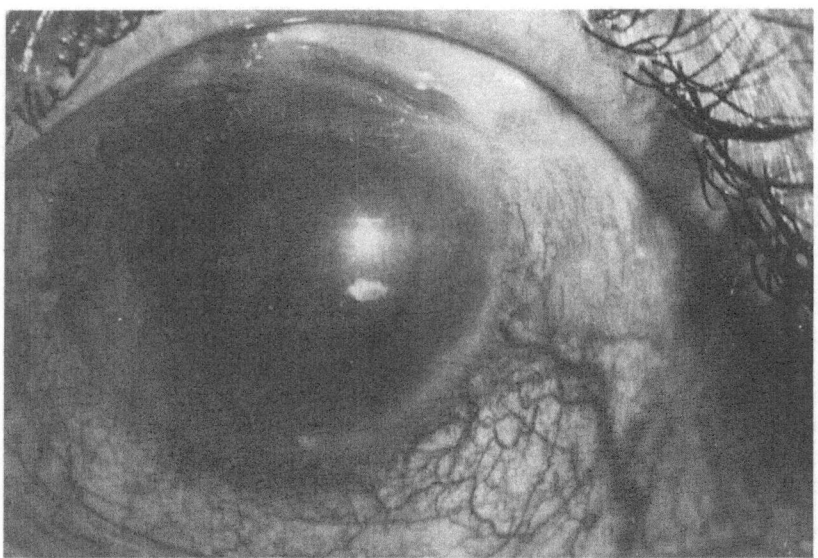

Fig. 2. Four months later, the same eye as shown in Figure 1, has more surface scarring and vascularization.

vascularization and surface scarring are more advanced. This inexorable superficial vascularization and scarring are optically troublesome. The use of topical corticosteroids to abort this vascularization has not been successful. Furthermore, chronic use of steroids increases the likelihood of infection, glaucoma, and cataract.

A secondary failure of normal resurfacing frequently occurs following keratoplasty after chemical injury. In the worst cases, the sequence of persistent epithelial defect, stromal ulceration, and possible perforation is all too familiar. This clinical course precludes the prolonged use of high dose corticosteroid therapy, leading to a very high incidence of immunologic graft reaction. A case of surface defect followed ultimately by graft failure is shown in the next Figures. Figure 3 shows the well apposed wound and smooth surface to a graft done 1 year after a thermal injury. Nine months later, the eye showed the characteristic epithelial defect which frequently develops in these cases (Fig. 4). In addition, regrowth of surface vessels is prominent. Despite all efforts, the defect persists, associated with stromal ulceration, making the continued use of corticosteroids quite hazardous. Finally, (Fig. 5) immunologic rejection leads to endothelial dysfunction, which when added to surface failure, results in a very unsatisfactory outcome.

'Surface graft failure' by itself, seemingly unrelated to any immunologic process in the epithelium or endothelium can also preclude useful vision following keratoplasty for chemical injury. In Figure 6, for example, an eye grafted for the second time following sulfur dioxide burns shows a satisfac-

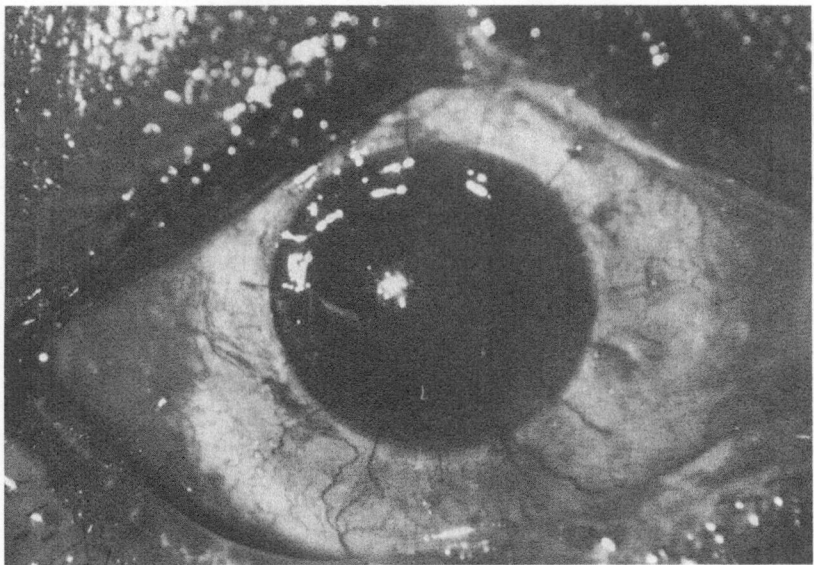

Fig. 3. Keratoplasty in an eye that had been thermally injured one year prior to the operation. The graft wound edges are well opposed and the surface smooth 2 weeks after the operation.

tory visual result. Slowly, however, progressive superficial vascularization and scarring occur without endothelial failure. After a total of 3 1/2 years

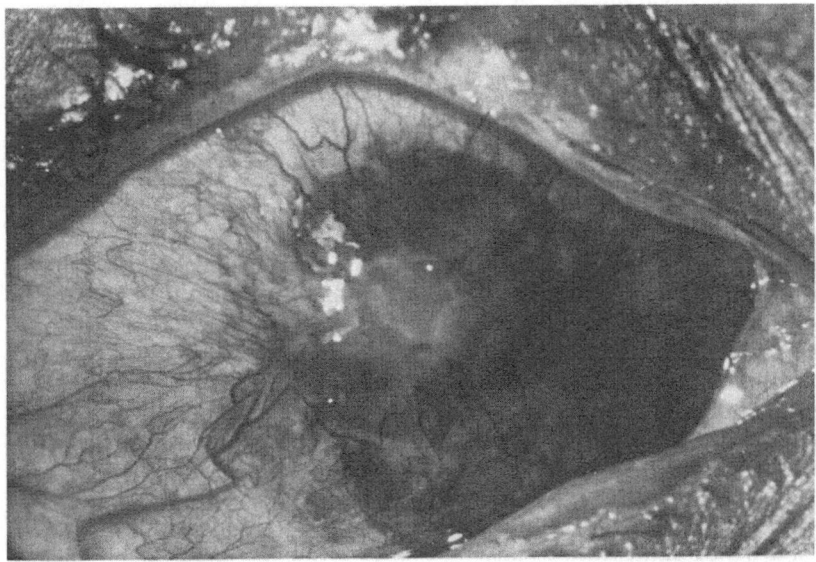

Fig. 4. Nine months later, the same eye as shown in Figure 3, had developed an epithelial defect and surface vascularization.

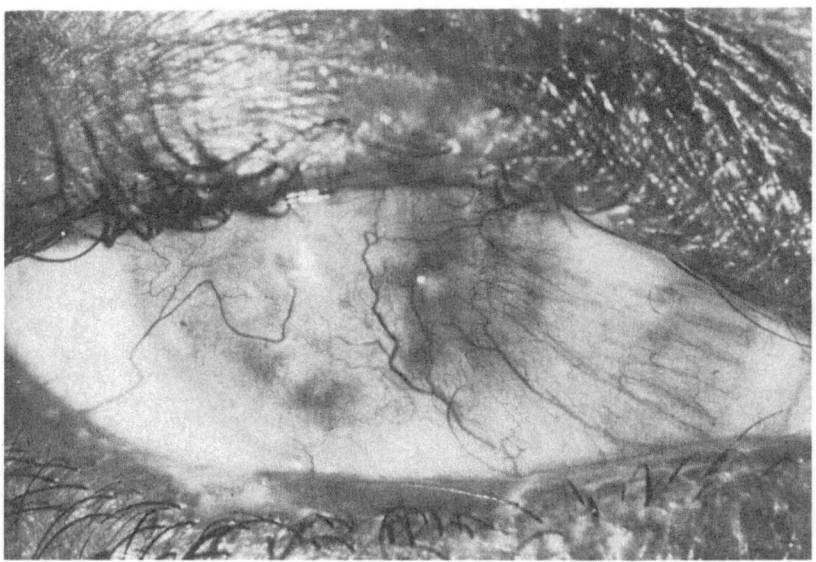

Fig. 5. One and one-half years later, the same eye as in Figures 3 and 4, underwent immunological rejection in addition to surface failure.

204

(Fig. 7), the vision in the eye has decreased so much that it is no longer adequate for ambulation. At the same time, however, the endothelium

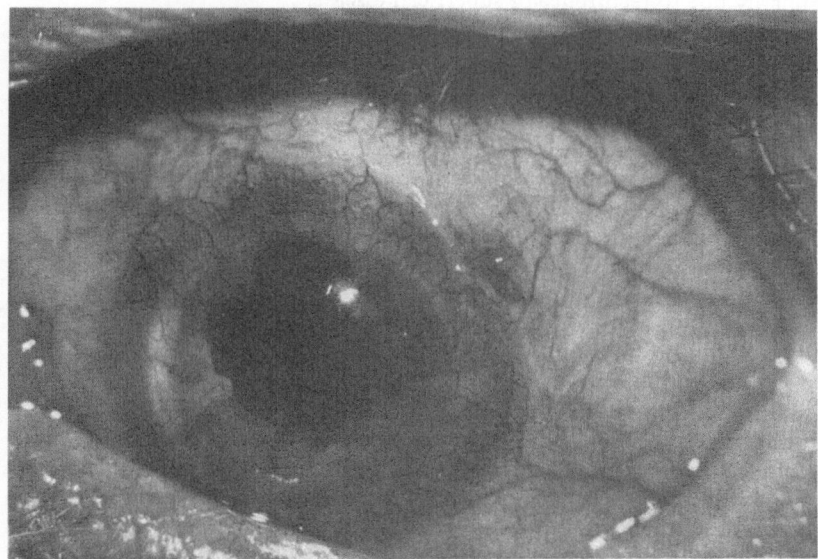

Fig. 6. A keratoplasty following a sulfur dioxide burn had satisfactory results for about 1 year.

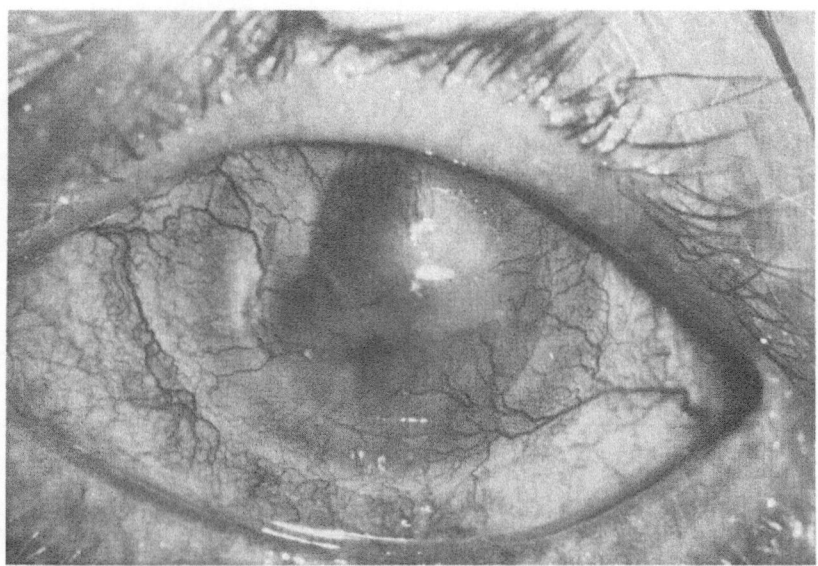

Fig. 7. Three and one-half years after the keratoplasty, the eye shown in Figure 6 had severe vascularization and scarring.

remains functioning, with no significant stromal edema. When a subsequent graft was done, histologic examination confirmed the presence of an intact endothelium in this particular cornea, indicating that the graft failure was primarily due to recurrence of superficial disease.

These experiences with inadequate resurfacing of the corneal surface by conjunctivally derived epithelium after chemical injury have led us to investigate methods by which we can identify, prior to surgery, those eyes whose conjunctival epithelium will be unlikely to make the usual transition from conjunctival to corneal cells.

By isolating conjunctiva, with subsequent incubation in nutrient media, we feel that we may have a technique which allows us to evaluate the viability and potential for replication and differentiation of this source of ocular surface cells. Since biopsies of conjunctiva are available clinically, such a method for evaluating ocular surface cells may be useful in patients.

METHODS

This method has been evolved using rabbit tissue. Sections of conjunctiva, approximately 6 mm in diameter, are removed and mounted on a three-prong holder (Fig. 8). This tissue is then immersed in 20 ml of incubation medium, which is TC-199 with Earle's salts and 25 mM Hepes buffer with l-glutamine. Rabbit serum is added to a final concentration of 20% in some of the incubations. To all samples, 500 U of penicillin and 500 mcg streptomycin are added. The medium is changed at 48 hour intervals. At various periods of time, histologic appearance, tritiated thymidine uptake, goblet cell counts and glycogen content are determined.

RESULTS

The results verify that incubation of isolated conjunctival samples maintains the viability of the epithelial cells for at least 48 hours. Regardless of the medium used, the histologic appearance of the cells is normal by light microscopy. By 72 hours, however, the epithelial layer begins to show loss of the normal architecture.

The mitotic activity of conjunctival epithelial cells shows a marked reduc-

Table 1. Mitotic activity in isolated conjunctival epithelium (tritiated thymidine-labelled cells per 100 epithelial cells).

Incubation Time	Without Serum	P*
1 hour	5.4 ± 0.5 (5)	
24 hours	1.5 ± 0.5 (4)	<0.005
48 hours	5.8 ± 1.9 (5)	
72 hours	1.6± 0.6 (7)	<0.005

*P values compare the number of labelled cells at 1 hour without serum to the 1 hour value and are given if $P < 0.005$ using the student T-test.

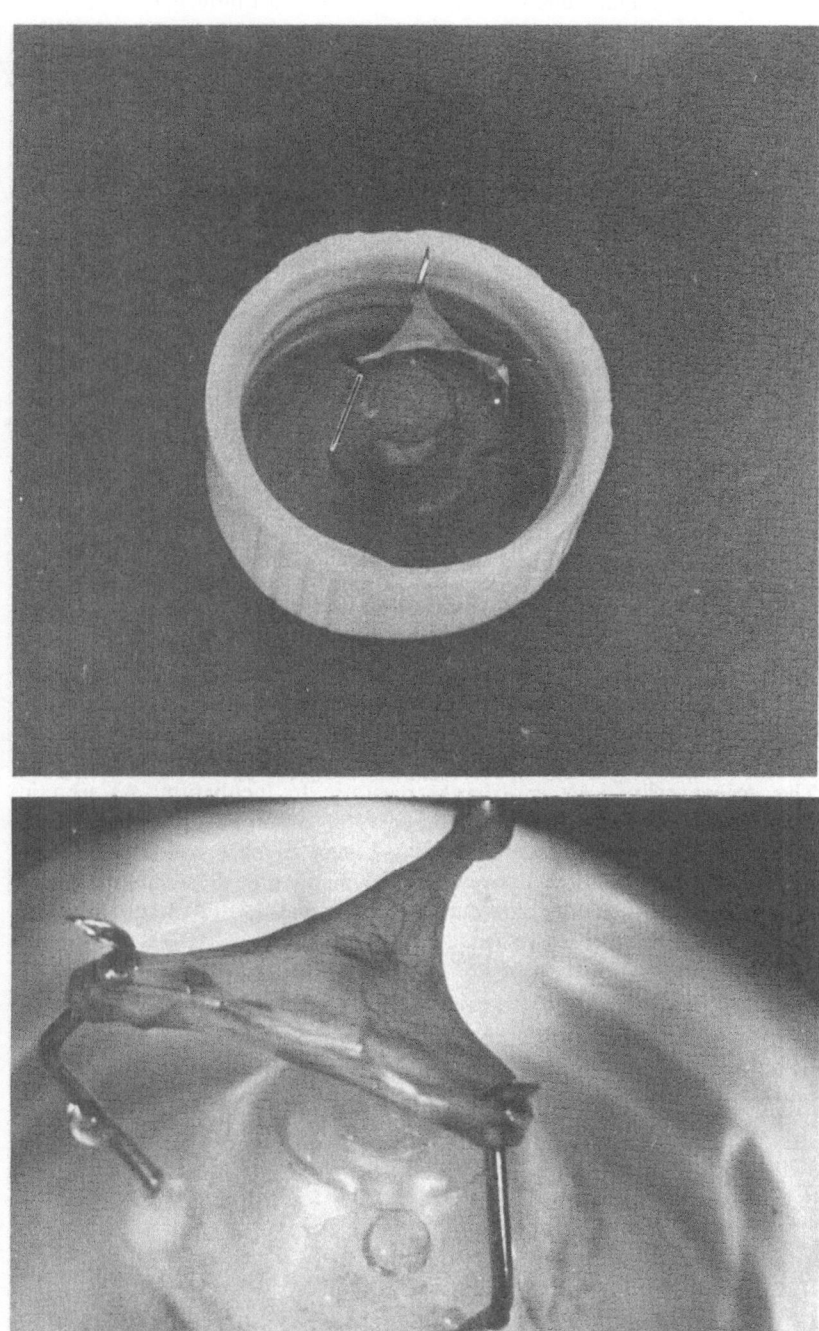

Fig. 8. Conjunctiva mounted on a 3-pronged holder for incubation.

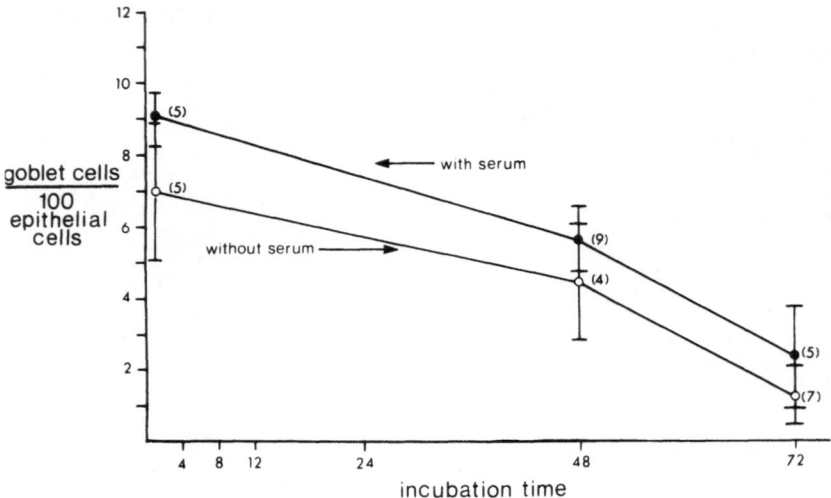

Fig. 9. Goblet cells in isolated conjunctival epithelium. The number of goblet cells per 100 epithelial cells, bracketed by the standard errors of the mean, is plotted against hours of incubation with and without serum in the medium.

tion in rate at 24 hours, followed by a resurgence of activity at 48 hours (Table 1). At 72 hours, the rate has fallen substantially again. The data in Table 1 show the results obtained in serumfree medium. The mitotic rates in serum-enriched medium were not significantly different.

The goblet cells show a different response to incubation. As seen in Figure 9, the number of goblet cells per 100 conjunctival epithelial cells drops significantly during the three day period of observation. No significant difference was noted between regular media and those enriched with the rabbit serum. At no point during the incubation did the conjunctival glycogen content increase (Table 2).

Table 2. Glycogen content of isolated conjunctiva.

	Glycogen (μM/gm dry weight)	P
Normal	8.8 ± 1.3 (7)	
Incubated		
48 hours	7.9 ± 1.8 (6)	NS
72 hours	10.7 ± 3.5 (5)	NS

DISCUSSION

By adding ^{3}H-thymidine to the incubation medium of our samples, it was possible to compare mitotic rates of samples subjected to different incubation techniques. Regardless of the medium used, the percent of cells showing mitotic activity is 5 to 6% for conjunctiva *in vitro*. Previous studies of normal corneal epithelium have shown a 0.4 to 1.3% of cells involved in mitotic activity at any one time, *in vivo* (Buschke *et al.*, 1943; Hanna and O'Brien, 1960). The rapid conjunctial epithelial cell turnover in isolated culture may not reflect the state found *in vivo*, but it is expected, nevertheless, that a comparision of rates obtained *in vitro* in various surface disease states will be of value.

Decreased goblet cell counts are found routinely in a number of diseases characterized by poor corneal epithelialization (Ralph, 1975) such as the dry eye conditions and Vitamin A deficiency.

It may be that the potential for differentiation into goblet cells, on the one hand, or into corneal epithelial cells, on the other hand, is lost when conjunctiva is primarily diseased or injured. The initial population of goblet cells in conjunctival samples, and the time course of goblet cell population changes in culture may then tell us something about the ease with which the bulk of conjunctival cells can make the complex biochemical transformation into corneal epithelial cells.

Even under circumstances which support the bulk of the conjunctival epithelial cells, as in the present experiments, the goblet cells seem to be more sensitive to the environment. Similarly, goblet cells disappear when conjunctiva is called upon to cover a defect in the conjunctiva itself, or when the conjunctiva begins to move across the denuded cornea (Friedenwald, 1951; Maumanee and Scholz, 1948). Only after the phase of sliding and mitosis is complete do goblet cells reappear. The stress of placing the tissue in culture may similarly turn off the mucus production, by which we recognize goblet cells histologically.

A second reason for the disappearance of goblet cells in culture may be more fundamentally related to the avascularity of this environment. In the case of re-epithelialization of the cornea from the conjunctiva, the reappearance of goblet cells after the initial closure of the defect is soon followed by permanent loss of goblet cells. The intriguing observation (Thoft *et al.*, 1979) that subsequent vascularization of a cornea covered by epithelium derived from conjunctiva causes a reappeareance of goblet cells has led us to believe that the presence of goblet cells in ocular surface epithelium is directly related to the presence of underlying vessels.

We would expect, therefore, that goblet cells would be lost in an avascular culture system. The rate of goblet cell loss in culture may be related to the capacity for complex cellular differentiation, and such rates are currently being investigated in normal and diseased human conjunctiva. The ultimate use of information derived from *in vitro* observation of cellular differentiation will require correlation of such data with the clinical behavior of the ocular surface in human disease.

In summary, (1) mitotic rates of conjunctival epithelial cells *in vitro* appear to be higher than that of corneal cells, (2) goblet cell proportion drops during incubation and (3) goblet cell frequency may indicate conjunctival health *in vitro* as *in vivo*.

REFERENCES

Buschke, W., J.S. Friedenwald & W. Fleischmann. Studies on the mitotic activity of the corneal epithelium. *Bull. Johns Hopkins Hosp.* 73:*143*, (1943).

Friedenwald, J.S. Growth pressure and metaplasia of conjunctival and corneal epithelium. *Doc. Ophthalmol.* 5–6: *184*, (1951).

Friend, J. & R.A. Thoft. Functional competence of ocular surface epithelium. *Invest. Ophthalmol. Vis. Sci.* 17:*134*, (1978).

Hanna, C. & J.E. O'Brien. Cell production and migration in the epithelial layer of the cornea. *Arch. Ophthalmol.* 64:*536*, (1960).

Maumanee, A.E. & R.O. Scholz, III. The histopathology of the ocular lesions produced by the sulfur and nitrogen mustards. *Bull. Johns Hopkins Hosp.* 82:*121*, (1948).

Ralph, R.A. Conjunctival goblet cell density in normal and dry eye syndromes. *Invest. Ophthalmol.* 14:*299*, (1975).

Thoft, R.A. Conjunctival transplantation. *Arch. Ophthalmol.* 95:*1425*, (1977).

Thoft, R.A. & J. Friend. Biochemical transformation of regenerating ocular surface epithelium. *Invest. Ophthalmol. Vis. Sci.* 17:*14*, (1977).

Thoft, R.A., J. Friend & H. Murphy. Ocular surface epithelium and corneal vascularization in rabbits. 1. The role of wounding. *Invest. Ophthalmol.* 18: *85*, (1979).

Author's address:
Eye Research Institute of
Retina Foundation
20 Staniford Street
Boston, Massachusetts 02114
U.S.A.

HISTOPATHOLOGICAL STUDY OF THE HUMAN HERPES SIMPLEX DENDRITIC AND PUNCTATE KERATITIS BY REPLICA TECHNIQUE

P.C. MAUDGAL AND L. MISSOTTEN

(Louvain, Belgium)

We developed an *in vivo* corneal replica technique for the histological examination of superficial keratitis (Missotten and Maudgal, 1977). This technique allowed us to study the replication and maturation of the virus and formation of disseminating inclusion bodies in experimental herpes simplex keratitis (Maudgal, 1976, Maudgal and Missotten, 1978). Histopathology of the human dendritic ulcers by this technique was first reported by us (Maudgal and Missotten, 1977a). An efficient therapeutic effect of this technique in herpes simplex keratitis has also been shown (Maudgal and Missotten, 1977b). In this paper we describe the histopathology of dendritic as well as punctate forms of herpes simplex keratitis.

SUBJECTS AND METHODS

Corneal replicas were made in 25 patients having superficial herpes simplex keratitis in one eye. One patient presented an unilateral granular punctate keratitis while the other showed typical dendritic ulcers. Herpes simplex virus was isolated in the cultures from conjunctival scrapings from the case of punctiform keratitis.

The tehnique of making corneal replicas and preparation of flat mounts has been described before (Missotten and Maudgal, 1977). The replicas and the unstained flat mounts were examined by the oblique illumination and phase contrast microscopy. Later the flat mounts were stained with heamatoxylin-eosin (HE) and Loves toluidine blue ammonium molybdate (TMB) method (Pearse, 1968) for light microscopy.

Some flat mounts were stained with acridine orange and examined by fluorescence microscopy. Afterwards these acridine orange stained slides were also stained by TBM technique, and examined by light microcopy.

RESULTS

Oblique illumination and phase contrast microscopy of the replicas showed rounded epithelial cells which fused to form syncytia of different sizes in the dendritic ulcers (Figs. 1 and 2). The nodular areas and the terminal bulbs of the dendrites contained larger syncytia. In the punctiform keratitis swollen and rounded epithelial cells were present in the clinically visible punctate lesions in the replica (Fig. 3). In the larger punctate lesions cell fusion was also observed but the syncytia were never as large as in the dendritic ulcers.

Studies of different stained and unstained preparations suggest that the syncytia are produced by the fusion of cells. Partly fused cells were seen at the periphery of syncytial masses (Fig. 4). Deformed nuclei of different sizes were observed in the syncytia. Usually they were small and rounded but could be irregular and elongated. In some parts of the syncytia the

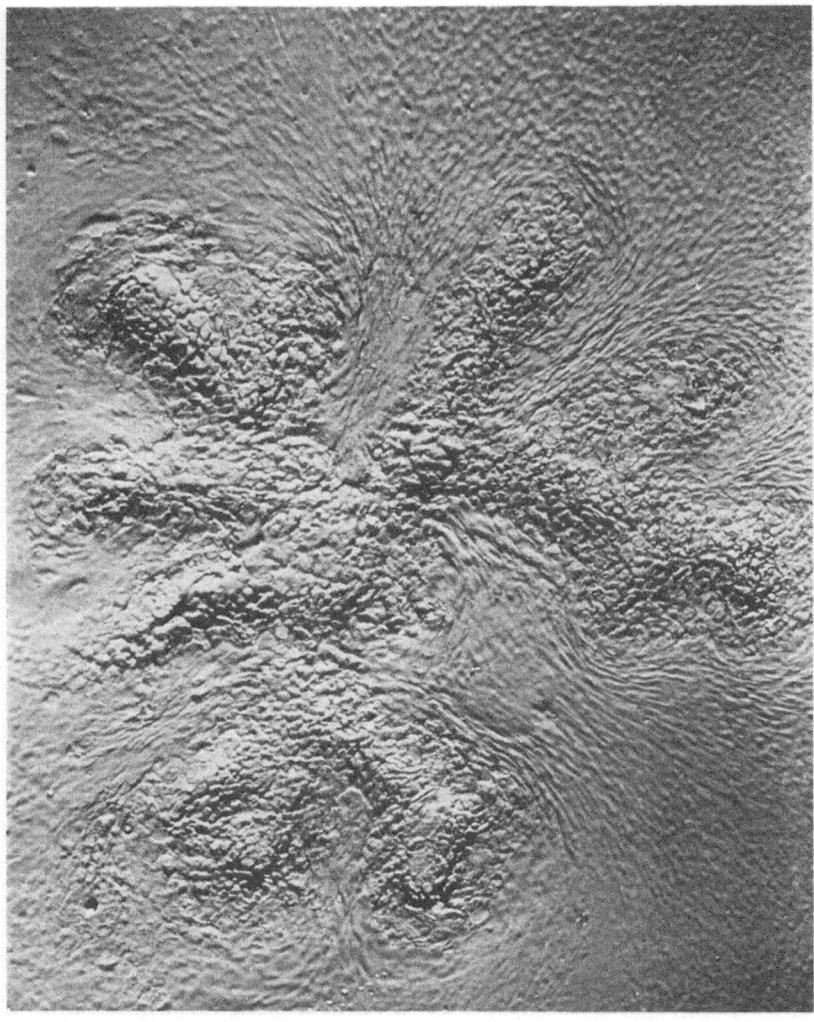

Fig. 1. Replica of a dendritic corneal ulcer. Rounded epithelial cells and syncytia are seen in the dendritic lesion. Note the elongated cells surrounding the ulcer. Oblique illumination microscopy X 52.

212

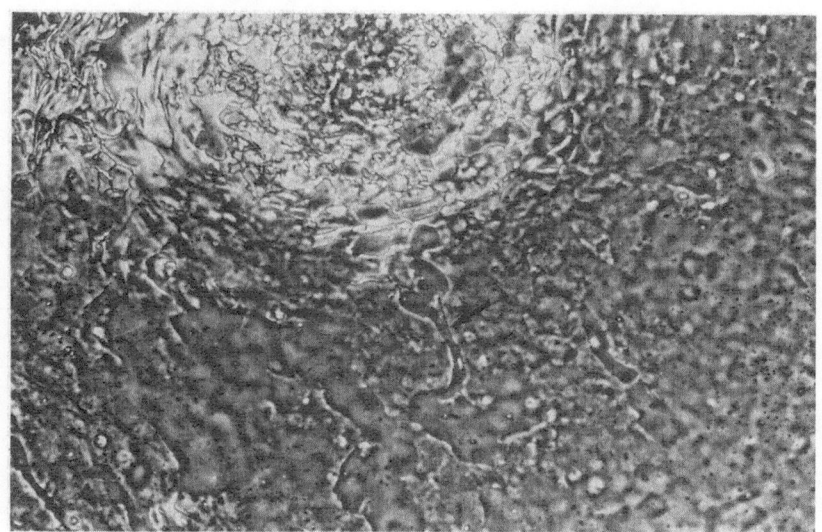

Fig. 2. Cell rounding and syncytia formation seen in a terminal bulb (partly shown above) of a dendrite. Extention of pseudopodia like process (arrow) to peripheral cells which have alse become fused. Corneal replica.
Phase contrast microscopy X 195.

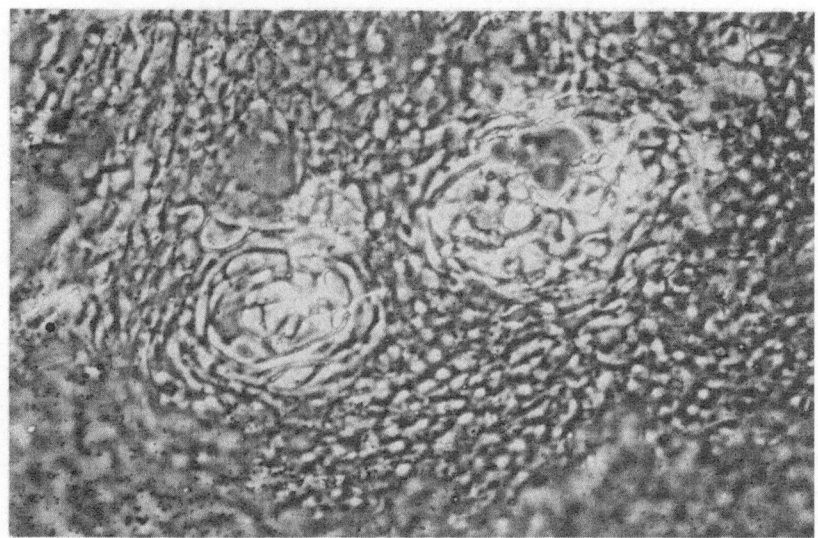

Fig. 3. Corneal replica from a punctiform herpes simplex keratitis. Rounding and fusion of epithelial cells in the punctate lesions is evident. Elongated cells surround the lesions. Peripheral cells are oedematous.
Phase contrast microscopy X 270.

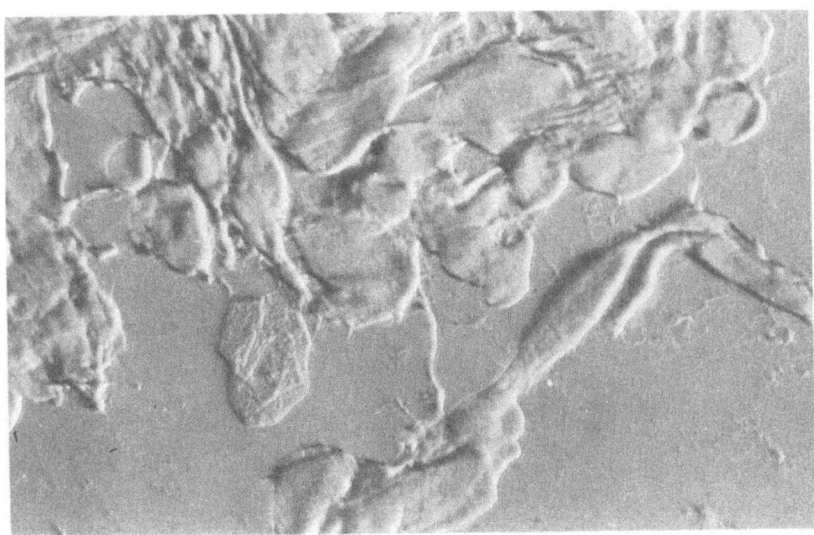

Fig. 4. Flat mount of the dendritic corneal ulcer. Partly fused cells are seen in the periphery of syncytium. Oblique illumination microscopy X 315.

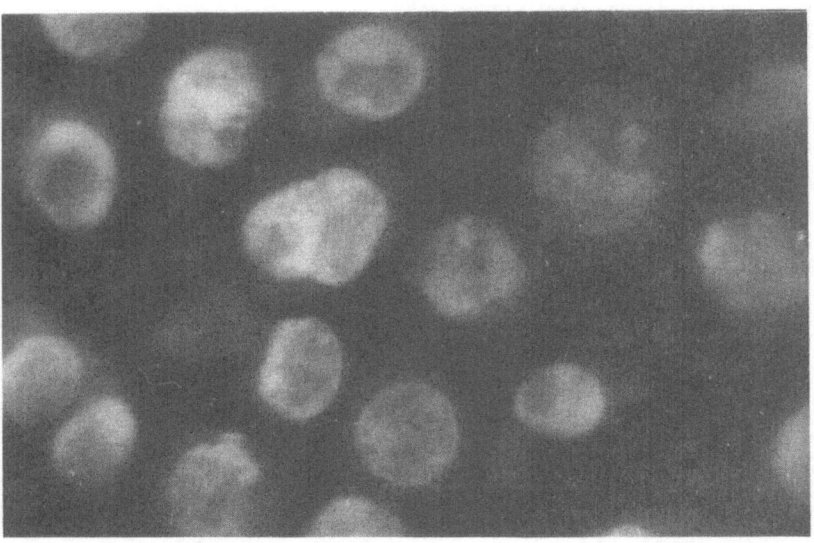

Fig. 5. Flat mount of the dendritic ulcer. Moth eaten appearance of nuclei after intensive IDU therapy. Acridine orange staining. Fluorescence microscopy X 755.

nuclei were not clearly defined and only faint basophillic masses or fragmented nuclear masses of different sizes were seen.

Acridine orange and TBM stainings showed the loss of nuclear DNA from these nuclei. The rounded and liquifying cells showed either an increase or decrease in the size of nuclei. Clumping and fragmentation of the nuclear material was also seen.

In the replicas of patients who were under intensive IDU therapy, irregular punched out areas or moth eaten appearance of some nuclei was seen by the acridine orange and TBM stainings (Fig. 5).

The cytoplasm of the rounded cells gave an intense red fluorescence of RNA by acradine orange staining. In some cells the cytoplasm formed only a marginal strip around the nuclei while in others it was present in large amounts, quite out of proportion to the size of nuclei. Occasionally, the large cells showed marked vacuolation and diffuse granules in the cytoplasm (Fig. 6).

Some fused and rounded cells showed diffuse granular green fluorescence of DNA in the cytoplasm (Fig. 7). On TBM staining of the same slides the areas of green fluorescence on acridine orange staining showed fine metachromatic particles, indicating that they contained DNA.

The partly fused cells adjacent to the syncytia also showed variations in the size of nuclei and the amount of cytoplasm. In addition to the clumping and fragmentation of the nuclear chromatin, these cells showed granular changes resembling 'A granules' of Love and Wildy (1963) and basophillic intranuclear inclusions surrounded by an area of rarefaction of nucleoplasm. Rarely a C-miotic lesion or failure of spindle formation was seen.

In the areas of necrosis fragmented nuclear masses were found scattered in the cell debris. Numerous ghost cells were seen in the necrosed parts of syncytia. The ghost cells possessed strongly eosinophillic homogenous cytoplasm and basophillic stellate nuclear material in the center. With TBM

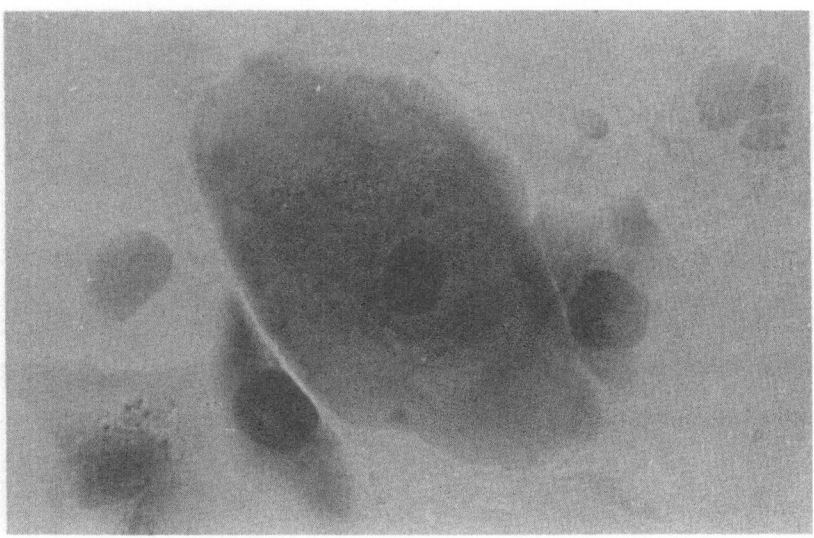

Fig. 6. A large cell showing vacuolation and granular change in the cytoplasm. Flat mount of dendritic ulcer.
H.E. Stain. X 630.

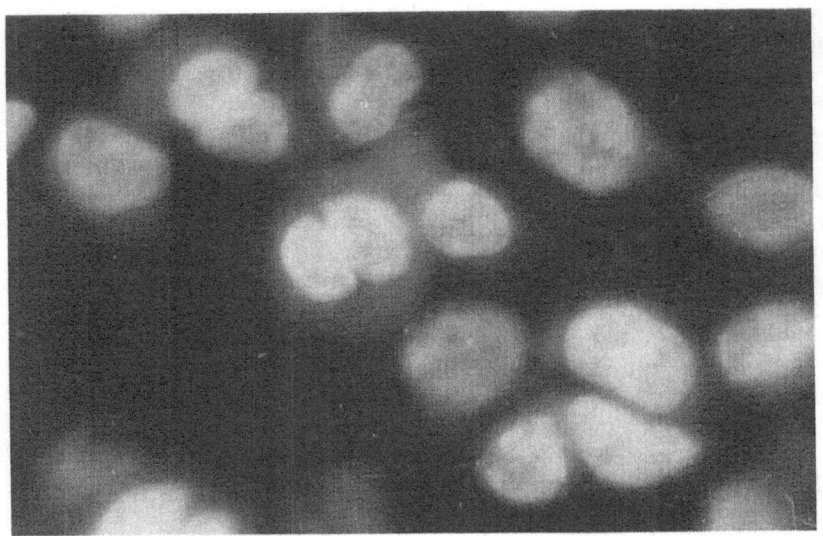

Fig. 7. Fusion of cells in the dendritic keratitis. Stronger fluorescence in the cytoplasm was due to DNA. Moth eaten appearance of some nuclei is due to IDU therapy. Acridine orange staining of the flat mount.
Fluorescence microscopy X 755.

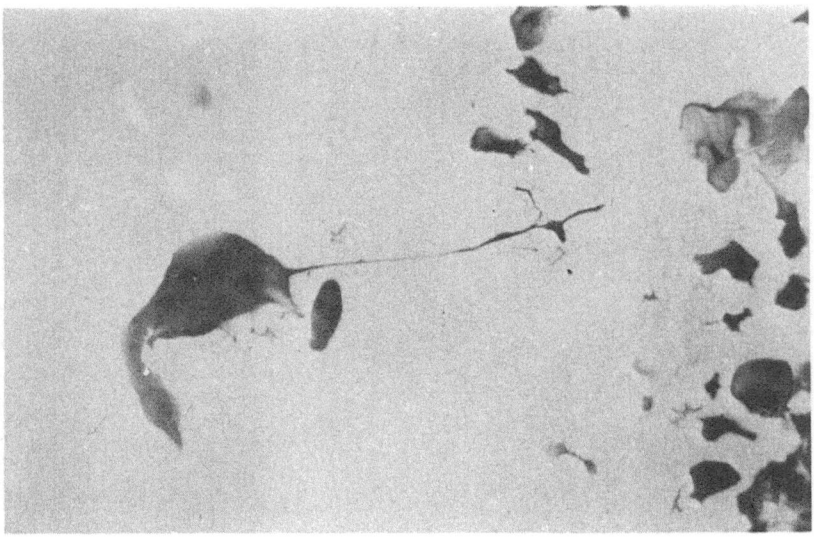

Fig. 8. Extension of pseudopodia like process from a small syncytium. Flat mount of a dendritic ulcer.
H.E. staining X 280.

staining the cytoplasm of these cells did not stain but the stellate nuclear material and the cell membranes gave metachromatic staining. The size of the stellate nuclei varied and sometimes this material was totally absent.

Apart from the ghost cells and areas of necrosis the cytoplasmic and nuclear changes described above were also observed in the specimen from punctate keratitis.

Pseudopodialike processes were often observed extending from the fused cells and syncytia in the dendrites towards the peripheral cells (Fig. 2). These processes were stained with TBM and HE stains (Fig. 8). Acridine orange staining showed the presence of RNA and DNA in the pseudopodia-like processes. They varied in length and thickness and were often seen extending across a few cells. The peripheral cells which came in contact with the tip of these processes had also become rounded, swollen and fused. These phenomena were also observed in the case of punctate keratitis.

Adjacent to the dendrites upto 4 layers of epithelial cells had become elongated and orientated parallel to the long axis of the finger-like projections of the dendrites (Fig. 1). They occupied the area between two adjacent projections and formed an arcuate pattern around the terminal bulbs. In the case of punctiform keratitis the elongated cells completely surrounded the lesions. Occasionally, cytoplasmic inclusions were found in these cells. These inclusions were situated near to nuclei and contained basophillic granular particles in an eosinophillic matrix surrounded by a halo.

The epithelial cells peripheral to the elongated cells were oedematous and larger and showed increased fluorescence of RNA and DNA. Such cells showed intranuclear lesions described above and could be found upto 2 mm away from the dendritic ulcers. These areas did not show any abnormalities on slit lamp examination of patients. The replicas of patients with diffuse epithelial oedema but no fluorescein staining clinically showed large number of swollen and rounded cells in extensive areas.

DISCUSSION

Clinically the dendritic corneal ulcers are known to contain swollen epithelial cells (Duke-Elder, 1965). Thygeson (1958) and Naib et al. (1967) showed characteristic polynucleate cells in the corneal scrapings of dendritic keratitis. Degeneration, clumping of nuclear material and epithelial cell rounding have been shown by Hudson et al. (1976) in experimental herpes simplex keratitis. The histological features of human dendritic ulcers by replica technique were first reported by us (Maudgal and Missotten, 1977).

Studies of the corneal replicas show that the dendritic ulcers and the punctiform lesions of herpes simplex keratitis are composed of different sized syncytia and the rounded liquefying cells. The syncytia arise due to the fusion of cells. Larger syncytia are present in the nodular areas and terminal bulbs of the dendrites. The giant polykaryocytes described by Thygeson (1958) and Naib et al. (1967) could have been the parts of syncytia broken during the scrapings or preparation of slides.

Another constant feature of the herpes simplex keratitis is the extensions of pseudopodialike processes from the fused cells towards the peripheral cells. The cells which come in contact with the tip of these processes also become rounded and seem to give rise to another syncytium. Thus the pseudopodialike processes appear to help in the extension of the dendritic lesions.

The granular particles detected in some nuclei resemble the A granules or maturing virus particles demonstrated by Love and Wildy (1963) in herpes virus infected Hela cell cultures and by us in experimental herpes simplex keratitis in rabbits (Maudgal, 1976; Maudgal and Missotten, 1978). The green fluorescence of DNA in the cytoplasm of some cells may be related to the release of these virus particles into the cytoplasm.

Although large swollen nuclei are seen in many cells balloon degeneration was absent. Deformed small nuclei in the rounded cells and bizarre shaped nuclei and the nuclear fragments in the syncytia formed a constant feature. However it was not possible to confirm if these nuclei or fragments contained virus particles. C-miotic lesions or colchicine-like effect, shown by Love and Wildy (1963) in Hela cell cultures and by us in human dendritic keratitis were infrequently seen. This could be due to the relatively inactive stage of the superficial epithelial cells which no longer divide. The basophillic granules in the cytoplasmic inclusions could be the replicating virus particles.

The stronger stainings of cytoplasm by TBM, HE and their selective differentiation by the acridine orange method show the increase in RNA and DNA in the infected cells. There is ample evidence that the virus specific RNA and DNA are synthesized in infected cells while the synthesis of cell specific ribonucleoproteins decreases (Rakusanova *et al.* 1972; Frenkel *et al.* 1973; and Bolden *et al.* 1975). This increase in the RNA and DNA suggests the stimulation of cell activity by the virus.

Moth eaten appearance of nuclei was seen only in the patients who were on intensive IDU therapy prior to making a corneal replica.

Surrounding the dendritic lesions the superficial epithelial cells are elongated and orientated parallel to the long axis of the lesion and in an arcuate pattern around the terminal bulbs. In the case of punctate keratitis such cells were seen surrounding the punctate lesions. The elongated cells appear to be characteristically present in keratitis herpetica as they were absent in other forms of superficial keratitis with punctiform lesions (personal observation).

Scattered diseased cells may be found upto 2 mm away from the dendritic lesions. Larger areas of involvement are present in the cases having superficial corneal oedema. It is noteworthy that such areas do not stain with fluorescein and appear clinically normal. Similarly lack of leucocytes is also an interesting finding.

SUMMARY

Dendritic ulcers or punctate lesions caused by herpes simplex virus show characteristic histological lesions unlike any other form of superficial keratitis we have studied upto now. The important features are: 1. the rounding and fusion of cells which results in syncytia formation; 2. the extension of pseudopodialike processes from the syncytia towards the peripheral cells; 3. the characteristic arrangement of the elongated cells around the dendrites and the punctate lesions; 4. intranuclear inclusions; 5. the release of virus particles into the cytoplasm and the cytoplasmic inclusions; 6. the formation of rounded ghost cells with stellate nuclei.

Although the biomicroscopic appearance of the herpetic punctate keratitis does not show any differentiating features from other forms of superficial punctate keratitis its histological picture is typical. Rounding of cells and the intranuclear inclusions are also found in the superficial epithelial cells in the areas which appear normal on clinical examination.

REFERENCES

Bolden, A., J. Aucker & A. Weissbach. Synthesis of herpes simplex virus, vaccinia virus, and adenovirus DNA in isolated Hela cell nuclei. *J. Virology* 16: *1584-1592,* (1975).

Duke-Elder, S. System of Ophthalmology, Vol. 8, Diseases of the outer eye. Kimpton, London, 1965.

Frenkel, N., S. Silverstein, E. Cassai & Roizman, B. RNA synthesis in cells infected with herpes simplex virus. VII. Control of transcription and of transcription abundancies of unique and common sequences of herpes simplex virus 1 and 2. *J. Virology* 11: *886-892,* (1973).

Hudson, J.B., M.J. Hollenberg, J.S. Wilkie & B.J. Lewis. Ultrastructural study of lesions induced in rabbit cornea by herpes simplex virus 1 and 2. *J. Infectious Diseases* 133: *367-381,* (1976).

Love, R., & P. Wildy. Cytochemical studies of nucleoproteins of Hela cells infected with herpes virus. *Journal of Cell Biology* 17: *237-254,* (1963).

Maudgal, P.C. The epithelial response in keratitis sicca and keratitis herpetica (an experimental and clinical study). Thesis for D. Sc (Ophth.) University of Louvain, 1976 (in press).

Maudgal, P.C. & L. Missotten. Histopathology of human superficial herpes simplex keratitis 1977(a) (in press).

Maudgal, P.C. & L. Missotten. Therapeutic effect of the corneal replicas in keratitis. 1977(b) (in press).

Maudgal, P.C. & L. Missotten. Development of the disseminating inclusion bodies in experimental herpes simplex keratitis. Read before the Soc. Belge d'Ophtal. 1978 (in press).

Missotten, L. & P.C. Maudgal. The corneal replica technique used to study the superifical corneal epithelium *in vivo. Amer. J. Ophthal.* 84: *104-111,* (1977).

Naib, Z. A. Clepper & S. Elliot. Exfoliative cytology as an aid in the diagnosis of ophthalmic lesions. *Acta cytologica* 11: *295-303,* (1967).

Pearse, G.A.E. Histochemistry: Theoretical and applied, Part I. Churchill Livingstone: Edinburgh 1968.

Rakusanova, T., T. Ben-Porat & S. Kaplan. Effect of herpes virus infection on the synthesis of cell specific RNA. *Virology* 49: *537-548,* (1972).

Thygeson, P. Cytological observations on herpetic keratitis. *Amer. J. Ophthal.* 45: *240-245,* (1958).

Author's address:
A.Z. St. Rafaël
Department of Ophthalmology
Kapucijnenvoer 7
3000 Louvain
Belgium.

219

SUPERFICIAL PUNCTATE KERATOPATHY:
EARLIEST CORNEAL MANIFESTATION OF XEROPHTHALMIA

ALFRED SOMMER, NANI EMRAN AND TIEN TAMBA

(Bandung, Indonesia)

Xerophthalmia remains a major cause of corneal destruction and blindness in many developing countries. The widely used clinical classification, shown in table 1, suggests a sharp distinction between cases with and without corneal disease (WHO/USAID Report, 1976). But few if any cases of mild xerophthalmia (XN, X1A, X1B) have undergone careful slit lamp examination; consequently little is known of the earliest manifestations of corneal involvement.

The Indonesian Nutritional Blindness Prevention Project is presently conducting clinical examinations of large numbers of xerophthalmic children. Preliminary results indicate punctate epithelial keratopathy is the earliest corneal manifestation of xerophthalmia, and is already present in the vast majority of cases classically considered free of corneal disease.

METHODS

All cases of xerophthalmia presenting to the Cicendo Eye Hospital, Bandung, or referred from outlying clinics were examined with a handlight and Haag Streit 900 slit-lamp (with and without fluorescein). Additional ophthalmologic, pediatric, bacteriologic, biochemical and histopathologic investigations were performed but are not germane to the present discussion.

Cases were enrolled in one of several treatment regimens depending upon the severity of their disease. Those with clear corneas by handlight examination were randomly chosen to receive either low dose (700 IU) or high dose (200,000 IU) vitamin A orally. Every attempt was made to reexamine all cases at frequent intervals, and low dose recipients received high dose therapy after 3 months, or sooner if their condition deteriorated significantly.

Table 1. Classification active xerophthalmia.

XN*	Night Blindness
X1A	Conjunctival Xerosis
X1B	Conjunctival Xerosis with Bitot's spot
X2	Corneal Xerosis
X3A	Corneal Xerosis with Ulceration
X3B	Keratomalacia

RESULTS

Corneal Xerosis (X2)

Corneal xerosis (X2) was the severest lesion in 30 cases. All 47 eyes with corneal xerosis presented with extensive punctate keratopathy: myriads of densly packed, tiny, brightly staining specks. Over 90% of the time they covered the entire cornea. In the remainder, and whenever the density of lesions varied, there was a striking predeliction for the inferior half of the cornea, especially the infero-nasal quadrant.

The lesions healed in a definite pattern. Superior and temperal aspects of the cornea cleared first, the infero-nasal last. Within one week of receiving vitamin A many of the lesions ceased to stain, leaving a mixture of staining and nonstaining white specks. By the second week many of the nonstaining specks had bcome lightly pigmented, and by the fourth week all staining had ceased, leaving residually pigmented specks, most apparent inferiorly.

Controls

Both eyes of twenty nine age/sex/locale matched controls of corneal cases were normal by handlight examination. Only 2 controls (4 eyes) had definite punctate keratopathy (7%). In each instance it was minimal and limited to the periphery of the infero-nasal quadrant.

Non-corneal xerophthalmia (XN, X1A, X1B)

If punctate keratopathy is an early manifestation of xerophthalmia, the proportion of individuals affected, and the extent and intensity of corneal involvement might be expected to increase with increasing evidence and severity of disease.

For convenience we graded the distribution of lesions 1 through 4, representing involvement of the infero-nasal quadrant, inferior half, inferior three-fourths, and the entire surface of the cornea. Intensity was graded 1 through 3, indicating mild, moderate and heavy concentrations of lesions respectively. All corneas appeared crystal clear by handlight exam, the basis

Table 2. Punctate keratopathy among patients classified XN, X1A, X1B.

Clinical classification		Number of eyes	Percent positive	Average extent*	Average density**
XN:	History Positive Exam Negative	18	22	1.0	1.0
XN:	History Positive Exam Positive	10	60	1.3	1.7
X1A, X1B		63	75	1.9	1.9

* Graded: 1=infero-nasal quadrant; 2=inferior 1/2 of cornea; 3=inferior 3/4 of cornea; 4=entire corneal surface.
** Graded: 1=mild; 2=moderate; 3=heavy.

222

for their clinical classification (Sommer, 1978). Results are shown in table 2.

Children presenting with a history of night blindness unconfirmed by clinical examination may be assumed to have the least evidence and mildest form of xerophthalmia. Of 9 cases (18 eyes) 22% had punctate keratopathy. Among affected corneas the average distribution and density of lesions was 1.0.

In 5 children (10 eyes) clinical examination confirmed the presence of night blindness. Sixty percent of cases and eyes had punctate keratopathy, with an average distribution of 1.33 and density of 1.67.

Thirty-four children had conjunctival xerosis (X1A, X1B) in at least 1 eye. Seventy-five percent of 63 involved eyes had punctate keratopathy, with an average distribution and intensity of 1.9.

Therapeutic Trial

The importance of vitamin A deficiency in the genesis of these lesions is confirmed by their response to therapy. Followup examinations are available on 18 cases (26 eyes) with punctate keratopathy treated with a single oral dose of 200,000 IU vitamin A. Results are shown in table 3.

Table 3. Punctate keratopathy among X1A, X1B patients*: response to 200,000 IU Vitamin A.

Duration since Treatment	Percent Improved	Percent Cured	Total Percent Improved or Cured
1–3 Days	40	0	40
4–7 Days	75	25	100
2 Weeks	20	80	100
1 Month	–	100	100

* 26 Eyes available for at least 1 follow-up examination.

Between 1 and 3 days following treatment 40% of involved corneas improved. By days 4–7 all showed improvement and 25% were entirely free of punctate staining ('cured'). The proportion free of staining rose to 80% at 2 weeks and 100% at 1 month.

In contrast the course of the disease in 10 low dose recipients (18 involved eyes) with punctate keratopathy was markedly different. By the end of the first month none of the corneas showed improvement, while 61% had actually deteriorated at some time in the interval, 4 of them alarmingly so. All 4 were treated with 200,000 IU vitamin A with subsequent improvement or cure within 9 days.

Both eyes of one low dose recipient eventually healed spontaneously, at 65 days.

DISCUSSION

Our observations leave little doubt that punctate epithelial keratopathy is an early manifestation of xerophthalmia, and already present in a majority of eyes usually considered free of corneal involvement. Sixty percent of confirmed cases of night blindness (XN) and 75% of eyes classified X1A or X1B (conjunctival xerosis), but only 7% of controls were affected. The latter may well represent incipient xerophthalmia. Serum vitamin A levels among locale matched controls were considerably below random sample norms (unpublished data).

Pathogenesis of the lesions and their predeliction for the infero-nasal quadrant remain uncertain. They may be the direct result of impaired vitamin A metabolism of the corneal epithelium, or secondary to instability of the tear film with local drying. But suggestions that they are due to loss of conjunctival mucous producing goblet cells (Dohlman and Kalevar, 1972) seem unlikely. All corneas improved within 7 days of therapy and 80% ceased to stain by two weeks, long before goblet cells reappear (Sommer *et al.*, 1978; Sullivan *et al.*, 1973; and unpublished data).

Both eyes of one low dose recipient healed spontaneously at 65 days, probably from improved diet or treatment outside the study. Preliminary results of our longitudinal field study indicate almost 50% of children with noncorneal xerophthalmia improve spontaneously over a 4 month period (unpublished data).

The presently accepted xerophthalmia classification, primarily derived from handlight examinations, is insufficiently precise for research purposes. Nonetheless it remains a useful clinical tool. Medical workers encountering the disease are unlikely to have more than a handlight available, and any child suspected of having active xerophthalmia deserves immediate treatment, whether or not subtle slit-lamp evidence of early corneal involvement is already present.

REFERENCES

Dohlman, C.H. & V. Kalevar. Cornea in Hypovitaminisosis A and protein deficiency. *Isr. J. Med. Sci.* 8: *1179–1183*, (1972).

Sommer, A. Field Guide to the Detection and Control of Xerophthalmia. World Health Organization, Geneva, (1978).

Sommer, A., T. Sugana, D. Edi & W.R. Green. Vitamin A responsive pan-ocular xerophthalmia in a healthy adult. *Arch. Ophthalmol.* 96: *1630–1634,* (1978).

Sullivan, W R., J.P. McCulley & C.H. Dohlman. Return of goblet cells after vitamin A therapy in xerosis of the conjunctiva. *Am. J. Ophthalmol.* 75: *720–725,* (1973).

Vitamin A Deficiency and Xerophthalmia. Report of a joint WHO/USAID Meeting. Technical Report Series 590, World Health Organization, Geneva, 1976.

Author's address:
P.O.B. 134
Bandung
Indonesia.

ADENOSINE TRIPHOSPHATE, ADENOSINE DIPHOSPHATE, ASCORBIC ACID, GLUTATHIONE AND LACTATE IN EXPERIMENTAL ULTRAVIOLET KERATITIS

M. REIM, E. SCHUETTE, G. SCHARSICH, M. SEIDL, H.G. KESTERNICH AND A.W. BUDI SANTOSO

(Aachen, Germany)

The superficial tissues of the eye are sensitive to UV irradiation. UV keratitis is the dramatic debridement of the corneal epithelium following UV irradiation. After a lag period of 6–10 hours, the disease begins with the onset of heavy pains, congestion of the conjunctiva and lacrimation.

According to a hypothesis of PIRIE (1946, 1965) it was postulated that the light produced peroxides in the transparent tissues of the eye. These peroxides were supposed to be toxic to cells, attacking primarily all membrane structures.

In the cornea the toxic peroxides may be eliminated by means of the glutathione peroxidase (GSHPX) and by direct non enzymatical reduction by ascorbic acid. The resulting dehydroascorbic acid as well as the oxidized glutathione obtain their reducing potentials from the glutathione reductase and further from the hexose phosphate shunt.

In rabbits it is possible to produce the UV keratitis in a model experiment (Duke-Elder, 1972). But the energy necessary is larger in rabbits than in man. Cogan and Kinsey (1946), Kinsey (1948) and Bachem (1956) found a spectral sensitivity of the cornea in the ultraviolet range from 280 to 310 nm and the maximum sensitivity at 288 nm.

METHODS

We used an analytical UV lamp to produce experimental UV keratitis (Original Hanau Fluotest forte, Typ 5261, 210 W, Original Hanau Quarzlampen GmbH, Hanau, Germany; Fig. 1). Rabbits of a grey german wild strain weighing 2,5–3,5 kg were operated on in general anesthesia by i.v. injection of Pentobarbital (35 mg/kg). The cornea of one eye was irradiated for 20 min in a distance of 30 cm. To avoid drying of the corneal surface, it was carefully rinsed with saline (four drops per minute). Then the lids were closed with adhesive tape as long as the animal was kept in general anesthesia. The other eye of the animal served as control. It was kept closed by adhesive tape during the irradiation of the experimental eye.

At different time intervals following the UV irradiation, again in general anesthesia the corneal epithelium was scraped and frozen in liquid nitrogen. The anterior chamber was punctered at the limbus with a 20 gauge needle and 0.2 ml of aqueous humour were aspirated. The stroma was excised at

225

Relative spectral energy of the Q 600 Quarz lamp

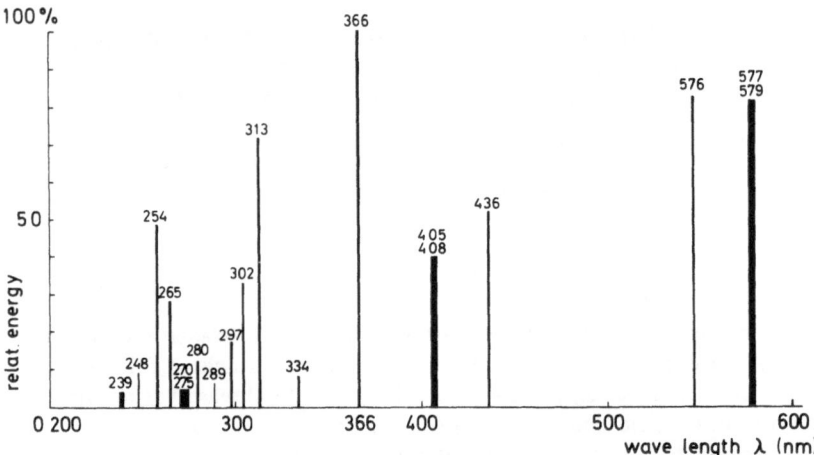

Fig. 1. Relative spectral energy of the UV lamp.

the limbus with scissors and crushed under liquid nitrogen in a mortar. Then the tissues and fluids were extracted in a glas in glas homogenizer using 1,0 and 0,5 ml of 0.5 N perchloric acid. The protein precipitate was separated from the homogenate by centrifugation at 2000 x g. The supernatants were neutralized with 10 N KOH to pH 3,0 and used for the assay of ascorbic acid (ASC), reduced (GSH), and oxidized (GSSG) glutathione. For the assay of the lactate and the adenosine phosphate levels, the supernatant was neutralized up to pH 6,5.

The reduced and oxidized glutathione were assayed in the combined optic enzymatic test using cristallysed glyoxalase I and glutathione reductase as described previously (Reim *et al.*, 1976). The lactate levels were determined enzymatically according to Hohorst *et al.* (1959). The ascorbic acid was assayed using the photometric test with 2,6 dichlorophenolindophenole as described by Reim *et al.* 1978.

The assay of the adenosine triphosphate (ATP) and the adenosine diphosphate (ADP) was performed in the enzymatic optical test according to Reim and Schmidt (1967). For the extraction of the corneal epithelium and endothelium, a newly developed modification of the rapid freezing method including freeze sawing and lyophilisation was used, which allowed the analyses of single epithelia and the pooled endothelia of one animal (Budi Santoso, 1978).

RESULTS

After UV irradiation, the cornea remained normal up to ten hours. Then the exposed area of the cornea epithelium developed punctate keratitis and some time later a superficial defect staining with fluorescein. The conjunctiva was red and swollen. 48 to 72 hours after the UV irradiation the epithelium was regenerated and looked quite normal. In semi thin sections, 3 hours after UV irradiation, the corneal epithelium showed a normal structure of the basal and intermediate cells, but slight intracellular edema.

Some of the superficial cells, however, were already swollen and debrided (Fig. 2). Besides, the scanning electron microscope revealed extrusion of nuclei.

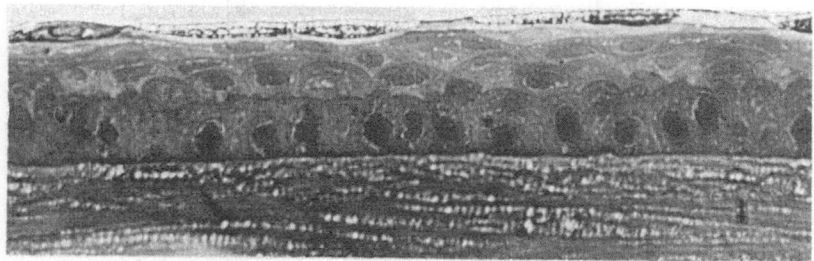

Fig. 2. Semi-thin section of the rabbit corneal epithelium 3 hours after UV irradiation. Toluidine blue stain, magnification of the Photograph 900 x.

The results of the glutathione assays were demonstrated in the diagram of Fig. 3. Initially, after UV irradiation both forms of the glutathione, the GSH and the GSSG were decreased. But the reduced glutathione decreased more slowly and later showed a transitory increase. Therefore, an increase of the GSG/GSSG was observed up to 14 hours after UV irradiation. At later stages of the UV keratitis, the GSH levels slightly decreased. But the GSH/GSSG ratios remained unchanged.

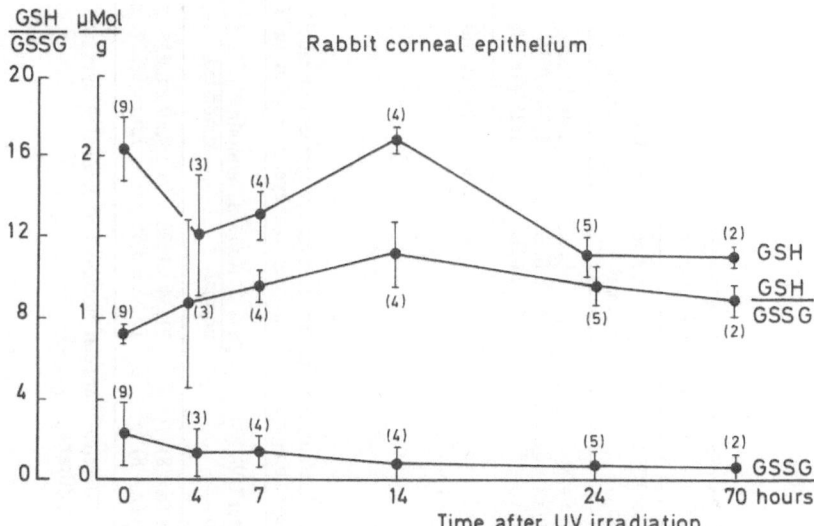

Fig. 3. Oxidized and reduced glutathione levels and GSH/GSSG ratio of the rabbit corneal epithelium after UV irradiation. Each symbol represents mean values ± s.e.m. (n = 8).

227

Table 1. Ascorbic acid levels in the anterior eye segment of rabbits after UV irradiation of the left eye compared to the normal right eye. m ± s.e.m. (μ Mol/g wet weight)

Time after UV irradiation	Aqueous humour		corneal stroma		corneal epithelium	
	normal	irradiated	normal	irradiated	normal	irradiated
30 min (n = 8)	1,42 ± 0,11	1,46 ± 0,24	3,78 ± 2,50	3,44 ± 2,59*	10,22 ± 0,86	11,04 ± 1,58
3 hours (n = 8)	1,49 ± 0,22	1,72 ± 0,36	4,78 ± 2,41	3,95 ± 1,39*	12,8 ± 2,33	9,64 ± 2,99*
24 hours (n = 8)	1,51 ± 0,31	1,25 ± 0,26*	5,60 ± 1,61	3,13 ± 1,25*	11,64 ± 1,82	7,40 ± 1,93*

* The difference between normal and irradiated eyes was statistically significant in paired samples.

Table 2. Lactate levels in the anterior eye segment of rabbits after UV irradiation of the left eye compared to the normal right eye. m ± s.e.m. (μ Mol/g wet weight)

Time after UV irradiation	Aqueous humour		corneal stroma		corneal epithelium	
	normal	irradiated	normal	irradiated	normal	irradiated
3 hours (n = 8)	11,34 ± 0,80	9,59 ± 0,41*	13,25 ± 0,62	12,22 ± 0,46*	26,04 ± 2,48	29,64 ± 2,49**
24 hours (n = 8)	10,56 ± 0,86	7,60 ± 0,52*	11,98 ± 0,16	8,70 ± 1,11*	24,21 ± 1,61	23,56 ± 1,34**

* The difference between normal and irradiated eyes was statistically significant
** not significant

Table 1 shows the results of the ascorbic acid assays. At 30 minutes after the UV irradiation the ASC levels of the corneal epithelium did not change, but the ASC levels of the stroma were slightly reduced. At 3 hours after the UV irradiation, the ASC levels of the epithelium and the stroma were statistically significantly decreased.

At 24 hours after the UV irradiation, the UV keratitis was fully developed. The decrease of the ASC levels in each of the compartments was surely a consequence of the visible damage to the epithelium.

In the incubation period of the UV keratitis, the lactate levels showed only slightly, but significantly decreased values (table 2). At later stages of the disease, the decrease of the lactate levels may be related of the destroyed corneal epithelium, the lactate production of which was certainly reduced. This observation was in correlation to previous results after freezing the corneal epithelium in vivo (Reim et al., 1971). Therefore, the lactate levels of the cornea did not seem to be primarily affected by UV irradiation.

During the incubation period of the UV keratitis, the ATP content of the corneal epithelium was reduced initially. A larger decrease was observed only 30 hours after the UV light exposure (Fig. 4).

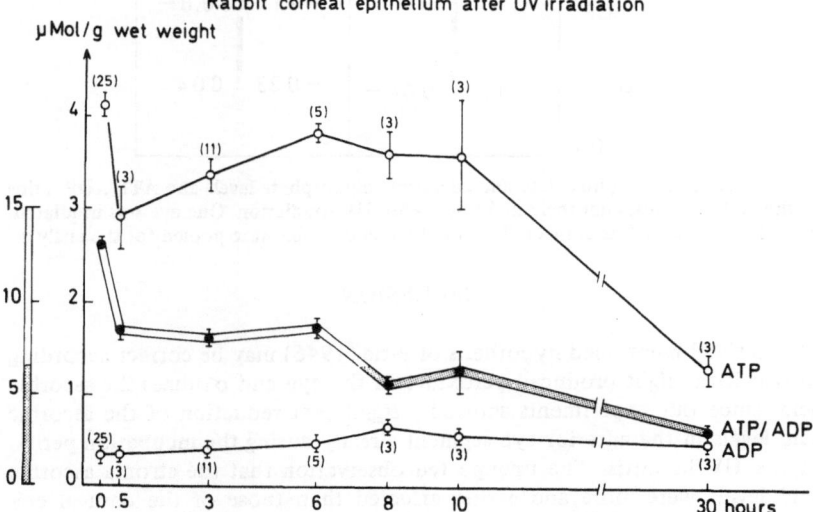

Fig. 4. Adenosine triphosphate, adenosine diphosphate levels and ATP/ADP ratios of rabbit corneal epithelium after UV irradiation. Each symbol represents mean values ± s.e.m. The number of experiments is given in parentheses.

But at that time, the epithelium was almost completely destroyed. The ADP levels were increased after UV irradiation showing a maximum level after 8 hours. Therefore, the ATP/ADP ratio was decreased from normal values at 13 to 8 within 6 hours. From 8 to 10 hours following the UV irradiation, the ATP/ADP ratio reached only 5–6, and after 30 hours, it was reduced to 3 (Fig. 4). The standard deviations of the mean were 3 to 8%. In the corneal endothelium 6 hours after the UV irradiation the ATP level was slightly but not significantly reduced. The ADP levels, however, were significantly elevated. Therefore, the ATP/ADP ratio of the corneal endothelium was decreased to half of the normal values (Fig. 5).

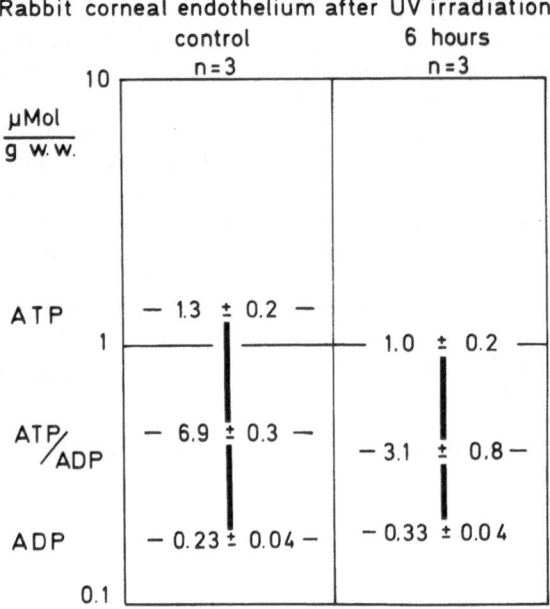

Fig. 5. Adenosine triphosphate and adenosine diphosphate levels and ATP/ADP ratios of the rabbit corneal endothelium 6 hours after UV irradiation. One eye was irradiated, the other eye served as control. Two or three endothelia were pooled for the analysis.

DISCUSSION

The initially mentioned hypothesis of Pirie (1946) may be correct according to which the light produced peroxides in the eye and oxidizes the ascorbic acid, since our experiments showed a significant reduction of the ascorbic acid levels in the anterior eye segment already during the incubation period of the UV keratitis. The unexpected observation that the stroma ascorbic acid levels were more and earlier affected than those of the corneal epithelium may be explained by the fact, that the compensation mechanisms of the epithelium are much stronger than those of the stroma. The corneal epithelium has the active hexose phosphate shunt and an efficient glutathione reducing system. These reactions are known to operate well under unfavourable conditions (Reim and Ashauer, 1975). Therefore, the glutathione levels and the GSH/GSSG ratios too, were more inclined to the reduced state in the epithelium during the incubation period of the UV keratitis. The well reduced state of the glutathione in the corneal epithelium may have effected a rapid reduction of dehydroascorbic acid possibly formed by the peroxides after UV irradiation. Apparently, the conditions for the reduction of the dehydroascorbic acid are not so favourable in the stroma than in the epithelium, since in the stroma the ascorbic acid occurs to a large extent in the extracellular space and therefore is not in immediate contact to the strictly intracellular reducing system of the glutathione and the hexose phosphate shunt.

The investigation of the glutathione and ascorbic acid levels in the cornea demonstrated that the reducing capacities of the hexose phosphate glutathione system were strong enough to compensate for the irradiation effect leading to UV keratitis as long as the epithelium was intact. It is known that after mechanical damage to the cornea the lactate levels were increased (Reim and Schmidt, 1967; Kilp, 1974). After UV irradiation however, the lactate levels of the cornea were rather reduced. This suggested an impairment of the glycolysis, possibly due to increased consumption of reducing capacities of the pyridine nucleotide coenzymes by the glutathione-hexosephosphate system.

In this context, it is remarkable that Foulks *et al.* (1977) discovered a decrease of the lactate dehydrogenase in the corneal epithelium 24 h after UV irradiation, while the activities of other enzymes of the energy producing metabolism were rather increased.

The decrease of ATP levels and more pronounced of the ATP/ADP ratios in the corneal epithelium after UV irradiation also demonstrated an early damage of the energy producing metabolism. After 30 min., already, the ATP levels and the ATP/ADP ratios were reduced by 29 and 38%, respectively. On the outbreak of the keratitis, these parameters decreased further. The same tendency was revealed in the corneal endothelium. The observation of changes of the ascorbic acid levels in the corneal stroma and of the adenosine phosphate content in the endothelium showed, that the irradition damage was not restricted the corneal epithelium, as experienced from clinical cases, but also affected the deeper layers of the anterior eye segment.

The reduced ATP levels in the corneal epithelium at later stages of the UV keratitis were found also by Foulks *et al.* (1977). The effect of UV irradiation on nucleotides was not unexpected since the spectral absorbance of these compounds lies mainly in the UV range of 260 nm.

The maximal UV absorption of the cornea between 280 and 310 nm as demonstrated by Cogan and Kinsey (1946) may lead further investigations to substances that show absorption bands in this region. Kinsey (1948) supposed that the UV irradiation may affect primarily the nucleoproteines. Therefore, the investigation of messenger RNA, transfer RNA or the enzymes catalyzing their reactions may help to find more biochemical lesions of the cornea by the absorption of UV light.

REFERENCES

Bachem, A. Ophthalmic Ultraviolet Action Spectra. *Amer. J. Ophthalmol.* 41: *969–975*, (1956).
Birch-Hirschfeld, A. Die Wirkung der ultravioletten Strahlen auf das Auge. *A. v. Graefes Arch. Ophthal.* 58: *469–562*, (1904).

Budi Santoso, A.W. Bestimmung der Adenosinphosphatspiegel in der Cornea bei der experimentellen Ultraviolett-Keratitis. Thesis, Aix la Chapelle, 1979).

Cogan, D.G. & E. Kinsey. Action Spectrum of Keratitis produced by Ultraviolet Radiation. *Arch. Opthal.* (Chicago), 35: *670–677* (1946).

Duke-Elder, W.S. Action on the outer eye. Photoophthalmia. System of Ophthalmology, Vol. IXX, Injuries Part. II, Chapter I, 918–928, (1972).

Foulks, G.N. J. Friend & R.A. Thoft. Effects of ultraviolet radiation on corneal epithelial metabolism. *Arch. Ophthal*, in press, (1977).

Hohorst, H.J. F.H. Kreutz & T.H. Bücher. Uber Metabolitgehalte und Metabolitkonzentrationen in der Leber der Ratte. *Biochem. Zeitschrift* 332: *18–46*, (1959).

Kilp, H. Einfluß von Kontaktlinsen auf Metabolite und Hydratation der Kaninchenhornhaut. *A. v. Graefes Arch.klin.exp.Ophthal.* 190: *275–280*, (1974).

Kinsey, V.E. Spectral Transmission of the Eye to Ultraviolet Radiations. *Arch. Ophthal.* (Chicago), 39: *508–513*, (1948).

Pirie, A. Glutathione peroxidase in lens and source of hydrogen peroxide in aqueous humour. *Biochem. J.* 96: *244–253*, (1965).

Pirie, A. Ascorbic acid content of the cornea. *Biochem. J.* 40: *96–99*, (1946).

Reim, M. & D. Ashauer. The glutathione of the cornea. *Arch. Opht.* (Paris), 35: *153–158*, (1975).

Reim, M., H.R. Beermann, P. Luthe & H. Cattepoel. The Redox State of the Glutathione in the Bovine Corneal Epithelium. *A. v. Graefex Arch. Ophthal.* 201: *143–148*, (1976).

Reim, M., B. Heuvels & H. Cattepoel. Glutathione Peroxidase in Some Ocular Tissues. *Ophthal. Res.* 6: *228–234*, (1974).

Reim, M., U. Hennighausen, D. Hildebrandt & R. Maier. Enzyme Activities in the Cornea Epithelium and Endothelium of Different Species. *Ophthal. Res.* 2:*171–182*, (1971).

Reim, M., H. Boeck, P. Krug & G. Venske. Aqueous Humour and Cornea Stroma Metabolite Levels under Various Conditions. *Ophthal. Res.* 3: *241–250*, (1972).

Reim, M. & F. Schmidt. Biochemische Veränderungen bei der Vereisung der Hornhaut in vivo. Ein Beitrag zur Kältetherapie. *Klin. Mbl. Augenheilk.* 150: *96–103*, (1967).

Reim, M., U. Lipp & G. Venske. Biochemical changes in the cornea after cryotherapy. Proc. XXI. Int. Congr. Ophthal. Mexico 1970, Excerpta Medica, Amsterdam 1971, pp. 550–554.

Reim, M. & P. Luthe. Compartmentation of Redox Metabolites in the Anterior Eye Segment? *A. v. Graefes Arch* 204: *135–140*, (1977).

Reim, M., E. Schuette, G. Scharsich, M. Seidl & H.G. Kesternich. Ascorbic acid, glutathione and lactate in experimental ultraviolet keratitis, *Doc. Ophthal.*, (in press).

This work was supported by the
Deutsche Forschungsgemeinschaft
53 Bonn – Bad Godesberg

Author's address:
Prof. Dr. med. M. Reim
Vorstand der Abteilung für Augenheilkunde
der Medizinischen Fakultät der HWTH
Goethestraße 27–29
5100 Aachen
Germany.

Docum. Ophthal. Proc. Series, Vol. 20

THE DARK CELLS OF CORNEAL EPITHELIUM IN A CASE OF LATTICE-LIKE DYSTROPHY*

P. VITTONE, R. BERTAGNO AND M. ZINGIRIAN

(Genova, Italy)

INTRODUCTION

As is known, between the basal cells of the corneal epithelium there are the so-called dark cells, whose nature and function are still under discussion (Iwamoto and De Voe, 1971; Segawa, 1964; Segawa, 1965; Sugiura, 1965; Teng, 1962; Vittone *et al.*, 1976).

We have found certain modifications of these cells in a patient suffering from corneal lattice dystrophy and who had undergone a perforating keratoplasty.

METHOD

The corneal flap, immediately after surgical removal, was fixed in 3% glutaraldehyde, buffered in Millonig's phosphate-buffer, post-fixed in 1% osmium tetroxide, deydrated in graded ethanol solution in the usual way, embedded in epoxy resin (Araldite-Epon) and sectioned on a LKB ultrotome. Thin sections were stained in 3% uranyl acetate in 50% ethanol, followed by lead citrate. A Simens Elmiskop 101 electron microscope was used to view and photograph the specimens.

RESULTS

The characteristics of the corneal epithelium under observation are as follows.

The superficial and intermediate layers of the corneal epithelium do not show substantial pathological changes. Conversely the basal layer presents important regressive alterations, even if irregularly distributed. In fact, while in some areas the typical basal cell structure remains absolutely unchanged, in other areas these cells show vacuolisation of the mitochondria and nuclear polymorphism.

Moreover between these cells and the basal membrane a thin, strongly electron-opaque band is inserted (Figs. 1 and 2). The aspect and the location of this electron-opaque band suggest that it represents the elongation of processes belonging to the so-called dark cells of the basal layer. In fact these cells appear particularly active and increased in number.

In some areas the clear basal cells are completely substituted by a contin-

*This work was supported by a grant of the Italian Research Council (C.N.R.).

233

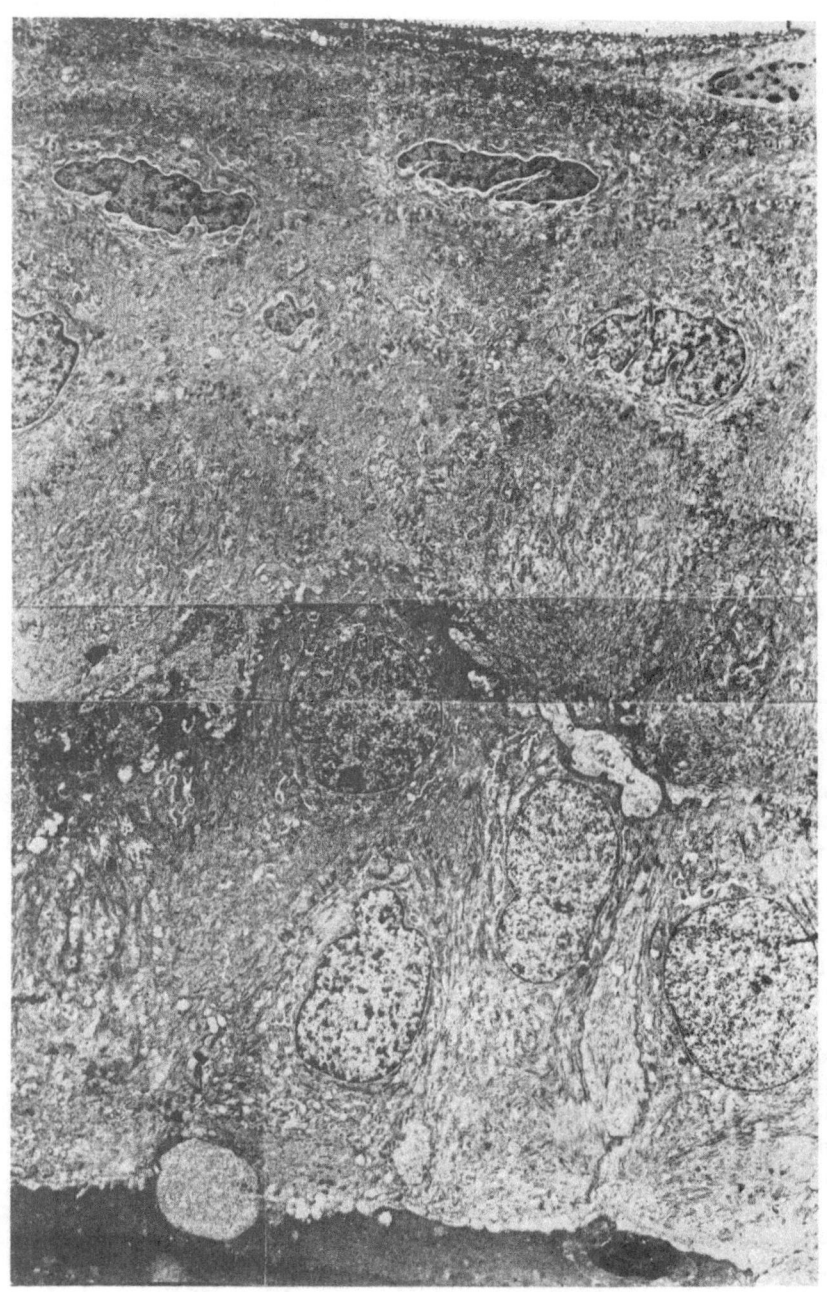

Fig. 1.

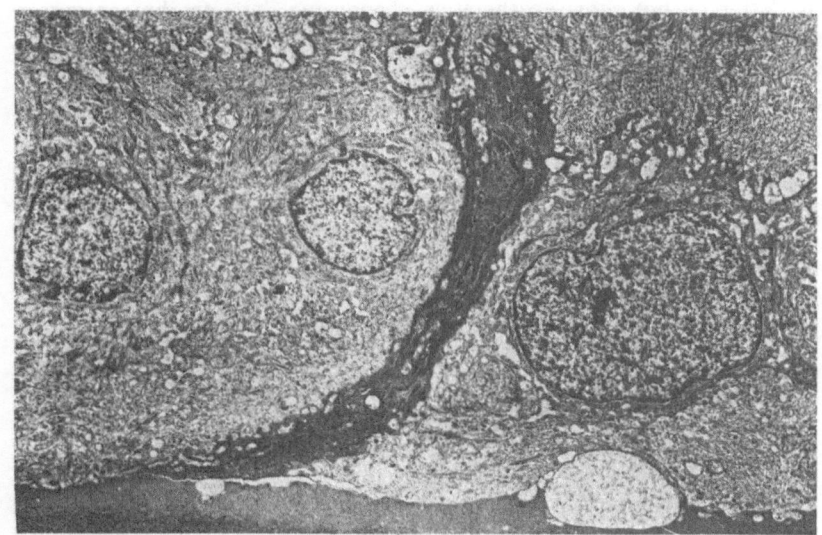

Fig. 2.

uous series of dark cells, in single or double rows, thus making an almost compact layer.

The dark cell elongations, growing upwards, tend to surround the clear basal cells which show initial cytoplasmatic degeneration (Fig. 3). Sometimes the clear basal cells are reduced to heavily degenerated residues, completely enclosed by dark cells (Figs. 3 and 4).

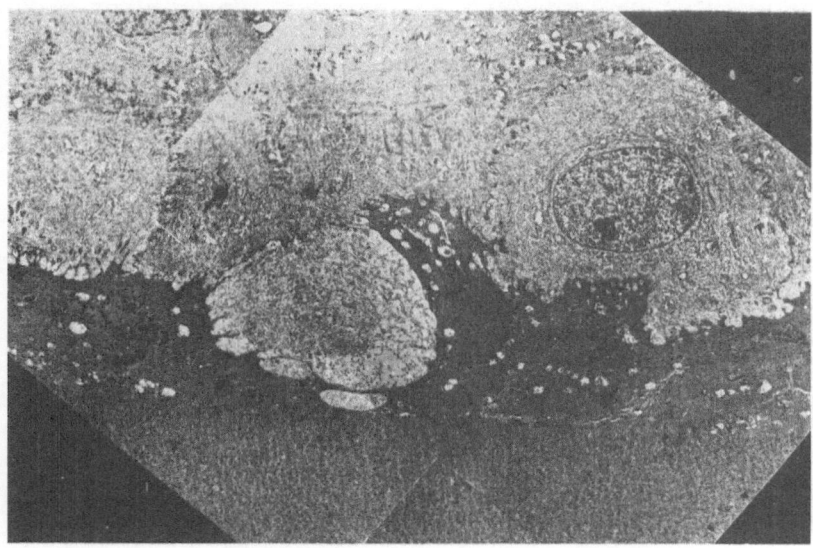

Fig. 3.

235

The latter do not show degenerative phenomena, but, on the contrary, a certain polymorphism and a marked abundance of nuclear chromatin, evidence of increased metabolic activity (Figs. 4 and 5).

The underlying basal membrane is normal in some areas, but in other it is hard to recognize.

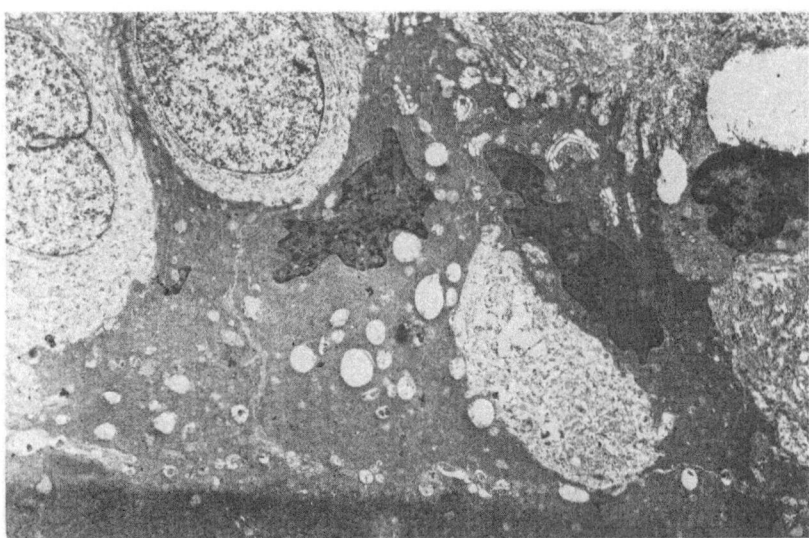

Fig. 4.

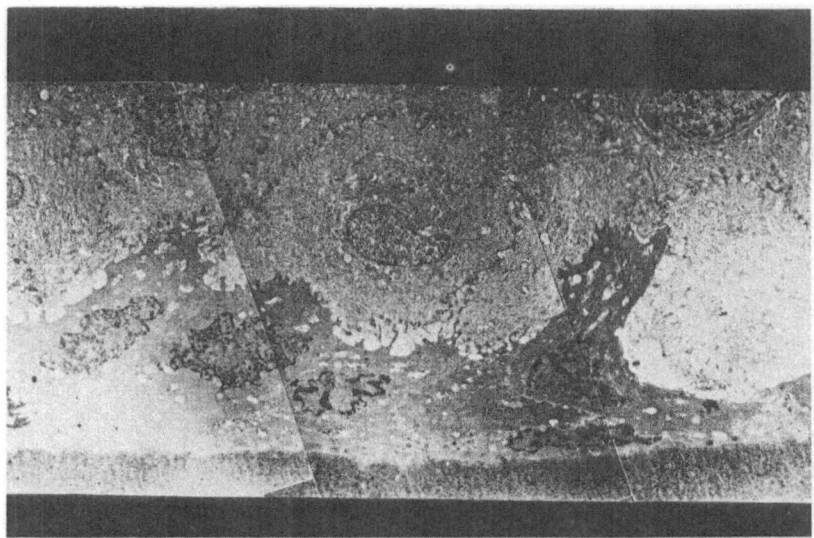

Fig. 5

CONCLUSIONS

From the observation of a case of corneal lattice dystrophy the normal relationship between clear and dark cells of the basal layer of the epithelium appears to change both in number and location.

The pathogenesis of such changes is controversial. There are two possible interpretations:

1. the primary changes consist of a degeneration of the clear cells which consequently would be substituted by dark cells;
2. the numerical increase and the hyperactivity of the dark cells are the primary phenomena, of which the suffering of the clear cells is a consequence.

The solution to this problem is rended difficult by our incomplete knowledge of the nature and function of the dark cells.

SUMMARY

The so-called dark basal cells of the corneal epithelium appear increased in number and exhibit a metabolic hyperactivity. Their elongations surround the clear basal cells, which show degenerative changes and sometimes are reduced to degenerated residues, completely enclosed by dark cells. The question, wether the primary change consistis of a degeneration of the clear cells or of an increased activity of the dark cells with a secondary suffering of the clear ones is at present controversial because of our incomplete knowleges about the nature and function of the dark cells.

REFERENCES

Iwamoto, T. & A.G. De Voe. Electron microscopy of Fuchs' dystrophy. Part 2. Anterior portion of the cornea. *Invest. Ophthal.* 10: *29*, (1971).

Segawa, K. Electron microscopic studies on the human corneal epithelium: dendritic cells. *A.M.A. Arch. Ophth.* 72: *650*, (1964).

Segawa, K. Electron microscopy of dendritic cells in the human corneal epithelium. *Invest. Opthal.* 4: *264*, (1965).

Sugiura, S. The polygonal cell system of corneal epithelium. In: 'The Structure of the Eye' II. Symposium Wiesbaden, 1965 Ed. J.W. Rohen. Stuttgard, F.K. Schattauer ed., pp. 463–479, 1965.

Sugiura, S. & H. Matsuda. Ultrastructure of Langerhans cell in human corneal limbus. *Jap. J. Ophthal.* 13: *197*, (1969).

Teng, C.C. Fine structure of the human cornea: epithelium and stroma. *Amer. J. Ophthal.* 54: *969*, (1962).

Vittone, P., R. Castellazzo, R. Bertagno, & M. Rolando. Osservazioni ultrastrutturali sulla distrofia a graticciata della cornea. *Boll. Oculist.* 55, 9–12: *437–449*, (1976).

Author's address:
University Eye Clinic
Viale Benedetto XV, 5
Genova 16132
Italy